Notes on Dental Materials

E. C. Combe MSc PhD DSc C Chem FRSC
Reader in Biomaterials Science
and Tutor to Dental Students,
University of Manchester,
and formerly Visiting Associate Professor
of Biological Materials at
Northwestern University Dental School,
Chicago, Illinois, USA
Fellow of the Academy of Dental
Materials.

FOREWORD BY

A. A. Grant DDSc MSc FRACDS
Pro-Vice Chancellor and Professor of
Restorative Dentistry
University of Manchester

FIFTH EDITION

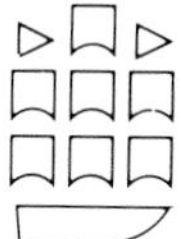

CHURCHILL LIVINGSTONE
EDINBURGH LONDON MELBOURNE AND NEW YORK 1986

CHURCHILL LIVINGSTONE

Medical Division of Longman Group UK Limited

Distributed in the United States of America by Churchill Livingstone Inc., 1560 Broadway, New York, N.Y. 10036, and by associated companies, branches and representatives throughout the world.

First edition 1972
Second edition 1975
Third edition 1977
Fourth edition 1981
Fifth edition 1986

ISBN 0 443 03112 6

British Library Cataloguing in Publication Data

Combe, E.C.
Notes on dental materials.—5th ed.
1. Dental materials
I. Title
617.6′95 RK652.5

Library of Congress Cataloguing-in-Publication Data

Combe, E.C. (Edward Charles)
Notes on dental materials.

Includes bibliographies and index.
1. Dental materials. I. Title. [DNLM: 1. Dental Materials. WU 190 C729n]
RK652.5.C66 1986 617.6′95 86-20754

Printed by Bell and Bain Limited, Glasgow.

Notes on Dental Materials

Foreword

The Dental School in the University of Manchester was one of the first in the United Kingdom to recognise the importance to the practising dentist of an understanding of the properties of dental materials.

Manchester's traditional strength in this field is evidenced by the large number of former associates of the Dental Materials Section who are now in charge of similar disciplines in other Universities.

Throughout his professional career, Dr Combe has been engaged in the teaching of dental materials at undergraduate and postgraduate levels. This, together with his leadership of an active and broadly based research group, has provided the experience and essential authoritative background for the production of the text.

The need for a fifth edition of this book within a period of some 14 years clearly demonstrates the special place it has come to occupy in the curriculum of many dental schools and the libraries of dental practitioners. Successive editions have introduced new features and updated existing information on traditional materials, and in this way have reflected the rapidity with which this field continues to expand. Indeed, the change in name of this well established teaching and research unit from Dental Materials to Biomaterials Science has itself been a response to the changing nature of the discipline.

This text will continue to be of benefit to all users of dental materials and others using materials in the biological environment.

Manchester, 1986 A.A.G.

Preface

As with earlier editions, this book is intended to accompany an instruction course in dental materials, to provide concise data for rapid revision of the subject and to give up-to-date information on the numerous new products that are becoming available. It is believed that the presentation of the subject matter in note form can help to fulfil these aims. As before, little emphasis is placed on details of techniques of using materials, where these are adequately covered in existing texts by clinical writers.

Compared to the fourth edition, the subject matter has been extended by the inclusion of discussion on the properties of enamel and dentine, resin-bonded bridges and some aspects of biomechanics. New chapters appear on thermal properties, optical properties and prefabricated pins and posts. Some re-arrangement of the structure of the book has been undertaken. Important contemporary aspects of the subject, such as light cured composites, and a discussion of resin-bonded bridges, are included. Currently available information on cermets has been incorporated.

It is hoped that this book will continue to be of benefit to all users of dental materials. Constructive comments on the book, for consideration for inclusion in future editions, will always be gratefully received and acknowledged.

Manchester, 1986 E.C.C.

Acknowledgements

The author is very grateful to all who have so willingly assisted in the preparation of this book. Professor Grant contributed the foreword, and has given his continual support and encouragement in this work. Dr D.C. Watts has given useful discussion on many sections of the text and kindly supplied the SEM pictures which appear for the first time in this edition.

Many others have given invaluable advice, including Professor M. Braden, Dr D. Brown, Mr C.J. Clark, Mr H.G. Kurer, Dr J.B. Moser, Mr M.J. Read and Mr G.A. Smith.

The author is grateful to Mrs T. Quinn and Mrs R. Durrell for typing the manuscript, to Miss A. Winstanley who drew the illustrations, and to his wife for assistance with proof reading and indexing.

The advice and assistance of the staff of Churchill Livingstone is also greatly appreciated.

Contents

Appendices

SECTION I

Basic scientific principles

1. Requirements of materials

1.1 INTRODUCTION

Two important questions must be asked about a material for use in the oral cavity:
(a) What effect will the material have on its environment? (Section 1.2)
(b) What effect will the oral environment have on the material? (Section 1.3)

Additional factors are important in the selection of a material, e.g. aesthetic properties, viscosity, adhesion, etc. (Section 1.4)

1.2 THE EFFECT OF MATERIALS ON THE ENVIRONMENT

It is of the utmost importance that dental materials should not have any harmful effects in the mouth, or on the body. In Chapter 3 biological properties are discussed, giving examples of potential hazards and summarising some of the techniques for the evaluation of materials.

1.3 THE EFFECT OF THE ENVIRONMENT ON MATERIALS

1.3.1 Chemical properties

A material in the mouth:
(a) should not dissolve in saliva, or in any fluid normally taken into the mouth,
(b) should not tarnish or corrode (Chapter 11).

1.3.2 Mechanical properties

For many dental applications, materials should possess suitable strength, rigidity, hardness, abrasion resistance, etc. The properties are considered in Chapter 4. Some time dependent properties are mentioned in Section 5.7.

1.3.3 Other physical properties

Other physical properties include density, thermal properties (Chapter 6) and optical properties (Chapter 7).

1.4 MISCELLANEOUS PROPERTIES

Other desirable properties include:

(a) Aesthetics, e.g. for dentures and certain restorative materials.
(b) Rheological or flow properties of materials (Chapter 5):
   (i) as supplied
   (ii) after mixing
   (iii) during setting
   (iv) of a set material
(c) Adhesion and surface properties (Chapter 15)

1.5 SUMMARY

Table 1.1 classifies the principal relevant properties of dental materials.

Table 1.1 Properties of dental materials

Biological properties (Chapter 3)		
Irritancy Toxicity		
Chemical properties (Section 1.3.1)	**Mechanical properties** (Chapter 4)	**Other physical properties** (Chapters 6 & 7)
Solubility Corrosion resistance	Stress-strain relationship Rigidity, elasticity Elastic limit Proof stress Tensile strength Compressive strength Impact strength Fatigue strength Ductility Resilience Toughness Hardness Abrasion resistance Time dependent properties (Section 5.7)	Density, specific gravity. Thermal properties — expansion — conductivity and diffusivity Optical properties — refractive index — opacity and translucency Aesthetics
Miscellaneous properties		
Rheological properties (Chapter 5) Surface properties and adhesion (Chapter 15) Availability, ease of use, safety of use Setting time and dimensional changes Stability on storage Special requirements for particular applications		

READING REFERENCE

Combe E C, Grant A A 1973 The selection and properties of materials for dental practice—1. Principles of selection. British Dental Journal 134: 16

This article considers biological, chemical, physical, mechanical and other properties of dental materials. Specific examples of the relevance of these properties to dental problems are given.

2. The structure of solids

2.1 INTRODUCTION

In solids, atoms are held together by a variety of forces. These are ionic, covalent and metallic bonds, and Van der Waals forces.

2.2 INTERATOMIC BONDING

Atoms can join together to form molecules. Combinations between atoms involve only the electrons in the outermost quantum shells—these are the *valency electrons*. In many molecules, the electrons are arranged to give a stable structure similar to an inert gas. To achieve a stable structure atoms may either receive or donate an extra electron or electrons, or share electrons.

2.2.1 Ionic bonds

Ionic bonds are formed by the transfer of an electron or electrons from one atom to another.

Example. Sodium chloride
If an atom of sodium lost an electron, it would acquire a stable structure similar to neon. It would also become positively charged, since it would have 11 protons and only 10 electrons. Such a species is known as an *ion*.

The process may be represented by:

$$Na \rightarrow Na^{+} + 1e^{-}$$

An atom of chlorine needs to gain only one electron to give it the same stable electronic structure as argon. Thus:

$$Cl + 1e^{-} \longrightarrow Cl^{-}$$

Positively charged ions such as Na^{+} are called *cations*. Cl^{-} is an example of an *anion*—a negatively charged ion.

Electrostatic attraction can occur between cations and anions. This is the principle of ionic bonding. For example, in sodium chloride, the ions exist in a cubic pattern. A two dimensional representation of this is:

$$\begin{array}{cccccccccc}
Na^{+} & Cl^{-} & Na^{+} & Cl^{-} & Na^{+} & Cl^{-} & Na^{+} & Cl^{-} & Na^{+} & Cl^{-} \\
Cl^{-} & Na^{+} & Cl^{-} & Na^{+} & Cl^{-} & Na^{+} & Cl^{-} & Na^{+} & Cl^{-} & Na^{+} \\
Na^{+} & Cl^{-} & Na^{+} & Cl^{-} & Na^{+} & Cl^{-} & Na^{+} & Cl^{-} & Na^{+} & Cl^{-} \\
Cl^{-} & Na^{+} & Cl^{-} & Na^{+} & Cl^{-} & Na^{+} & Cl^{-} & Na^{+} & Cl^{-} & Na^{+}
\end{array}$$

These bonds are non-directional and strong. Ionic solids are heat resistant and insoluble in organic solvents. They can generally be dissolved in ionising solvents such as water, acids and alkalies. In solution they *dissociate* into their constituent ions. Such solutions can conduct an electric current easily.

2.2.2 Covalent bonds

These are formed, not by the transfer of electrons as above, but by the sharing of electrons.

Example 1. A hydrogen atom may be written $H\cdot$, where the dot represents the valence electron. Two such atoms can share their electrons, $H:H$, so that each has a stable structure similar to helium.

Example 2. Similarly chlorine can form covalently bonded molecules:

$$:\ddot{\underset{\cdot\cdot}{Cl}}\cdot + :\ddot{\underset{\cdot\cdot}{Cl}}\cdot \longrightarrow :\ddot{\underset{\cdot\cdot}{Cl}}:\ddot{\underset{\cdot\cdot}{Cl}}:$$

(Again, the dots represent the valence electrons; the other electrons are not shown.)

Example 3. Carbon compounds are covalently bonded, e.g. methane:

$$\cdot\dot{\underset{\cdot}{C}}\cdot \quad + \quad 4H\cdot \quad \longrightarrow \quad H:\overset{H}{\underset{H}{\ddot{\underset{\cdot\cdot}{C}}}}:H$$

Example 4. Double and triple covalent bonds are possible, where two or three pairs of electrons respectively are shared between atoms. Ethylene (C_2H_4) may be written:

$$\begin{array}{ccc} H & & H \\ \ddot{\underset{\cdot\cdot}{C}} & : & \ddot{\underset{\cdot\cdot}{C}} \\ H & & H \end{array} \quad \text{or} \quad \begin{array}{ccc} H & & H \\ | & & | \\ C & = & C \\ | & & | \\ H & & H \end{array}$$

Similarly, acetylene (C_2H_2) is:

$$H{:}C\vdots\vdots C{:}H \quad \text{or} \quad H{-}C{\equiv}C{-}H$$

Example 5. Co-ordinate bonds can be formed, where both electrons to be shared by the two combining atoms are supplied by one of them. Ammonium ions, NH_4^+, are an example of this:

Ammonia (NH_3) has 3 covalent bonds:

$$\begin{array}{c} H{:}\ddot{\underset{\cdot\cdot}{N}}{:}H \\ H \end{array}$$

It also contains a *lone pair* of electrons, not shared by any of the hydrogen atoms. Such a species can combine with a hydrogen ion. H^+ which has no electrons, thus:

$$\begin{array}{c} H{:}\ddot{\underset{\cdot\cdot}{N}}{:}H \\ H \end{array} + H^+ \longrightarrow \left[\begin{array}{c} H \\ H{:}\ddot{\underset{\cdot\cdot}{N}}{:}H \\ H \end{array}\right]^+$$

Properties. Covalent bonds are directional in character. Such compounds are generally water-insoluble. Other properties of covalent compounds are illustrated by two contrasting examples:

(a) Diamond consists entirely of C atoms bonded together by covalent links in a three dimensional structure. The strength of these bonds is illustrated by the fact that diamond is the hardest known naturally occurring material, and can withstand temperatures of over 3000°C without breaking down.

(b) Polymers, where the atoms in a polymer chain are held together by covalent bonds (Ch. 8).

2.2.3 Metallic bonds

An atom of a metal can easily lose some of its outer shell electrons to give a positive ion. A solid metal may be considered to consist of positive ions, held together by a 'cloud' of free electrons (Fig. 2.1). The mobility of such electrons contributes to the well-known ability of metals to conduct heat and electricity.

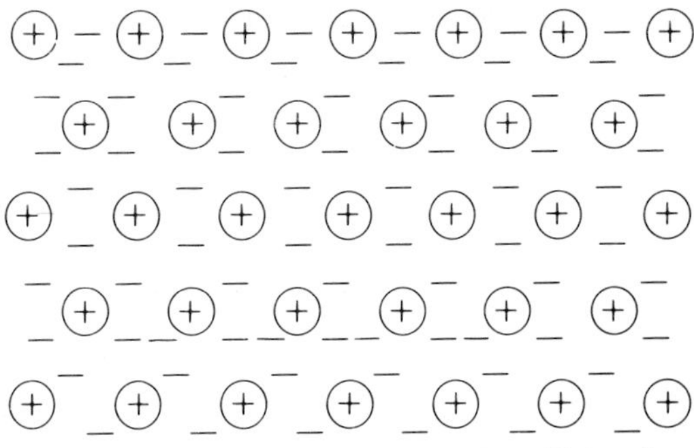

Fig. 2.1 Diagrammatic representation of metallic bonding.

2.2.4 Van der Waals forces

These physical forces are much weaker than the bonding between atoms described above. They arise due to electrostatic attraction between molecules or atoms which may arise in one of two ways:

(a) Molecules such as H_2O are asymmetrical, so the centres of the positive and negative charges do not coincide. This may be written:

$\delta+$ $\delta+$
H H
O
$\delta-$

where $\delta+$ and $\delta-$ represent small electric charges. Such molecules are termed *permanent dipoles*: the electrostatic forces may be represented diagrammatically by:

$\delta+$ $\delta+$ $\delta+$ $\delta+$
H H H H
O O
$\delta-$ $\delta-$

$\delta+$ $\delta+$
H H
O
$\delta-$

(b) Atoms of inert gases, and symmetrical molecules (e.g. CH_4) can form *fluctuating dipoles* due to the random motion of electrons: the resulting forces between such dipoles are very weak.

A solid whose molecules are bonded together by Van der Waals forces in general has a low modulus of elasticity, high thermal expansion and a low melting point, due to the comparative weakness of Van der Waals forces.

2.2.5 General comments

(a) More than one type of bond can exist in a material—for

example, calcium sulphate ($CaSO_4$) has ionic and covalent bonds.

$$Ca^{++}\left[\begin{array}{ccc} & :\ddot{O}: & \\ :\ddot{\underset{..}{O}} & :\ddot{\underset{..}{S}}: & \ddot{\underset{..}{O}}: \\ & :\underset{..}{O}: & \end{array}\right]^{=}$$

(b) Some substances can be bonded in more than one way—for example HCl may be written as:

$$H\ :\ddot{\underset{..}{Cl}}:\quad \text{or}\quad H^{+}\ :\ddot{\underset{..}{Cl}}:^{-}$$

The former structure is predominant in HCl gas, the latter in aqueous solution.

(c) Distinction should be made between:

- (i) atomic solids, such as diamond, and,
- (ii) molecular solids, such as polymers, where the covalently bonded molecules are held together by Van der Waals forces, and these latter forces dominate the mechanical properties (Ch. 8).

2.3 SPACING OF ATOMS

Two factors influence the distance between atoms in a solid (Fig. 2.2):

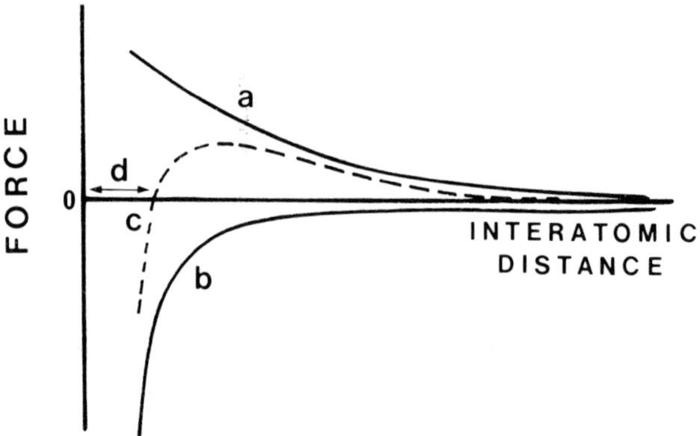

Fig. 2.2 Factors influencing the distance between atoms in a solid: (a) forces of attraction; (b) forces of repulsion; (c) resultant force, the sum of (a) and (b); (d) equilibrium interatomic distance.

(a) Forces of attraction, due to interatomic bonding, as discussed above.

(b) In addition, forces of repulsion occur between the electrons of neighbouring atoms. These forces increase rapidly with decreasing interatomic distance.

When two atoms are spaced such that these forces are equal and opposite, the atoms are in their equilibrium position. Application of an external force to a solid can displace atoms from this position. At the equilibrium position, the potential energy of the system is a minimum.

2.4 CRYSTALLINE SOLIDS

In many solids, the constituent atoms are regularly arranged in a *crystal lattice*. The atoms may be held together by ionic bonds (as in NaCl), covalent bonds (for example, diamond) or metallic bonds. Such materials are crystalline.

2.4.1 Types of crystal lattice

Different configurations of crystal lattices are possible; the simplest way to study these is to consider a *unit cell*—this is defined as the smallest repeating unit that is contained in a crystal. There are some 14 different possible crystal lattices; only three of dental interest are considered here:

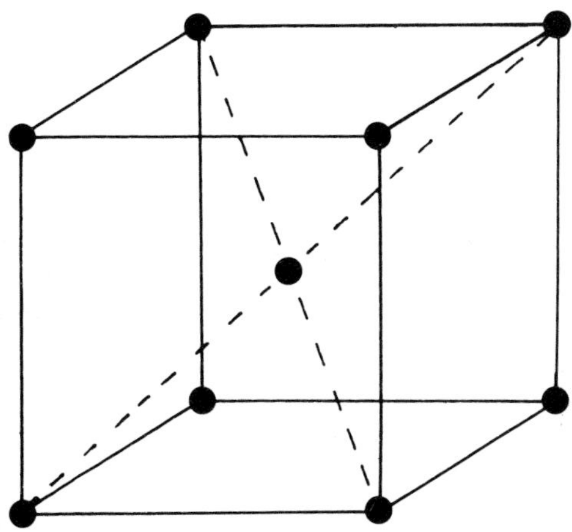

Fig. 2.3 Unit cell of a body centred cubic (b.c.c.) crystal lattice. The dots represent the positions of the atoms.

(a) Body centred cubic (b.c.c.)—as in some metals, e.g. iron below 910°C. Figure 2.3 shows the unit cell, with an atom at each corner of the cube, and one in the centre.

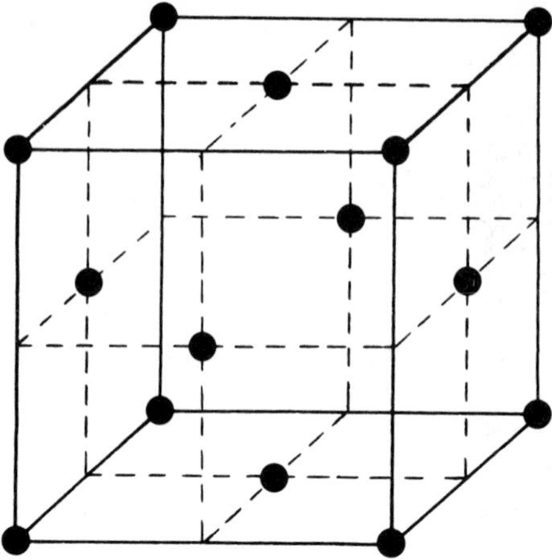

Fig. 2.4 Unit cell of a face centred cubic (f.c.c.) crystal lattice.

(b) Face centred cube (f.c.c.)—as in gold, silver, copper, platinum, palladium; also iron above 910°C. The unit cell is a cube with an atom at each of the eight corners, and one in the centre of each of the six faces, but none in the centre of the cube (Fig. 2.4).

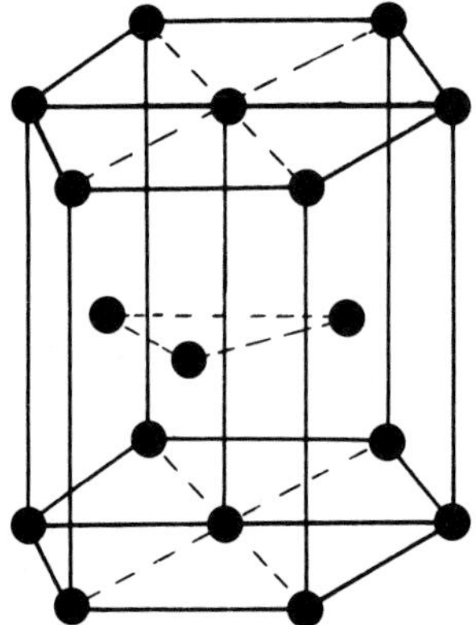

Fig. 2.5 Unit cell of a hexagonal close packed structure (h.c.p.).

(c) Hexagonal close packed structure (h.c.p.)—as in zinc and magnesium. This is depicted in Figure 2.5.

2.4.2 Crystal imperfections

The above are structures of ideal crystals. In practice imperfections occur, which have a considerable effect on the properties of a material. There are the following possibilities:

(a) Point defects, such as:

(i) Impurities—see Figure 2.6. These can cause distortion of the crystal lattice,

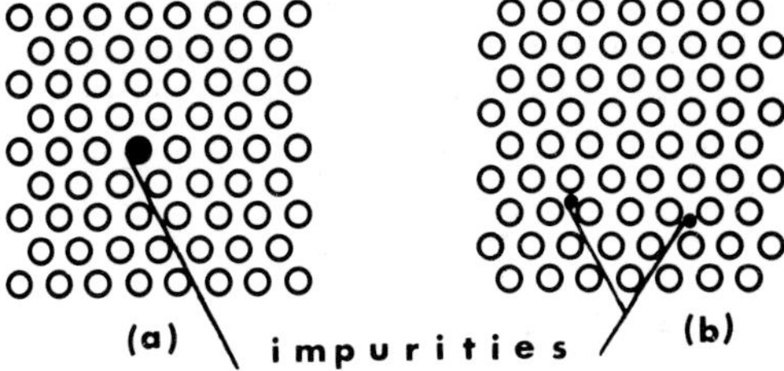

Fig. 2.6 Two dimensional representation of impurities in a crystal: (a) impurity substituted in crystal lattice, (b) impurities in interstitial positions.

(ii) Vacancies—see Figure 2.7. In this case also, distortion can occur. Vacancies provide the means whereby atoms can move in a crystal, hence solid state diffusion (Section 10.4.3, for example).

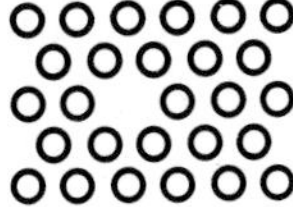

Fig. 2.7 Two dimensional representation of a vacancy in a crystal lattice.

(b) Line defects, particularly dislocations may be present (Fig. 2.8). These contribute to the liability of ceramic materials to fracture (Section 12.9.2). Plastic deformation in metals occurs by motion of dislocations (Section 9.6).

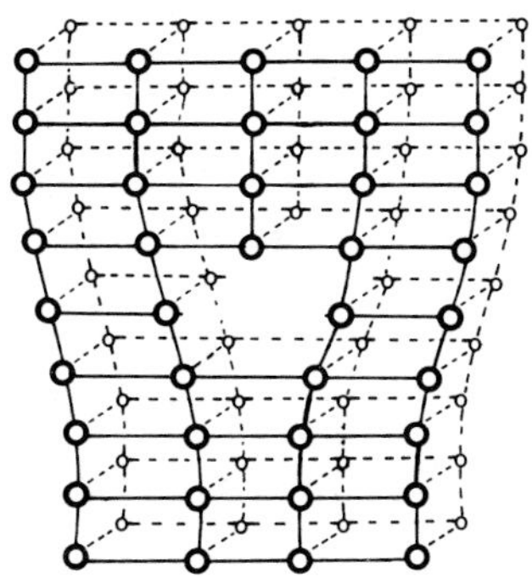

Fig. 2.8 A dislocation in a crystal.

Crystalline materials with few flaws and dislocations can be extremely strong (Section 13.3.1).

(c) Planar defects, such as grain boundaries in metals (Section 9.4.3).

2.5 AMORPHOUS SOLIDS

Amorphous means literally 'without form'. Gases, liquids and some solids, particularly glasses and many polymers, may be considered under this category. In such materials there is no long-range repeating structure, but merely a random arrangement of atoms or groups of atoms.

2.6 CLASSIFICATION OF SOLIDS

Solids may be generally classified into three types on the basis of their properties and behaviour:

(a) Polymers—long chain molecules, consisting of many repeating units (Chapter 8).

(b) Metallic materials, with their characteristic properties of, for example, thermal and electrical conductivity (Chapters 9–11).

(c) Ceramic materials, which are compounds of metallic and non-metallic elements (Chapter 12).

All these classes of material find many dental applications. Additionally, composite materials, such as polymer-ceramic composites (Chapter 13) are becoming increasingly important.

READING REFERENCE

Van Vlack L H 1985 Elements of materials science and engineering 5th edn. Addison-Wesley, Reading, Massachussetts

For greater depth of study, Chapters 2, 3 & 4 of this book are highly recommended.

3. Biological properties

3.1 INTRODUCTION

Dental materials should:
(a) be non-toxic; this is important not only for patients, but also for dental surgeons and ancillary staff.
(b) be non-irritant to the oral or other tissues.
(c) not produce allergic reactions, and,
(d) not be mutagenic or carcinogenic.

3.2 CLASSIFICATION OF MATERIALS

Materials may be classified into the following types from the perspective of biological compatibility:
(a) those which contact the soft tissues within the mouth.
(b) those which could affect the health or vitality of the dental pulp,
(c) those which are used as root canal filling materials,
(d) those which affect the hard tissues of the teeth, and,
(e) those used in the dental laboratory, which, though not used in the mouth, are handled and may be accidentally ingested or inhaled.

3.3 EXAMPLES OF HAZARDS

(a) Some dental cement components are acidic and may cause irritation (Ch. 17, 18).
(b) Phosphoric acid is used as an etchant for enamel (Ch. 20).
(c) Some periodontal dressing materials have contained asbestos fibres (Ch. 21).
(d) Mercury is used in dental amalgam, and mercury vapour is toxic (Ch. 22).
(e) Dust from alginate impression materials may be inhaled; some products contained lead compounds (Ch. 26).
(f) Metallic compounds (e.g. of lead and tin) are used in elastomeric impression materials (Ch. 27).

(g) Monomer in denture base materials can be irritant if present in excess (Ch. 33).
(h) Some dental porcelain powders used to contain uranium.
(i) Some people show allergic reactions to alloys containing nickel (Ch. 30).
(j) Laboratory materials have their hazards, such as: cyanide solution for electroplating (Ch. 40), vapours from low fusing metal dies (Ch. 40), siliceous particles in investment materials (Ch. 42) and fluxes containing fluorides (Ch. 44).

3.4 BIOLOGICAL EVALUATION

Methods used for evaluation of materials include tests for:
(a) Acute systematic toxicity. This can be achieved by animal experimentation, e.g. using rats, and the material administered either:
  (i) by an oral route, or
  (ii) intraveneously.
(b) Skin irritation, using, for example, albino rabbits, and assessing the skin for erythema and oedema.
(c) Skin sensitization, using guinea pigs.
(d) Oral mucosal irritation, e.g. by inserting the material into the cheek pouches of hamsters.
(e) Mutagenicity and carcinogenicity.

Additionally, in-use tests can be carried out for dental filling materials and root canal filling materials, using non-rodent animals such as monkeys, dogs, cats or ferrets.

In vitro tests, using tissue culture techniques, are becoming of increasing importance.

Only after satisfactory biological evaluation of materials can they be introduced into controlled clinical trials.

READING REFERENCE

Stanley H R 1985 Toxicity testing of dental materials. CRC Press, Boca Raton, Florida

This book provides a valuable compendium of methods of toxicity testing, classified as: initial tests (Ch. 3), secondary tests (Ch. 4) and usage tests (Ch. 5).

4. Mechanical properties

4.1 STRAIN

When an external force or load is applied to a material the phenomenon of *strain* occurs—this is a change in dimensions of the material, usually measured by its change in length (either an increase or decrease, depending on whether the material is in tension or compression, Fig. 4.1) per unit length. Thus strain is equal to e/L, where e is the change in length and L is the original length. Strain may also be expressed as a percentage of the original length, that is 100 e/L. Strain may be either *elastic* or *plastic*. If the material returns to its original length after removal of its load, its deformation has

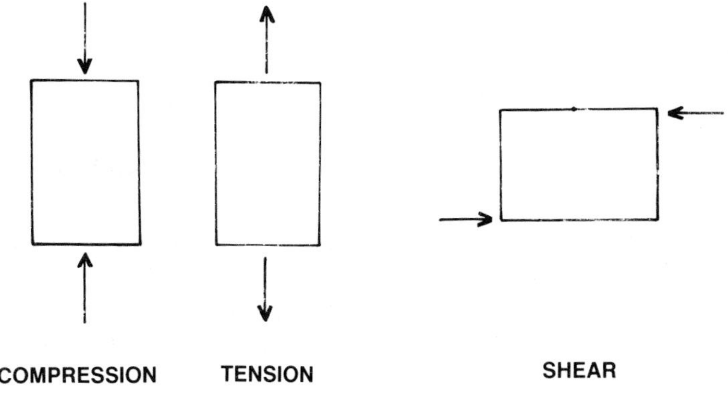

Fig. 4.1 Types of stress.

been elastic. If there is a permanent change in shape this is a plastic deformation.

4.2 STRESS

Associated with strain is the phenomenon of *stress*—this is an internal force/unit area in a material, equal and opposite to the applied load or force/unit area.

Stress is measured in units of force per unit area (e.g. N/m^2, kN/m^2, MN/m^2; see Appendix I for explanation of these SI units). Thus the stress $S = F/A$, where F is the load or force applied, and A is the cross-sectional area of the material over which the load is applied.

A material may be stressed in *compression*, *tension* or *shear* (Fig. 4.1). In practice, the stresses within a material are complex. Thus if a beam is bent as shown in Figure 4.2 (3-point loading, as used in measuring *transverse strength*), the lower portion of the beam is in tension, and the top is in compression. Shear stresses may also be present in this case, particularly in thick beams.

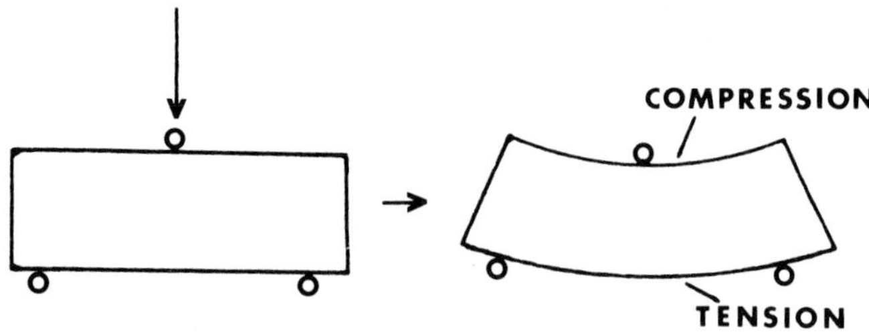

Fig. 4.2 Three-point loading of a beam.

In materials with cracks, notches, grooves, inclusions, surface scratches, or marked changes in contour due to design, *stress concentration* can occur. This is clearly to be avoided as far as possible in the construction of dental appliances, as it can lead to failure of the material.

4.3 TENSILE AND COMPRESSIVE PROPERTIES

4.3.1 Stress-strain relationship

If stress is plotted against strain for a material in tension or compression, a graph such as Figure 4.3 can result. Figures 4.4–4.6 are typical graphs for a ductile metal, a brittle ceramic and a polymer respectively. From such data many useful properties can be determined, as detailed below.

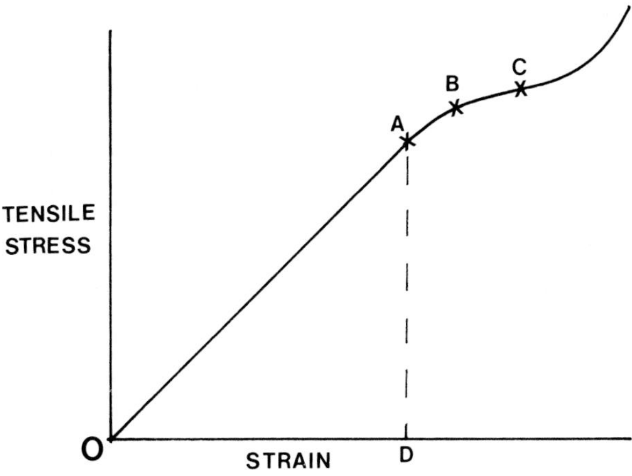

Fig. 4.3 Tensile stress-strain diagram.

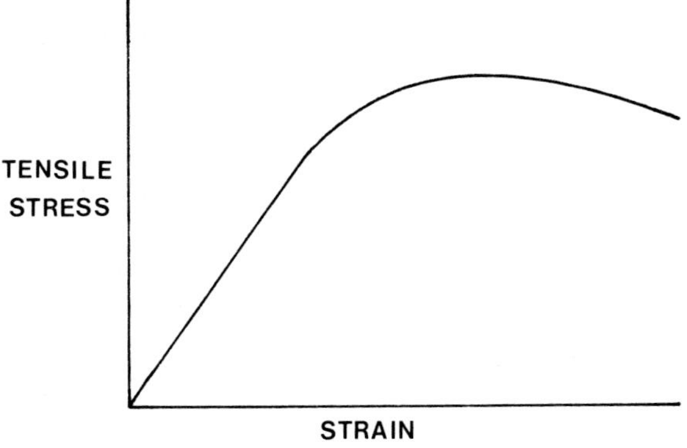

Fig. 4.4 Typical tensile stress-strain diagram for a ductile metal.

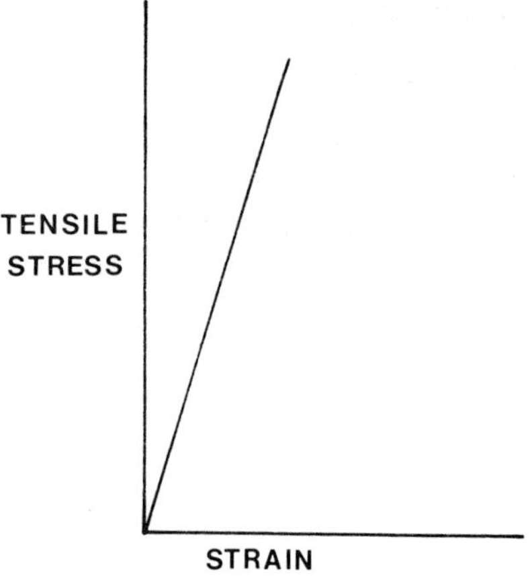

Fig. 4.5 Typical tensile stress-strain diagram for a brittle material e.g. a ceramic.

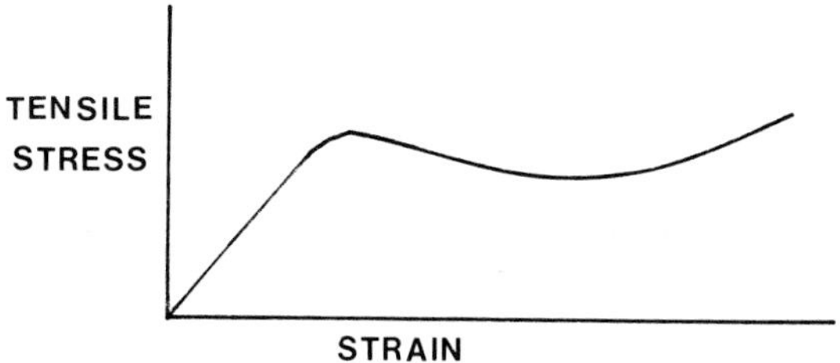

Fig. 4.6 Typical tensile stress-diagram for a polymer.

4.3.2 Modulus of elasticity

From Figure 4.3, it can be seen that between points 0 and A, stress is proportional to strain—this is an example where *Hooke's law* is obeyed. The slope of this linear portion is a measure of the rigidity of the material and is termed the modulus of elasticity. For example, portions of the stress-strain graphs of two materials are in Figure 4.7. Material I has a modulus of elasticity of 200 GN/m^2 and for material II the modulus is 100 GN/m^2. For a stress of 200 MN/m^2, I is strained by 0.1%, and II by 0.2%. Material I, with a higher modulus is more rigid; material II is more flexibile. The tensile modulus is often called *Young's modulus*, and is usually given the symbol E. The other corresponding moduli are the shear or elastic modulus (G) and the bulk modulus (k).

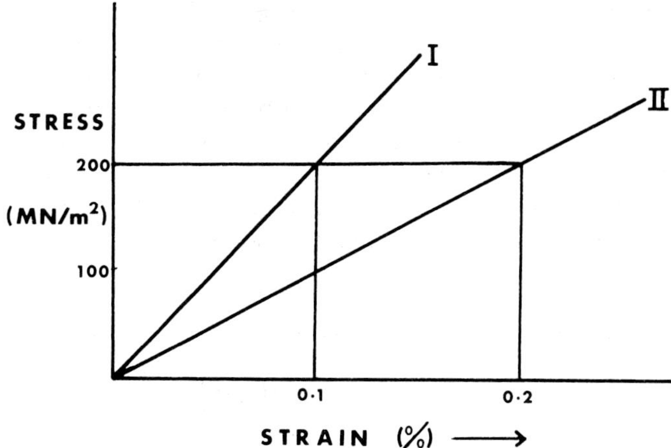

Fig. 4.7 Portions of the stress-strain graphs of two materials below the proportional limit.

4.3.3 Proportional limit

In Figure 4.3 this is represented by point A—the maximum stress at which stress is proportional to strain. Ceramic materials often break in the linear region of the graph (Fig. 4.5).

4.3.4 Elastic limit

Quite commonly, a material may be stressed above its proportional limit, yet behave elastically—that is, on removal of the load, the specimen returns to its original length. The *elastic limit* is the maximum stress which a material can endure without undergoing permanent deformation; it is represented by point B in Figure 4.3.

4.3.5 Yield point

A material reaches a *yield point* (C in Figure 4.3) when there is a rapid increase in strain without a corresponding increase in stress; the deformation is now completely plastic. In some instances there is a drop in stress (e.g. Figure 4.6). This decrease in stress can be accounted for by the contraction in cross-section (termed *necking*) which accompanies the elongation of the specimen, consequent on the material not changing in volume when it deforms plastically.

4.3.6 Proof stress

In practice it is very difficult to determine the proportional limit and yield point. Often, the data obtained depend on the accuracy and sensitivity of the testing machine. To overcome this, values of *proof stress* are often quoted, particularly in the tensile testing of metals. For example, the 0.1% proof stress is the stress corresponding to a 0.1% permanent (or plastic) strain (Fig. 4.8). A construction line is drawn from the 0.1% strain on the horizontal axis, parallel to the straight line portion of the stress-strain curve. The 0.1% proof stress is at the point of intersection of this line with the stress-strain graph.

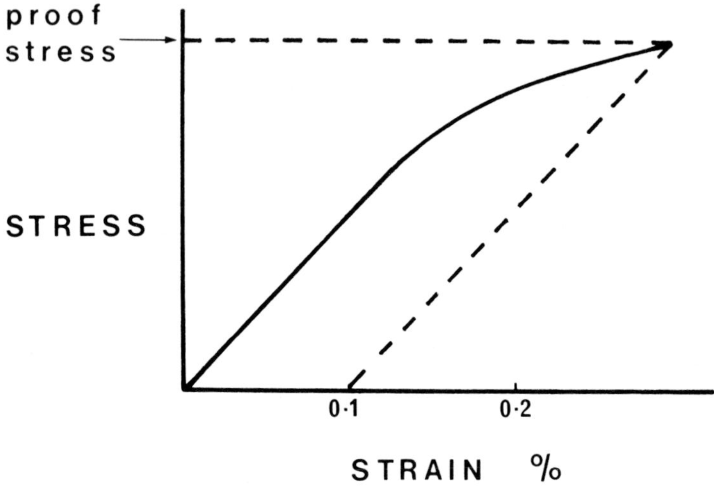

Fig. 4.8 0.1% proof stress.

4.3.7 Ductility and malleability

Many metals can be drawn out into the form of a wire—this property is termed *ductility*. *Malleability* is closely associated with ductility—it is the ability of a metallic material to be deformed to make thin sheets, without breaking or cracking. For example, gold can be rolled and beaten into sheets which are so thin that they can transmit light—it is thus a highly malleable metal.

These properties can be measured by:

(a) percentage elongation. After a metal specimen of known length has been fractured in a tensile test, the broken fragments are pieced together and the new length measured. A high percentage increase in length indicates a very ductile material.

(b) reduction in area of cross-section. The greater the malleability, the bigger is the reduction in cross-sectional area.

4.3.8 Poisson's ratio

Associated with the increase in length of material under tension (axial strain) there is also a decrease in cross-sectional area (lateral or transverse strain). Poisson's ration (μ) is defined as

$$\mu = \frac{\text{lateral strain}}{\text{axial strain}}$$

4.3.9 Compressive and tensile strength

Compressive and tensile strength is maximum stress that a material can undergo in compression or tension without fracture. The tensile strength is sometimes written as the U.T.S., or ultimate tensile strength. It is often measured by direct application of a tensile load to a specimen. In order to ensure good gripping of the specimen, its ends are often enlarged in relation to its central portion. Materials with little ductility (*brittle* materials) are liable to fracture at the gripped ends of the specimen.

An alternative method of measuring the tensile strength of brittle materials is to use the diametral compression test. A cylinder or disk of the material is compressed diametrically. A tensile stress is set up at right angles to the direction of the applied load (Fig. 4.9).

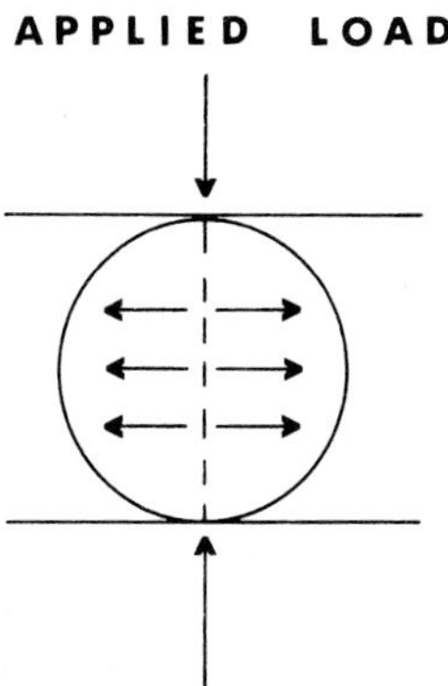

Fig. 4.9 Diametral compression test—a tensile stress is set up at right angles to the direction of the applied load.

The tensile strength is calculated from the formula:

$$\text{T.S.} = \frac{2P}{\pi t d},$$

where P is the load to fracture the material and t and d are the thickness and diameter of the specimen. The material must be Hookean up to fracture for this formula to be valid.

4.3.10 Resilience and toughness

The *modulus of resilience* is the maximum amount of energy a material can absorb without undergoing permanent deformation. It is measured by the area of the triangle OAD in Figure 4.3, and can be expressed by the formula $R = P^2/2E$, where P is the proportional limit and E the modulus of elasticity. R is expressed in terms of energy per unit volume, e.g. J/m^3 (Appendix I).

The *toughness* of a material is its ability to absorb energy without fracture. It is measured by the total area under a stress-strain graph. This can also be expressed in the units J/m^3.

4.4 IMPACT STRENGTH

In the previous section we have been considering the effects of applying a gradual increase in load to a material until fracture occurred. In practice, it is also desirable to know the effects of the application of a sudden force to a material because under these conditions materials are often more brittle.

This can be measured by making a specimen of known dimensions, clamping it firmly in position and breaking it with a swinging pendulum. The resulting reduction in amplitude of swing of the pendulum is measured. From this the energy to break a material can be calculated.

Two types of impact tester are available. In the *Charpy* tester the specimen is supported horizontally at the ends, and in an *Izod* instrument the material is clamped at one end and held vertically.

A problem of impact testing is that inconsistent results can be obtained, because specimens break in different places. In order to ensure more consistent results, specimens are notched. The material fractures at the notch, since this is its weakest part (Fig. 4.10). A notch also makes the material more brittle, hence this is a severe test of the toughness of a material. Impact strength varies markedly with the angle of the notch.

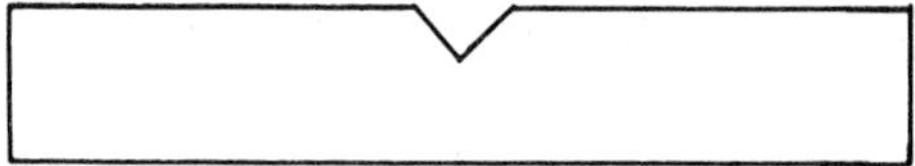

Fig. 4.10 Notched specimen for impact testing.

4.5 FATIGUE STRENGTH

The repetitive application of a small load to a material can sometimes cause its fracture. This is the phenomenon of fatigue. It is often encountered in the engineering industry. Dental appliances and restorations are also prone to this type of failure.

It is tested in the laboratory by giving many bending or twisting movements to a specimen, and counting the number of cycles (N) a material can withstand at a known stress (S). A graph of S versus log N is plotted, as in Figure 4.11. From the graph the *endurance limit* can be found; stresses below this limit will not cause fatigue fracture.

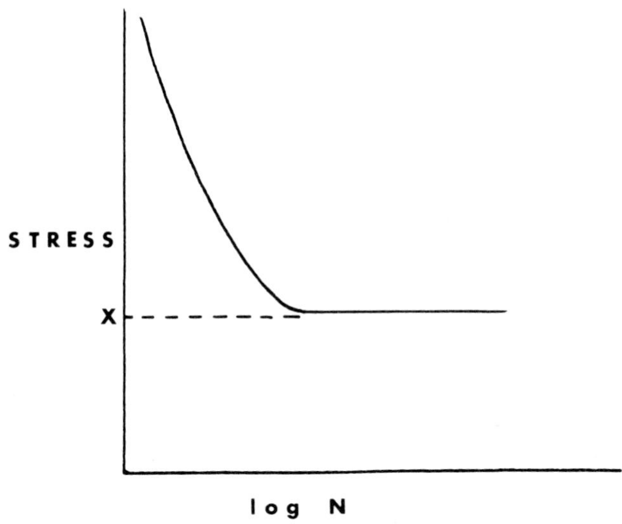

Fig. 4.11 S–N curve for a material, where S is the stress and N the number of cycles. X is the endurance limit (observed mainly for ferrous alloys; the S–N curve does not necessarily have a horizontal portion.)

4.6 HARDNESS

Hardness is the ability of a material to withstand indentation. An indentor of known dimensions is pressed into a material under a known load for a measured length of time. The hardness is calculated either from the depth or area of indentation. A small indentation indicates a hard material, and *vice versa*. Several types of tester are available (Table 4.1 and Fig. 4.12). With metals, the indentation is permanent, and the hardness number is related to the yield stress in compression. However, some problems are encountered with the use of steel ball indentors:

(a) it may shatter a brittle material:
(b) it may itself be deformed by a hard material, and
(c) it may cause elastic deformation rather than indentation.

Rubber hardness testing in fact utilises this, and rubber hardness is related to modulus.

Table 4.1 Hardness testers

Test	Indentor	Measurement	Results expressed in
Brinell	Steel ball	Area of indentation	BHN
Knoop	Diamond	Area of indentation	KHN
Rockwell	Steel ball or diamond point	Depth of indentation	Rockwell*
Vickers	Diamond	Area of indentation	VHN

*Rockwell hardness is expressed as a letter and a number, e.g. M105. The letter indicates the condition of testing, such as the load on the indentor, and the number indicates the hardness. For other testers, only a number is quoted.

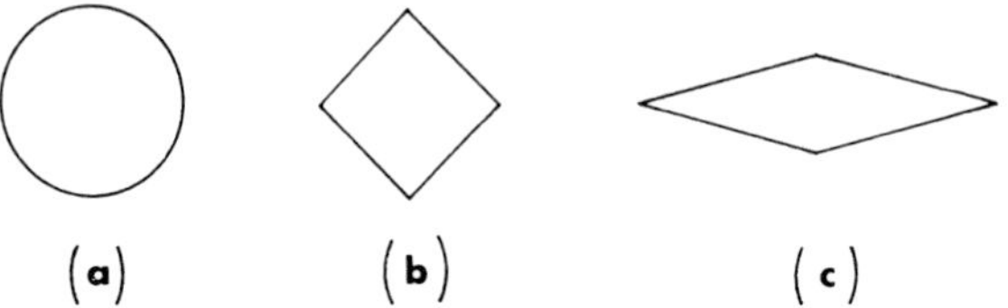

Fig. 4.12 Shape of indentations produced by hardness testers. (a) Brinell and Rockwell, (b) Vickers, (c) Knoop.

4.7 ABRASION RESISTANCE

Tests can be carried out to abrade or scratch the surface of a material under controlled conditions. Either the depth of the scratch, or the weight of material removed under reproducible conditions, can be measured.

4.8 TIME-DEPENDENT PROPERTIES

In some materials, particularly polymers, application or removal of a load produces a deformation, the magnitude of which is time-dependent. The apparent modulus of elasticity will depend on the time at which the strain is measured. The elastic modulus measured after a short time is relatively high compared with the modulus at infinite time, owing to the relaxation which can occur over a period of time. This phenomenon is termed *viscoelasticity*, because of the similarity of the behaviour of such a solid to a viscous fluid (Section 5.7).

READING REFERENCE

Van Vlack L H 1985 Elements of materials science and engineering 5th edn. Addison-Wesley, Reading, Massachussetts

This book provides excellent instruction for the student who requires study of materials science in greater depth. Section 1–5 deals specifically with selected properties of materials, including mechanical properties.

5. Rheological properties

5.1 INTRODUCTION

The science of the study of flow and deformation of matter is termed *rheology*. This is of importance in dental materials in the following instances:

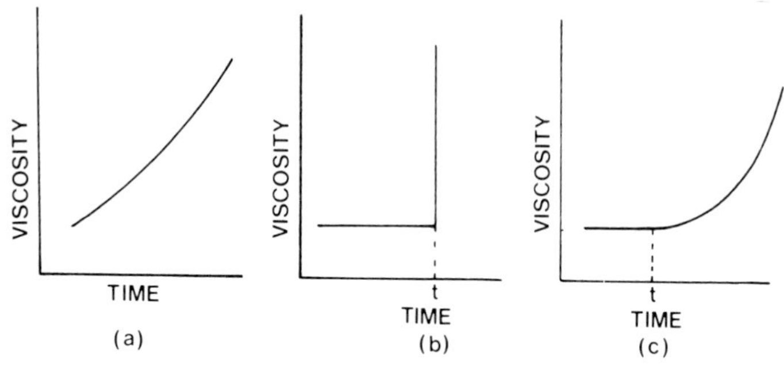

Fig. 5.1 Change in viscosity with time for setting materials:
(a) poor rheological characteristics from a manipulative viewpoint, showing no well defined working time.
(b) ideal properties—a well defined working time t followed by sudden setting.
(c) good properties, showing a working time t followed by gradual setting.

(a) Many dental materials are mixed as fluid pastes, which subsequently solidify.
(b) The mixed pastes are adapted to the required shape.
(c) The setting of such materials initially involves a change in viscosity with time, and then the development of an elastic modulus as solidification proceeds. From the physical analysis of these properties a *working time* and *setting time* can be defined. The working time is the period during which the material can be manipulated, ideally with no thickening taking place (Fig. 5.1). The

setting time is the time when the material has reached a given degree of rigidity.

(d) Flow and deformation of solids is also important. In chapter 4 the deformation of solids is presented as being either plastic or elastic. In practice, some solids asre *viscoelastic.* Such materials combine both viscous flow and elasticity, and their properties are time-dependent (Section 5.7).

5.2 VISCOSITY: NEWTONIAN BEHAVIOUR

The viscosity of a fluid is its resistance to flow. Consider a liquid as consisting of many parallel layers, or laminae, of material (Fig. 5.2).

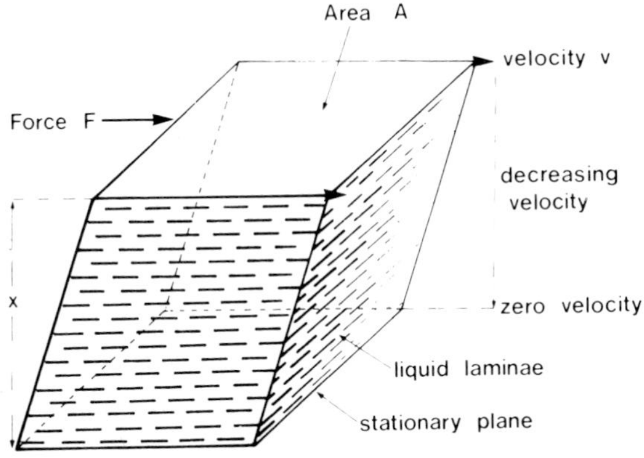

Fig. 5.2 Laminae of liquid.

A tangential force F is applied to the upper layer, of area A, in a plane perpendicular to that of the flow, so that it moves with velocity v. The layer in contact with the retaining surface is assumed to have zero velocity. Throughout the material there is a velocity gradient, that is, the velocity changes from one layer to another. The slope of the velocity-distance curve is the *velocity gradient* or *shear rate*, D, of the material, where D = dv/dx, and x is the distance from the retaining surface. D is expressed in units of velocity/distance (e.g., sec^{-1}). The *shear stress*, τ, is the force per unit area = F/A.

According to Newton's Law, τ and D are proportional to each other, and the constant of proportionality is equal to the coefficient of viscosity, thus:

$$\tau/D = \text{constant} = \eta \text{ (coefficient of viscosity)}$$

where τ is in dynes/cm^2 and D in sec^{-1}, η will have units dyne.sec/cm^2. 1 dyne.sec/cm^2 = 1 poise. Viscosities are often expressed in centipoise, where 100 centipoise = 1 poise. In S.I. units, 1 Pa.s = Nsm^{-2} = 10 poise.

The viscosity of a fluid depends on a number of factors, including:

(a) The nature of the substance.

(b) The temperature—the viscosity decreases with increasing temperature.

(c) Pressure—at very high pressures viscosity is greater.

(d) Shear rate (D)—fewer than 10% of all liquids are Newtonian. For most fluids τ/D is not a constant, but will vary with D (see Section 5.3). In these instances τ/D is termed the *apparent viscosity*.

(e) Shear history—for example, the structure of some materials is broken down on shearing.

5.3 NON-NEWTONIAN FLOW

For Newtonian behaviour, a plot of shear stress *versus* shear rate is a straight line through the origin (Fig. 5.3a). Non-Newtonian fluids are of the following types:

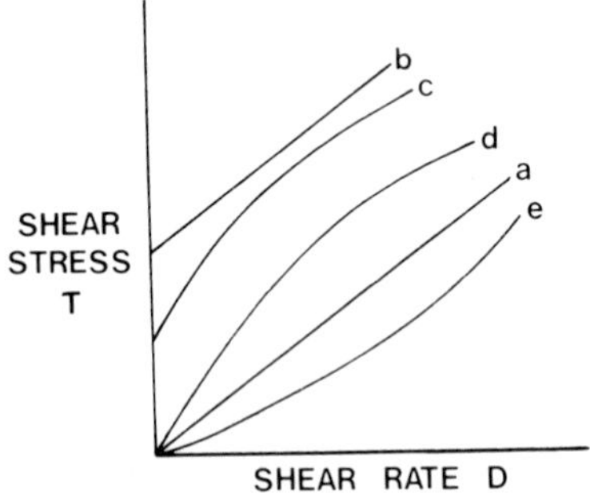

Fig. 5.3 Types of flow behaviour
(a) Newtonian flow
(b) Bingham flow
(c) Plastic flow
(d) Pseudoplastic flow
(e) Dilatant flow

(a) *Bingham flow* occurs when the shear stress—shear rate plot is linear, but has an intercept on the shear stress axis (Fig. 5.3b). This is termed the *yield stress*: below this stress the material will not flow.

Example: clay suspensions in water, composite filling materials (Section 19.8).

(b) Some fluids which show a yield stress also show a curvature in their D – τ curves—this is plastic flow (Fig. 5.3c).

(c) Some materials have a non-linear relationship between D and τ, but show no yield stress. These are termed *pseudoplastic* or *dilatant* (Fig. 5.3.d and e). For pseudoplastic materials the apparent viscosity decreases with increasing shear rate (shear thinning)—see Fig. 5.4.

Examples: many polymers, natural resins, blood, saliva, impression materials (Section 27.5), fluoride gels (Section 48.3) and viscous oils are pseudoplastic; wet sand with low water content is dilatant.

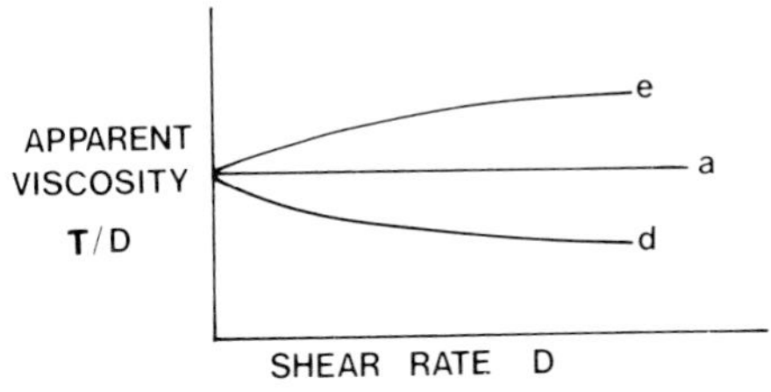

Fig. 5.4 Effect of shear rate on apparent viscosity
(a) Newtonian (d) Pseudoplastic (e) Dilatant

Some fluids have been found empirically to obey the following law:

$$\tau = kD^n, \text{ where k and n are constants.}$$

Thus: $$\log \tau = \log k + n \log D$$

Thus a plot of log τ *versus* log D is linear, with intercept log k, and slope n which is termed the flow index. If n = 1, the material is Newtonian; if n is less than 1, it is pseudoplastic; if n is greater than 1, it is dilatant. These are called *power law fluids*.

5.4 EFFECT OF SHEAR HISTORY

When some fluids are sheared at a steady rate, viscosity decreases with time. On standing the fluid regains its original viscosity. This is defined as *thixotropy* and is caused by structural breakdown and re-formation. Example: some type of paint.

5.5 ELASTO-VISCOUS LIQUIDS

Some fluids, although they flow, show some elastic recovery after being sheared, e.g. sputum.

5.6 MEASUREMENT OF RHEOLOGICAL PROPERTIES

The apparatus used may be classified into various principal types:
(a) Capillary viscometers:
  (i) The viscosity of Newtonian fluids can be determined by timing their flow in a capillary tube.
  (ii) Rheological characteristics can be determined by extrusion of the material under pressure through a capillary. Viscosity can be calculated from data for force of extrusion, volumetric flow rate through the capillary and capillary dimensions. It is important that the material should flow in laminar fashion; there should be no turbulence in the fluid.

(b) Falling body viscometers. Viscosity can be calculated from the time taken for a sphere to fall or roll through a fluid.

(c) Rotational viscometers
  (i) Coaxial cylinder viscometers—the fluid is placed between two coaxial cylinders, either of which is rotated, depending

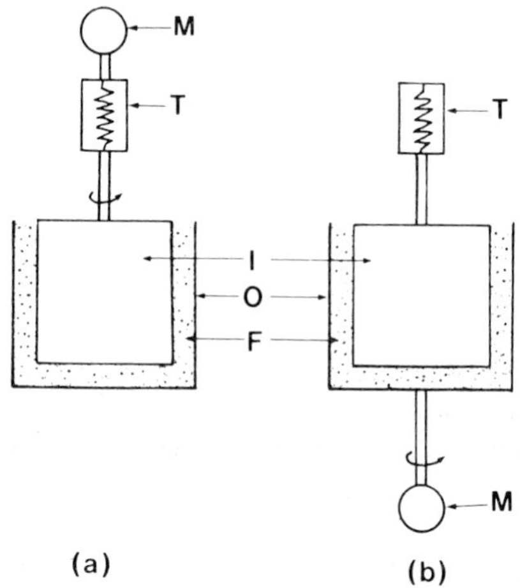

Fig. 5.5 Coaxial cylinder viscometers
(a) inner cylinder driven by motor
(b) outer cylinder driven by motor

M = motor; T = torque meter; F = fluid;
I = inner cylinder; O = outer cylinder

on the equipment design (Fig. 5.5). The shear rate is derived from the speed of rotation, and shear stress is obtained from a meter, which determines the torque transmitted through the liquid.

(ii) Cone-plate viscometers—in some instruments the fluid is sheared in the gap between a stationary plate and a rotating cone (Fig. 5.6). In all the viscometers described above, Newton's law is assumed in order to calculate the results. However, in the cone and plate viscometer, the shear rate is constant throughout the material, and depends only on the cone angle and speed of rotation. Shear stress can be calculated from torque and instrument dimensions. Hence shear stress and shear rate are independently measured. Thus this instrument is very suitable for the study of non-Newtonian fluids.

With an alternative instrument, the cone is fixed and the plate rotates or oscillates. Oscillatory shear tests can be used to measure elastic and viscous components of the deformation of fluids.

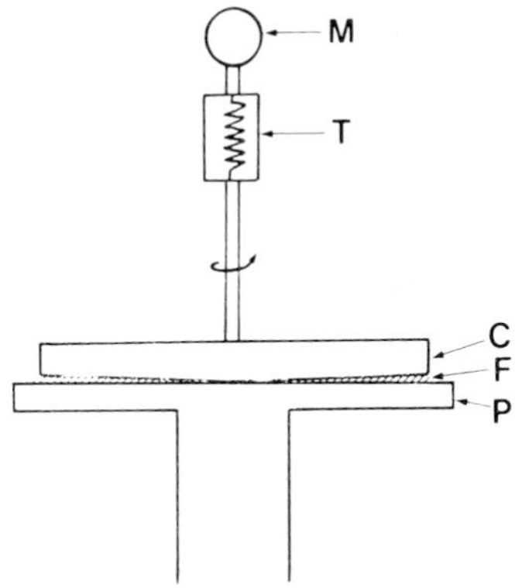

Fig. 5.6 Cone-plate viscometer
M = motor; T = torque meter; C = cone; F = fluid
P = plate

(iii) Rotating spindle viscometers—a spindle is made to rotate in the fluid, and viscous traction is measured.

(d) Parallel plate plastometer. This has two discs of the same size, between which the fluid is placed. One plate is made to move towards the other, and viscosity calculated from the force applied to move the plate and rate of movement.

(e) Qualitative instruments:

(i) Orifice viscometers consist of a fluid reservoir and an orifice. The time for a given volume of fluid to flow through the orifice is measured.

(ii) A penetrometer is a rod with a needle or cone which drops on to a sample and depth of penetration is measured.

(iii) Oscillating or reciprocating rheometers are frequently used in dental specifications. A platen oscillates in the material and the decrease in amplitude of oscillation is recorded as setting of the material occurs. Thus working and setting times are obtained.

Note: All rheological measurements require good temperature control.

5.7 VISCOELASTICITY

Reference has already been made to the use of oscillatory shear tests for measurement of elastic and viscous components of the deformation and fluids (Section 5.6(c)(ii)).

For studies of the viscoelastic behaviour of solids, two types of technique are of importance: (i) time-dependent techniques—creep and stress relaxation, and (ii) oscillatory techniques. Viscoelastic properties are of major importance in, for example, soft lining materials (Chapter 34) and denture base polymers (Fig. 33.1).

5.7.1 Time-dependent methods

(a) Creep

Creep is the slow deformation of a material under constant stress.

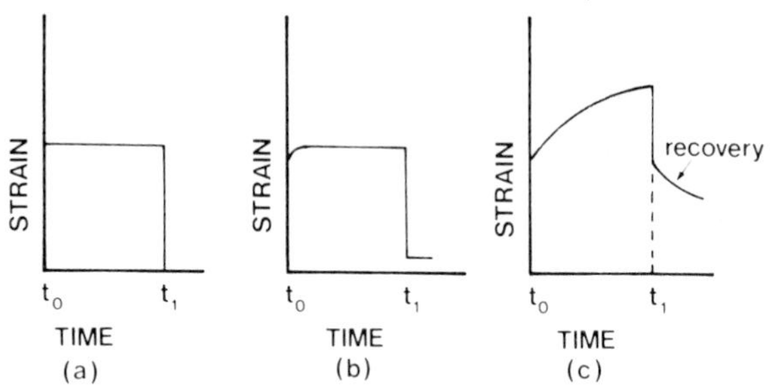

Fig. 5.7 Strain-time curves: load applied at t_0; load removed at t_1
(a) elastic material; no permanent strain.
(b) plastic material; permanent deformation at t_1
(c) viscoelastic behaviour; at t_1 recovery of the material commences.

The magnitude of deformation depends on the material, the temperature, the load, and the time of application of the load. Figure 5.7 illustrates the strain-time behaviour of material showing creep, in contrast to elastic and plastic deformations.

(b) Stress relaxation

When a viscoelastic material is given a constant strain, a gradual reduction in stress is observed (Fig. 5.8).

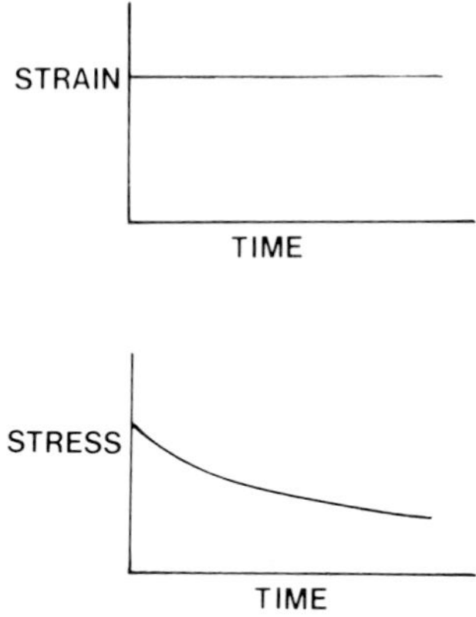

Fig. 5.8 Stress relaxation at constant strain.

5.7.2 Oscillatory techniques

Viscoelastic measurements can also be made by applying sinusoidal stresses or strains; the techniques include the torsion pendulum (free oscillations), vibrating reed techniques and wave propagation methods (fixed vibrations). It is possible theoretically to interrelate oscillatory and time-dependent methods.

READING REFERENCE

Sherman P 1970 Industrial rheology. Academic Press, London and New York

This book gives the general theory of rheology and details of experimental methods of determining rheological properties.

6. Thermal properties

6.1 INTRODUCTION

Materials in the mouth are subjected to variations in temperature because of the intake of hot foods and drinks. It is important to know about the transmission of heat by the materials (Sections 6.2 and 6.3) and also dimensional changes associated with thermal changes (Section 6.4).

6.2 THERMAL CONDUCTIVITY

Consider a lagged bar of materials, length d, surface area of cross-section A, the ends of which are kept at different temperatures, θ_1 and θ_2 (Fig. 6.1). The quantity of heat passing per second, Q, from one end to the other is given by:

$$Q = KA\,\frac{(\theta_1 - \theta_2)}{d},$$

where K is a constant, termed the *thermal conductivity* of the material. This may be defined as the quantity of heat passing per second between the opposite faces of a unit cube when the difference

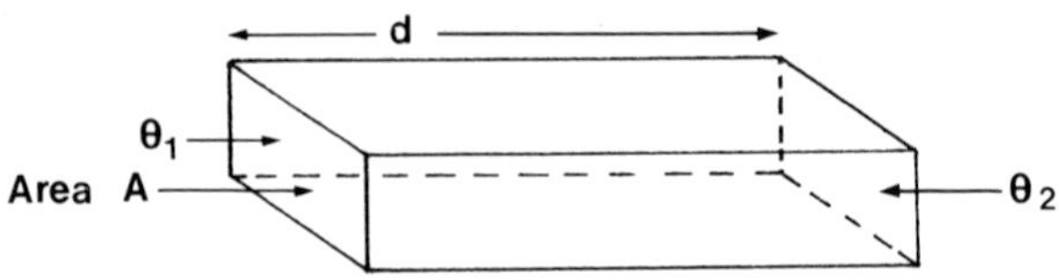

Fig. 6.1 Thermal conductivity

in temperature is unity. Thermal conductivity is expressed in units of W/mk.

6.3 THERMAL DIFFUSIVITY

The above discussion assumes steady state heat conditions. However, in the mouth, temperature changes are transient. To express the rapidity with which a material warms up before reaching the steady state, the *thermal diffusivity* is important. This is related to other properties as follows:

$$\text{Thermal diffusivity} = \frac{\text{Thermal conductivity}}{\text{Density} \times \text{specific heat}}$$

The units for diffusivity are mm^2/s.

6.4 THERMAL EXPANSION

The linear coefficient of thermal expanson of a material is the change in length per unit length when its temperature is lowered or raised by 1°C. This can be expressed as parts per million/°C.

6.5 DENTAL CONSIDERATIONS

(a) Temperature changes
- (i) It would be desirable for denture base materials to transmit some heat to the mucosal surfaces, so that denture wearers have the sensation of hot and cold foods (Section 33.3.5)
- (ii) In contrast, filling materials should not transmit heat to the pulp of the tooth (Section 19.2). Cements which have low thermal diffusivity are used for pulpal protection (Section 16.4).

(b) Dimensional changes
- (i) Ideally, filling materials should have similar coefficients of thermal expansion to enamel and dentine (Sections 14.5 and 19.9).
- (ii) Denture base materials and synthetic tooth materials should have similar coefficients (Section 33.3.5 and 37.2).
- (iii) Thermoplastic materials such as waxes often have a large coefficient of thermal expansion.

Numerical example: Calculate the percentage shrinkage of a wax of coefficient of thermal expansion 350 ppm/°C, on cooling from 55°C to 35°C.

Answer. For 1°C drop, shrinkage = 350 parts/million
= 0.035%

For 20°C drop, shrinkage $= 20 \times 0.035 = 0.7\%$

7. Light, colour and aesthetics

7.1 THE NATURE OF LIGHT

Visible light is a very small part of the electromagnetic spectrum (Table 7.1), being that region of the spectrum of wavelength approximately 380 nm to 780 nm. White light is made up of mixtures of colour (Table 7.2) as can be demonstrated by the well known experiment of Newton, in which light is dispersed by a prism (Fig. 7.1).

Table 7.1 The electromagnetic spectrum

Nomenclature	Frequency Hz	Approximate Wavelength m
Gamma rays	$3 \times 10^{22} - 3 \times 10^{19}$	$10^{-14} - 10^{-11}$
X-rays	$3 \times 10^{19} - 3 \times 10^{16}$	$10^{-11} - 10^{-8}$
Ultraviolet	$3 \times 10^{6} - 6 \times 10^{14}$	$10^{-8} - 5 \times 10^{-7}$
Visible light	$6 \times 10^{14} - 3 \times 10^{14}$	$4 \times 10^{-7} - 8 \times 10^{-7}$
Infra-red	$3 \times 10^{14} - 3 \times 10^{12}$	$10^{-6} - 10^{-4}$
Microwaves	$3 \times 10^{12} - 3 \times 10^{8}$	$10^{-3} - 1$
Radio waves	$<3 \times 10^{8}$	>1

To characterise a source of visible light, it is essential to know how much light is emitted at each wavelength. When energy *versus* wavelength is plotted., a *spectral energy distribution curve* is obtained. Figure 7.2 shows a typical curve for daylight, and Figure 7.3 is for blue light, with a peak wavelength of about 470–480 nm (of the type used for photopolymerisation of dental restorative materials, see Section 19.4).

Table 7.2 Wavelength of different regions of the visible spectrum

Colour	Approximate Wavelength nm
Violet	380–430
Blue	430–460
Blue-green	460–500
Green	500–570
Yellow	570–590
Orange	590–610
Red	610–780

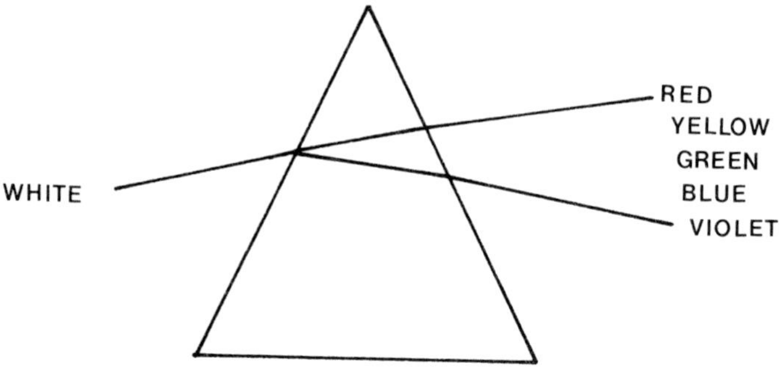

Fig. 7.1 Dispersion of white light as it passes through a prism.

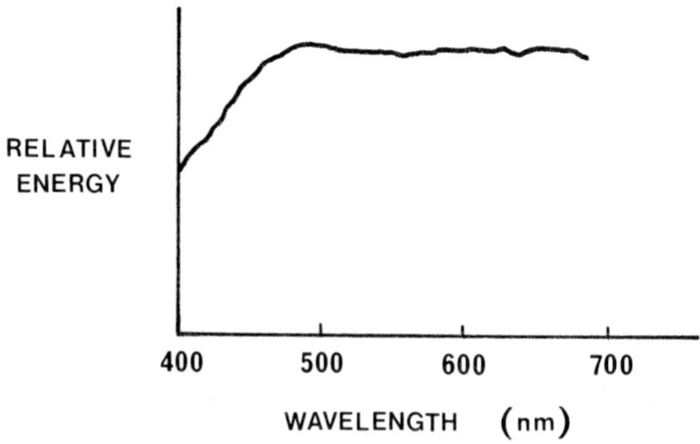

Fig. 7.2 Spectral energy distribution curve for sunlight.

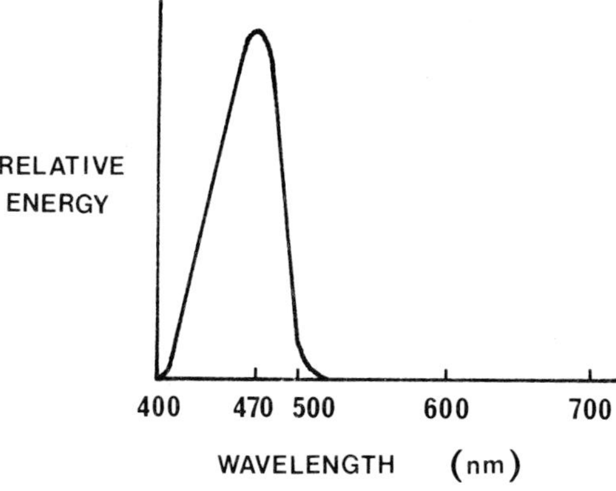

Fig. 7.3 Spectral energy distribution curve for blue light.

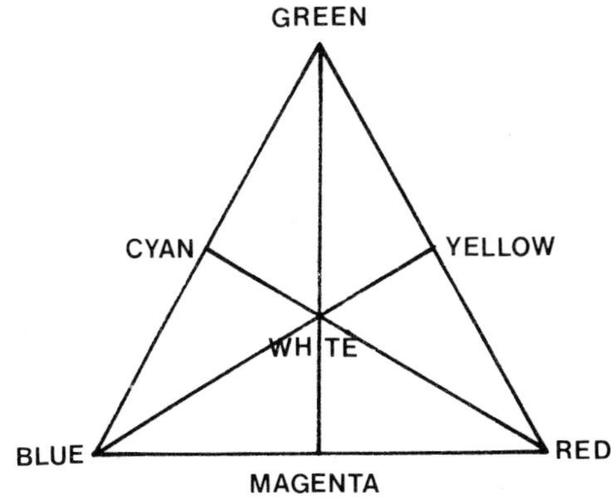

Fig. 7.4 Representation of colour addition.

7.2 COLOURS

There are three additive *primary* colours, namely, blue, green and red. If lights of these colours are added in the correct proportions, white light is produced.

A *secondary* colour is obtained by the addition of two primary colours, e.g. blue + green = cyan; green + red = yellow; red + blue = magenta.

Colour addition can be represented by an equilateral triangle, with the primary colours at the corners, and secondary colours at the mid-point of the sides (Fig. 7.4).

Two colours are said to be *complementary* if they combine to produce white. Examples (see Fig. 7.4): blue + yellow; green + magenta; red + cyan.

7.3 LIGHT AND MATTER

When a beam of light strikes an object, one of three things can happen: (a) transmisson, (b) absorption, (c) scattering of light.

7.3.1 Transmission of light

Substances which are *transparent* can transmit light. A beam of light changes direction at the boundary between materials, unless the angle of incidence is 90°. The refractive index n of a substance is given by:

$$n = \sin i / \sin r,$$

where i = the angle of incidence of light entering the material from air

and r = the angle of refraction of the light (Fig. 7.5)

Note that as well as refraction some light is reflected from the surface of the material.

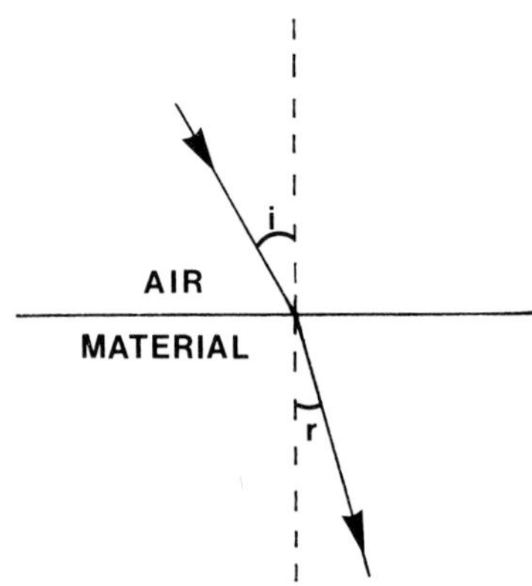

Fig. 7.5 Refractive index.

7.3.2 Absorption of light

Opaque materials absorb light. Lambert's law of absorption states that each successive layer of a substance absorbs an equal fraction of the light passing through it. This may be expressed as:

$$I_x/I_o = e^{-Kx},$$

where I_o = initial intensity of light
I_x = intensity of light after passage through distance x of the material
K = the *absorption coefficient* of the material

7.3.3 Scattering of light

In certain circumstances light can be scattered by matter. This will occur with a material which contains small particles of different refractive index from the bulk of the substance (Fig 7.6). If some light is transmitted, and some scattered, the substance is said to be *translucent*.

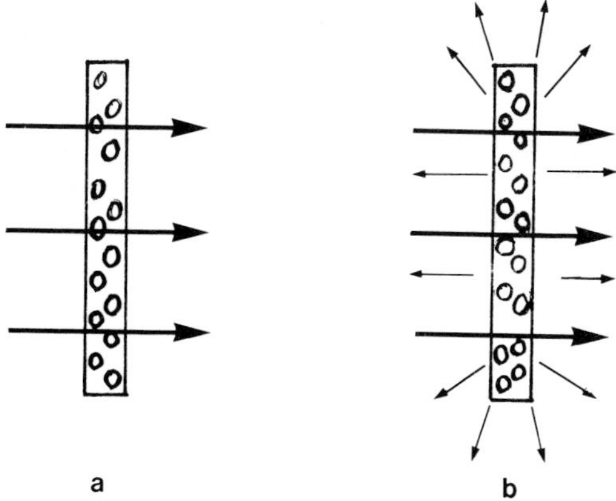

Fig. 7.6 (a) 2 components with same refractive index; no light scattering. (b) 2 components with different refractive indices; light scattering occurs.

7.4 COLOUR : PHYSICAL ASPECTS

The colour of an object will depend on a number of physical factors:
(a) The colour of the light source—in particular, the spectral energy distribution curve—affects the colour appearance of an object. For example, materials may appear to be different when viewed under different conditions, e.g. fluorescent light *versus*

daylight. Also, the colour of the surroundings may alter the light source.

(b) The nature of the object

- (i) If the object transmits coloured light (Section 7.3.1), some light energy is absorbed by the material. For example, a green filter absorbs blue and red light.
- (ii) For objects which reflect light: if it appears white, it reflects all colours; if it is black, it absorbs all colours; if it is coloured, that colour is reflected and all others are absorbed by the material.
- (iii) A translucent material appears lighter in colour than an opaque object.
- (iv) A substance which appears to have a high gloss reflects a large amount of light at the surface.
- (v) With mixed pigments, *subtractive* colour mixing occurs (distinguish from addition of colours as happens with light sources, Section 7.2). Thus yellow + cyan gives green, cyan + magenta gives blue; magenta + yellow gives red.
- (vi) Colour matching is important. *Metamerism* is said to occur when objects appear to match under one light source but not another (see Section (a) above).
- (vii) Some materials have the property of *fluorescence*. This is defined as the ability to absorb light of one wavelength and emit light of a different wavelength or colour. For example, natural teeth absorb ultra-violet radiation (400 nm wavelength) and emit light of 400–450 nm wavelength.

7.5 COLOUR : PHYSIOLOGICAL AND PSYCHOLOGICAL ASPECTS

(a) The retina of the eye contains specialised cells, which are called rods and cones. Stimuli received by the cones result in detection of colour.

(b) Some people have defective colour vision; this is caused by cell abnormalities.

(c) The eye is not equally sensitive to all colours; the greatest sensitivity is to green (wavelength c. 550 nm).

(d) Colour fatigue can occur. After seeing one colour constantly for a long period, the response of the eye to that colour is diminished.

(e) Psychological aspects are important, since optical illusions can occur. For example, the appearance of an object depends on its background; darker backgrounds make materials appear lighter.

7.6 COLOUR MEASUREMENT

To define a colour unambiguously, three parameters are important:
(a) *Hue* The hue is the colour—e.g. blue, red, green.
(b) *Value* is the darkness or lightness of the colour
(c) *Chroma* or *saturation* measures the intensity of the colour; e.g. low values of chroma indicate a weak colour.

One frequently used method of specifying colours is the *Munsell colour co-ordinate system* (Fig. 7.7). On the vertical axis is plotted the value. The hue is represented by a circle. The chroma is the distance from the centre.

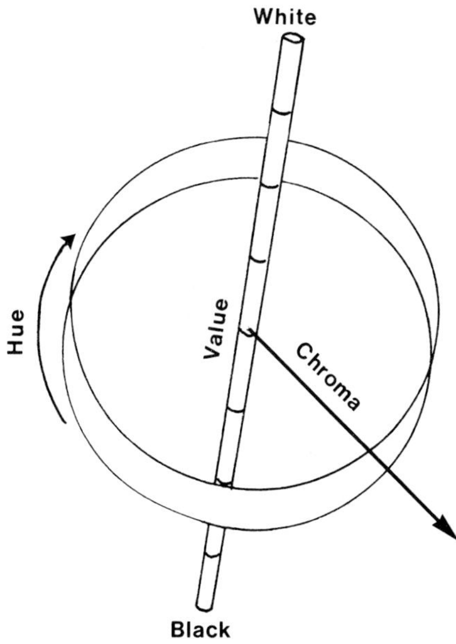

Fig. 7.7 Munsell colour co-ordinate system.

7.7 DENTAL CONSIDERATIONS

In many aspects of restorative dentistry, aesthetic considerations are important, for example, dentures, porcelain restorations, anterior restorative materials. The following factors are of relevance:
(a) Materials are pigmented by the manufacturer, and care should be taken in choosing a shade of material to give colour matching. Shade guides are often provided for this purpose. It is important to match colours under appropriate conditions of lighting.

(b) Aesthetic materials should be permanent in colour, neither showing staining (caused by external factors, e.g. constituents of diet) nor discolouration (caused by internal factors, such as chemical changes in components of the material).
(c) For best aesthetic effects, materials should be translucent.
(d) In some instance, dental materials (e.g. dental porcelain) contain fluorescing agents to enhance aesthetic appeal.

READING REFERENCE

Billmeyer F W Jr Saltzman M 1981 Principles of colour technology 2nd edn. Wiley, New York

A comprehensive treatise on the topic of colour.

8. Polymers

8.1 INTRODUCTION

Polymers are long chain molecules, consisting of many repeating units. A *monomer* is the smallest repeating unit in the polymer chain.

Polymerisation is the reaction by which polymers are prepared from monomers.

Polymers may be classified into (a) natural and (b) synthetic materials.

(a) Natural polymers include:

- (i) Proteins (or polyamides or polypeptides), containing the chemical group $(-\overset{\overset{\displaystyle O}{\|}}{C}-NH-)$ — this is known as an amide or peptide link (see Appendix III).
- (ii) Polyisoprenes, such as rubber and gutta percha (Appendix III).
- (iii) Polysaccharides, e.g. starch, cellulose, agar and alginates (Appendix III).
- (iv) Polynucleic acids, such as deoxyribonucleic acids (DNA) and ribonucleic acids (RNA).

(b) Synthetic polymers are produced industrially, or in the laboratory, by chemical reactions. Many such materials have become familiar to everyone, e.g. 'Bakelite', 'Nylon', 'Terylene' 'Polythene', 'Perpex', poly-(vinyl chloride). Not suprisingly, many of these have been used for dentures, and in other dental applications. In this chapter we were primarily concerned with synthetic polymers (including some inorganic materials), the reactions by which they can be made, how they are moulded, and their structure and properties.

Two types of chemical reaction, which result in polymers of dental interest, are considered: (a) condensation and (b) addition reactions.

8.2 CONDENSATION REACTIONS

Definition: this is a reaction between two molecules to form a larger molecule, with the elimination of a smaller molecule (this is often, but not always, water).

Some examples of interest:

(a) 'Nylon.' An organic acid (with a —COOH group) can react under appropriate conditions with an amine (with a —NH_2 group), to give a material with an amide linkage (as in proteins, Section 8.1).

$$R-\overset{O}{\overset{\|}{C}}-OH + H-\underset{H}{N}-R' \longrightarrow R-\overset{O}{\overset{\|}{C}}-NH-R' + H_2O$$

where R and R′ are organic groups.

Similarly a di-acid (molecule with 2 —COOH groups) can react with a di-amine(2 —NH_2 groups) to yield a polymer, called 'Nylon' (Appendix III, no. 25).

(b) 'Bakelite' is formed by the reaction of phenol with formaldehyde, to give molecules with a complex three-dimensional network (Appendix III, no. 4).

(c) Polycarbonates have the structure

$$—O-R-O-\overset{O}{\overset{\|}{C}}-O-R-O-\overset{O}{\overset{\|}{C}}—$$

where R is an organic group. Two reactions by which such compounds can be produced are discussed in Appendix III, no. 30.

(d) Epoxy compounds contain the group:

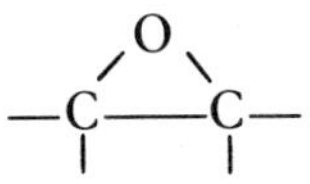

$$
\begin{array}{c}
\quad O \\
\diagup \quad \diagdown \\
-\underset{|}{C}—\underset{|}{C}-
\end{array}
$$

They are very important, for example, as adhesives. Some of their chemical reactions are listed in Appendix III, no. 15.

(e) Polysulphides—the basic constituents of some synthetic rubber materials—are formed as follows:

$$Cl—R—Cl + Na_2S_x \longrightarrow —R—S_x— + 2NaCl$$

(where x > 2).

(f) Silicones are inorganic polymers, formed by the condensation of silanols:

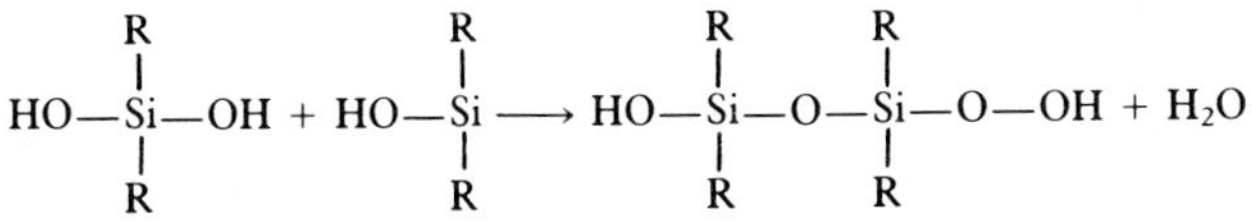

$$HO—\underset{R}{\overset{R}{\underset{|}{\overset{|}{Si}}}}—OH + HO—\underset{R}{\overset{R}{\underset{|}{\overset{|}{Si}}}} \longrightarrow HO—\underset{R}{\overset{R}{\underset{|}{\overset{|}{Si}}}}—O—\underset{R}{\overset{R}{\underset{|}{\overset{|}{Si}}}}—O—OH + H_2O$$

leading to the formation of a polymer chain:

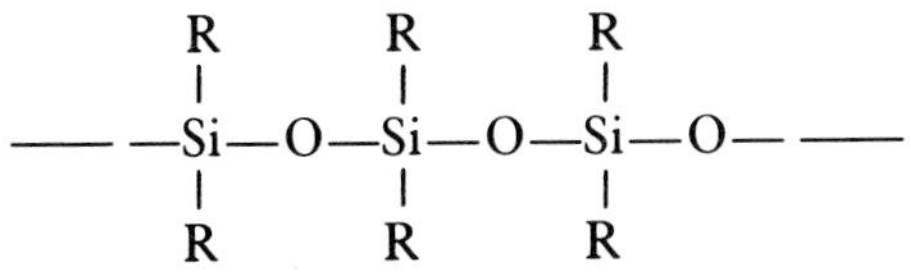

$$—\;—\underset{R}{\overset{R}{\underset{|}{\overset{|}{Si}}}}—O—\underset{R}{\overset{R}{\underset{|}{\overset{|}{Si}}}}—O—\underset{R}{\overset{R}{\underset{|}{\overset{|}{Si}}}}—O—\;—$$

8.3 FREE-RADICAL ADDITION REACTIONS

Definition: An addition reaction occurs between two molecules (either the same or dissimilar) to give a larger molecule without the elimination of a smaller molecule such as water. This type of reaction takes place for *vinyl* compounds—these are reactive organic compounds containing carbon-carbon double bonds. Some examples are listed in Table 8.1.

8.3.1 Activation and initiation

The polymerisation of a vinyl compound requires the presence of *free radicals*—these are very reactive chemical species having an odd (unpaired) electron. Such free radicals are formed, for example, in the decomposition of a peroxide. Thus under appropriate conditions, a molecule of benzoyl peroxide can yield two free radicals:

$$C_6H_5COO{-}OOCC_6H_5 \longrightarrow 2(C_6H_5COO\cdot)$$

These in turn can decompose to give other free radicals:

$$C_6H_5COO\cdot \longrightarrow C_6H_5\cdot + CO_2$$

Table 8.1 Vinyl monomers and their corresponding polymers.

Name of monomer	Formula of monomer	Corresponding polymer	Name of polymer
Ethylene	$H_2C{=}CH_2$	$\ldots{-}CH_2{-}CH_2{-}CH_2{-}CH_2{-}{-}$	Poly(ethylene) or polythene)
Vinyl chloride	$H_2C{=}CH{-}Cl$	$\ldots{-}CH_2{-}CHCl{-}CH_2{-}CHCl{-}{-}$	Poly(vinyl chloride) (or P.V.C.)
Styrene	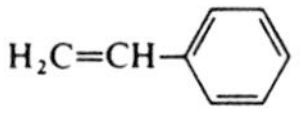 $H_2C{=}CH{-}C_6H_5$	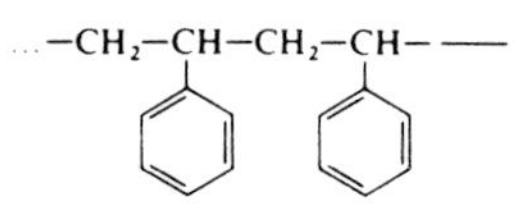 $\ldots{-}CH_2{-}CH(C_6H_5){-}CH_2{-}CH(C_6H_5){-}{-}$	Polystyrene
Acrylic acid	$H_2C{=}CH{-}C({=}O){-}OH$	$\ldots{-}CH_2{-}CH(COOH){-}CH_2{-}CH(COOH){-}{-}{-}$	Poly(acrylic acid)
Methacrylic acid	$H_2C{=}C(CH_3){-}C({=}O){-}OH$	$\ldots{-}CH_2{-}C(CH_3)(COOH){-}CH_2{-}C(CH_3)(COOH){-}{-}$	Poly(methacrylic acid)
Methyl methacrylate	$H_2C{=}C(CH_3){-}C({=}O){-}O{-}CH_3$	$\ldots{-}CH_2{-}C(CH_3)(COOCH_3){-}CH_2{-}C(CH_3)(COOCH_3){-}{-}{-}$	Poly(methyl methacrylate), (or acrylic)

Such chemical species are able to initiate vinyl polymerisation; they will be designated R•.

Before initiation occurs, however, the initiator requires to be activated. Activation is achieved by decomposition of the peroxide, either by (a) ultra-violet light, visible light or other electromagnetic radiation such as γ-rays, (b) heat, or (c) other chemicals, such as tertiary amines (e.g. N, N-dimethyl-p-toluidine, Appendix III, no. 13), or mercaptans (e.g. lauryl mercaptan, Appendix III, no. 22). In practice, methods (b) and (c) above are widely used for dental acrylic polymers, thus these are 'heat-cured' and 'self-cured' acrylics (Sections 33.3 and 33.4). Important dental examples in the use of visible light activation are given in Sections 19.3.6 and 33.7.

Instead of using a two-component system for activation and initiation, such as peroxide and amine, as in (c) above, a chemical such as p-toluene sulphinic acid (Appendix III, no. 46) may be employed. This produces free radicals which can initiate the polymerisation.

8.3.2 Propagation

Free radicals can react with monomer as follows:

$$\underset{\text{(free radical)}}{R\cdot} + \underset{\text{(methyl methacrylate)}}{CH_2{=}\overset{\overset{\displaystyle CH_3}{|}}{\underset{\underset{\displaystyle COOCH_3}{|}}{C}}} \longrightarrow R{-}CH_2{-}\overset{\overset{\displaystyle CH_3}{|}}{\underset{\underset{\displaystyle COOCH_3}{|}}{C}}\cdot$$

This free radical in turn can react with another molecule of monomer:

$$R{-}CH_2{-}\overset{\overset{\displaystyle CH_3}{|}}{\underset{\underset{\displaystyle COOCH_3}{|}}{C}}\cdot + CH_2{=}\overset{\overset{\displaystyle CH_3}{|}}{\underset{\underset{\displaystyle COOCH_3}{|}}{C}} \longrightarrow R{-}CH_2{-}\overset{\overset{\displaystyle CH_3}{|}}{\underset{\underset{\displaystyle COOCH_3}{|}}{C}}{-}CH_2{-}\overset{\overset{\displaystyle CH_3}{|}}{\underset{\underset{\displaystyle COOCH_3}{|}}{C}}\cdot$$

Thus the reaction proceeds, leading to the formation of a polymer chain.

These equations may be written in a simplified form, where M represents a molecule of monomer:

$$R\cdot + M \longrightarrow R{-}M\cdot, \text{ and,}$$

$$R{-}M\cdot + M \longrightarrow R{-}M{-}M\cdot, \text{ and so on.}$$

8.3.3 Termination

This occurs when two free radicals react to form a stable molecule:

$$R{+}CH_2{-}\overset{\overset{\displaystyle CH_3}{|}}{\underset{\underset{\underset{\underset{\underset{\underset{\displaystyle CH_3}{|}}{O}}{|}}{C{=}O}}{|}}{C}}{+}_n CH_2{-}\overset{\overset{\displaystyle CH_3}{|}}{\underset{\underset{\underset{\underset{\underset{\underset{\displaystyle CH_3}{|}}{O}}{|}}{C{=}O}}{|}}{C}}\cdot + R\cdot \longrightarrow R{+}CH_2{-}\overset{\overset{\displaystyle CH_3}{|}}{\underset{\underset{\underset{\underset{\underset{\underset{\displaystyle CH_3}{|}}{O}}{|}}{C{=}O}}{|}}{C}}{+}_{n+1}R$$

or by a transfer process:

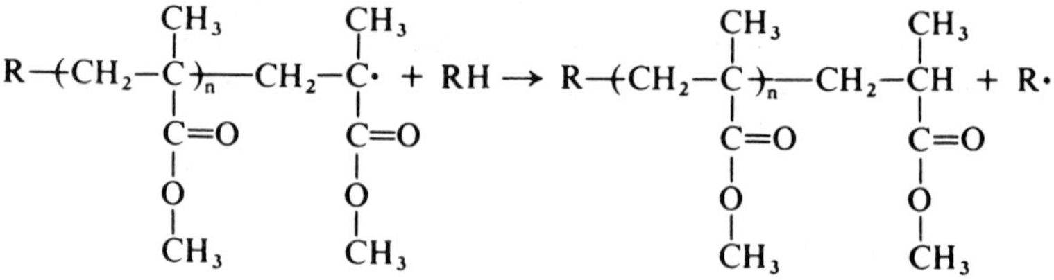

$$R\!-\!\left(CH_2-\underset{\substack{|\\ C=O\\ |\\ O\\ |\\ CH_3}}{\overset{\substack{CH_3\\ |}}{C}}\right)_n\!-CH_2-\underset{\substack{|\\ C=O\\ |\\ O\\ |\\ CH_3}}{\overset{\substack{CH_3\\ |}}{C}}\cdot + RH \rightarrow R\!-\!\left(CH_2-\underset{\substack{|\\ C=O\\ |\\ O\\ |\\ CH_3}}{\overset{\substack{CH_3\\ |}}{C}}\right)_n\!-CH_2-\underset{\substack{|\\ C=O\\ |\\ O\\ |\\ CH_3}}{\overset{\substack{CH_3\\ |}}{CH}} + R\cdot$$

Simplified form:

$$R{-}M_n{-}M\cdot + R\cdot \longrightarrow R{-}M_{n+1}{-}R, \text{ and,}$$
$$R{-}M_n{-}M\cdot + RH \longrightarrow R{-}M_{n+1}{-}H + R\cdot$$

8.4 IONIC POLYMERISATION

Addition polymerisation can occur by ionic as well as by free radical mechanisms.

8.4.1 Anionic polymerisation

Example: The polymerisation of cyanoacrylates:

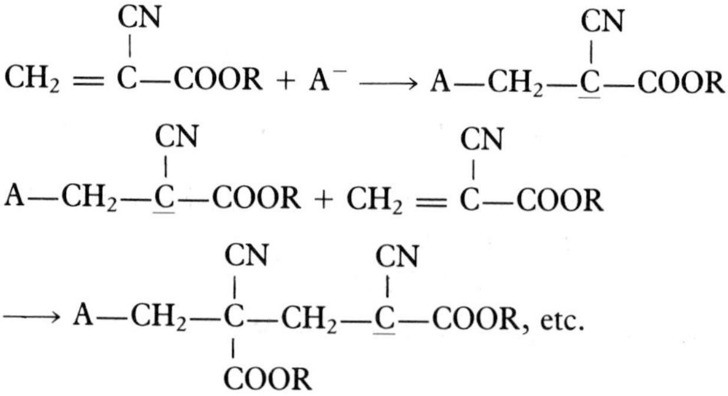

$$CH_2 = \overset{\substack{CN\\ |}}{C}{-}COOR + A^- \longrightarrow A{-}CH_2{-}\overset{\substack{CN\\ |}}{\underline{C}}{-}COOR$$

$$A{-}CH_2{-}\overset{\substack{CN\\ |}}{\underline{C}}{-}COOR + CH_2 = \overset{\substack{CN\\ |}}{C}{-}COOR$$

$$\longrightarrow A{-}CH_2{-}\underset{\substack{|\\ COOR}}{\overset{\substack{CN\\ |}}{C}}{-}CH_2{-}\overset{\substack{CN\\ |}}{\underline{C}}{-}COOR, \text{ etc.}$$

where R may be methyl, ethyl, propyl or butyl group, and A^- may be, for example, OH^-.

8.4.2 Cationic polymerisation

Example: Epimine compounds contain the group:

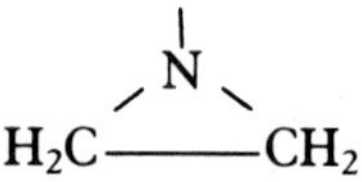

$$\begin{array}{c} | \\ N \\ \diagup \quad \diagdown \\ H_2C{-\!-\!-\!-}CH_2 \end{array}$$

A material such as benzene sulphonate ester:

$$C_6H_5—SO_3R$$

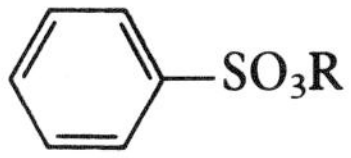

can supply cations, R^+ which can add to an epimine group causing ring opening:

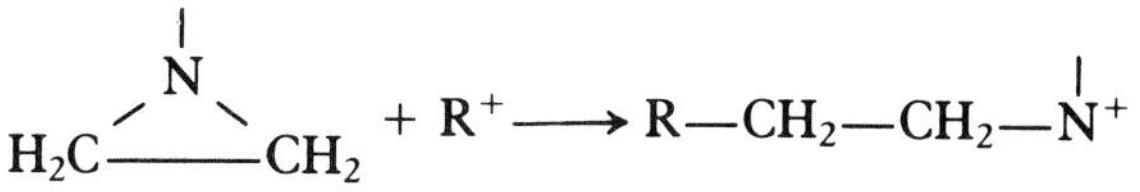

$$\underset{H_2C—CH_2}{\overset{|}{N}} + R^+ \longrightarrow R—CH_2—CH_2—\overset{|}{N}^+$$

In this type of reaction, molecules with two epimine groups can be cross-linked (Section 8.5).

8.5 CROSS-LINKING

Many reactions can be used to prepare polymers with chemical bonds between different chains. These materials are said to be *cross-linked.*

Examples:

(a) Some condensation polymers, such as phenol-formaldehyde (Appendix III, no. 4).
(b) Dimethacrylate compounds can undergo similar free-radical addition reactions to methyl methacrylate. These dimethacrylates may be:

(i) aliphatic, such as ethylene glycol dimethacrylate:

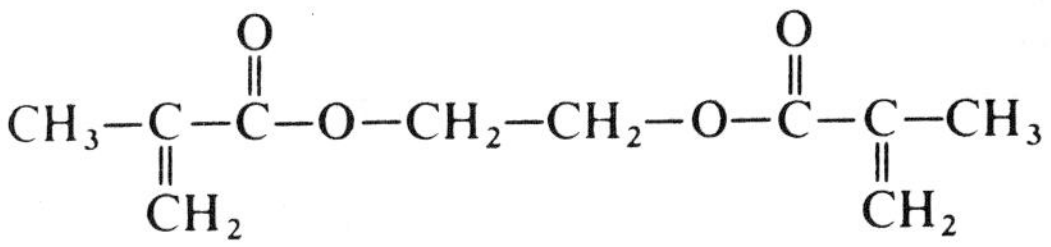

$$CH_3—\underset{\underset{CH_2}{\|}}{C}—\overset{\overset{O}{\|}}{C}—O—CH_2—CH_2—O—\overset{\overset{O}{\|}}{C}—\underset{\underset{CH_2}{\|}}{C}—CH_3$$

(ii) aromatic, such as Bowen's resin (Appendix III, no. 7).
(iii) alicyclic.

(c) Compounds with two epimine groups can be cross-linked by a benzene sulphonate ester (Section 8.4).
(d) Elastomers are also cross-linked (Section 8.6.2).

8.6 POLYMER STRUCTURE AND PROPERTIES

8.6.1 Degree of polymerisation and molecular weight

The *degree of polymerisation* (D.P.) may be defined as the number of repeating units in a polymer, i.e. the number of monomer units joined together. The *molecular weight* (mol.wt) is equal to the degree of polymerisation multiplied by the molecular weight of the repeating units.

It should be noted that the growth of polymer chains is a random process—some chains grow faster than others, some are terminated before others. Thus not all chains have the same length—that is, they have a distribution of molecular weights. The quoted molecular weight for a polymer is an average value.

8.6.2 Physical state

In terms of physical state, polymers exist as:
(a) elastomers or rubbers,
(b) hard amorphous polymers (organic glasses), for example, poly(methyl methacrylate),
(c) hard partially crystalline polymers, for example, polyethylene, and
(d) fibres; for example, nylon can exist in this form.

The first two of the above are considered here, as they are the most relevant to dentistry.

Rubbers consist of long chain molecules that are coiled and in random thermal motion. These molecules may be linked on to one another at relatively isolated points by covalent bonds (cross-links, Section 8.5). The specific feature of a rubbery polymer is that when the material is stretched the only work done is in uncoiling the molecules. Thus such materials are easy to deform, the deformation being largely reversible.

Although these materials are rubbery at room temperature, the effect of intermolecular forces will increase as temperature decreases, and at a reasonably well defined temperature (T_g, the *glass transition temperature*) the forces become so large as to inhibit uncoiling. Below the glass transition temperature the material will therefore be rigid just like polymers of type (b) above.

If a polymer of type (b) is heated, it is found to lose rigidity at a well defined temperature *above* room temperature, and become rubbery. In fact the difference between polymers of types (a) and (b) is that the former have a T_g well *below* room temperature, whereas the T_g of the latter is above room temperature.

8.6.3 Effect of molecular weight on properties

In many polymers the chains are held together by secondary, or Van der Waals forces, and molecular entanglement. Materials of high mol.wt have a greater degree of molecular entanglement, and have greater rigidity and strength and higher values of T_g and T_m (the melting temperature) than low mol.wt polymers.

8.6.4 The effect of cross-linking on physical properties

Cross-linking affects the physical properties of a polymer. A small degree of cross-linking limits the amount of movement of the polymer chains relative to each other when the material is stressed. Thus the deformation is elastic rather than plastic. Also, the polymer may have a higher value of T_g. Extensively cross-linked polymers are harder, more brittle and more resistant to the action of solvents than non-cross-linked materials.

8.6.5 Plasticisers

Liquids are able to penetrate between the randomly orientated chains of a polymer. As a result the molecules are further apart, and the forces between them are less. Such liquids are *plasticisers*. They soften the material and make it more flexible by lowering its T_g. If sufficient plasticiser is added, a polymer which is normally glassy at room temperature can have its T_g depressed to below room temperature, thus making it flexible and rubbery. This principle is used in producing acrylic soft lining materials (Ch. 34).

8.6.6 Co-polymers

Polymer chains which contain two or more different types of monomeric units can be prepared—these are termed *co-polymers*.

Several types of co-polymer are possible, for example, as below, where A and B represent different monomer units:

(a) alternating co-polymer

—A—B—A—B—A—B—A—B—A—B—A—B—A—B—

(b) random co-polymer

—A—B—A—A—B—B—A—B—A—A—A—B—B—A—

(c) block co-polymer

—A—A—A—A—A—A—A—B—B—B—B—B—B—B—

(d) graft co-polymer

```
—A—A—A—A—A—A—A—A—A—A—A—A—A—A—
   |                           |
   B                           B
   |                           |
   B                           B
   |                           |
```

Co-polymerisation processes have enabled chemists to 'tailor-make' molecules of predicted properties for special applications.

8.7 METHOD OF FABRICATING POLYMERS

8.7.1 Condensation polymers

When these were used dentally, they were supplied in an intermediate stage of condensation, and moulded by the application of heat and pressure to the required shape; during this process the condensation process continued.

8.7.2 Compression moulding

The products of addition polymerisation are usually *thermoplastic*; that is, they soften on heating and harden on cooling, without chemical change, (contrast to *thermosetting* polymers, which do not soften, but burn or decompose on heating). Thermoplastic polymers can be moulded by the application of heat and pressure.

8.7.3 Injection moulding

Industrially, thermoplastic materials are often moulded by heating the polymer until it is soft enough to be injected into a mould of the required shape. This method is used dentally, though not frequently (Section 33.2.2(f)).

8.7.4 Dough technique

This method is widely used dentally in the moulding of poly(methyl methacrylate) for dentures (Ch. 33). A dough is formed from a mixture of the monomer (liquid) and polymer (powder); this is packed into a mould and the monomer is polymerised under the appropriate conditions of activation and initiation (Section 8.3.1) to give a solid material.

8.8 DENTAL APPLICATIONS OF POLYMERS

The following list mentions polymers in the order in which they are considered in the following sections of this book; they are not necessarily placed in order of importance.

(a) Cements—polyacrylic acid is a constituent of zinc polycarboxylate cements (Section 17.3) and glass-ionomer cements (Section 18.3).
(b) Restorative materials—composite materials (Ch. 19).
(c) Polymers used in the so-called adhesive techniques (Ch. 20).
(d) Varnishes contain natural resins such as copal or rosin (Section 21.2).
(e) Impression materials—agar and alginates (Ch. 26) and polysulphide, silicone and polyether elastomers (Ch. 27).
(f) Polymeric crown and bridge materials (Ch. 32).
(g) Denture base materials (Ch. 33).
(h) Soft linings—plasticised polymers, higher methacrylates and silicone rubbers (Ch. 34).
(i) Acrylic tooth materials (Ch. 37).
(j) Orthodontic base polymers (Section 38.2).
(k) Die materials—filled polymers (Section 40.3.3).
(l) Some pattern materials for partial denture construction can be made of polymers such as polyethylene (Table 8.1, Section 41.4.2).
(m) Mouth protectors are made of polymeric materials (Ch. 49).

READING REFERENCES

Billmeyer F W 1971 Textbook of polymer science, 2nd edn. Wiley, New York & London

This is a comprehensive textbook on polymer science, dealing with many aspects of the physics, chemistry and properties of polymers.

McCabe J F, Wilson H J 1974 Polymers in dentistry. Journal of Oral Rehabilitation 1: 335

This is an extensive review of most of the polymers in current dental use.

9. Metals

9.1 CHARACTERISTIC PROPERTIES

Metals are usually:

(a) hard,
(b) lustrous,
(c) dense—the density is related to the atomic weight of the element, and to the type of lattice structure, which determines how closely the atoms are packed,
(d) good conductors of heat and electricity, due to the nature of the metallic bonds (Section 2.2.3),
(e) opaque, since the free electrons absorb the electromagnetic energy of light, and,
(f) ductile and malleable (Section 4.3.7).

Metals are also *electropositive*; that is, they give positive ions in solution.

Of over 100 elements in the periodic table, some 68 are metals; 8 are *metalloids* (for example, silicon, arsenic and boron)—these are similar to metals in some respects. All the remaining elements are non-metals.

9.2 OCCURRENCE AND EXTRACTION

Metals can occur either as the pure elements, or in compounds with other elements in ores. Examples:
gold occurs as the pure metal
silver occurs as the pure metal, or as Ag_2S or AgCl
copper seldom occurs as pure metal; is obtained as Cu_2S, CuS and oxides
iron—as Fe_2O_3.

An *ore* contains the compound of the metal, together with unwanted earthy material. Ores often go through the following processes before conversion to the metal: grinding, grading according to size and quality, and concentrating. The following methods of production of metals are available:

(a) Thermal methods—some oxides can be readily converted to metals in the presence of a reducing agent, for example:

$$Fe_2O_3 + 3C \xrightarrow{\text{heat}} 2Fe + 3CO$$

(b) Hydro-metallurgical methods—the ore is soaked in a dilute aqueous solvent such as sulphuric acid. Electrolysis of such a solution can yield the metal in a very pure state. Examples—silver, zinc and copper.

(c) Thermo-electrolytic—this is done by electrolysis of the molten mineral, and is used for aluminium, calcium, sodium, etc.

9.3 FORMING AND SHAPING

9.3.1 Casting

This involves melting the metal (or alloy, see Ch. 10), and shaping it in a mould. For example, steel, bronze, aluminium, etc., can be poured into moulds of sand and clay. The clay bonds the sand together. Such moulds are destroyed after use. *Die-casting* uses

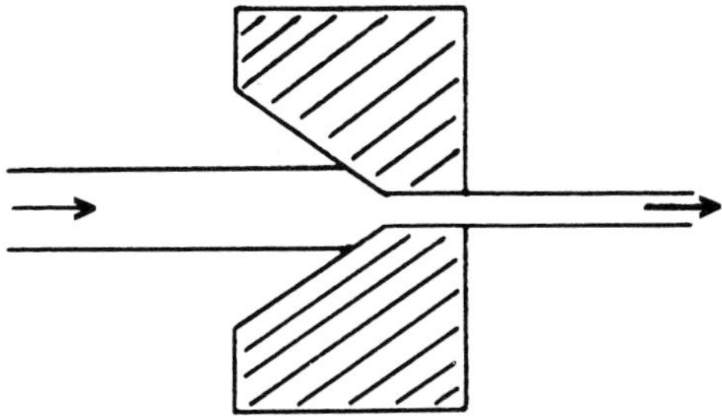

Fig. 9.1 Drawing a wire through a die.

permanent metal moulds. In dentistry investment casting is very important where an investment mould is made from a wax pattern; the principles of this are discussed in Chapter 43.

9.3.2 Cold working

In general, metals can be hammered into a sheet, extruded, or rolled. They can be pulled through dies to form wires (Fig. 9.1—see Section 38.4.1).

9.3.3 Powder metallurgy

A metal powder can be pressed under high pressure to produce a formed object. The product of this process is weak as there is little adhesion between the particles. Improved strength results on *sintering*, in which the pressing is heated in a non-oxidising atmosphere below the melting point, and the particles agglomerate. This technique is used to make tungsten carbide burs (Section 46.3). Sintering can also occur on heating certain oxide powders (Section 17.2.4)

9.3.4 Electroforming

Using the process of electrolysis, a metal can be plated on to a conducting surface; for the principles, and dental examples, see Section 40.3.5

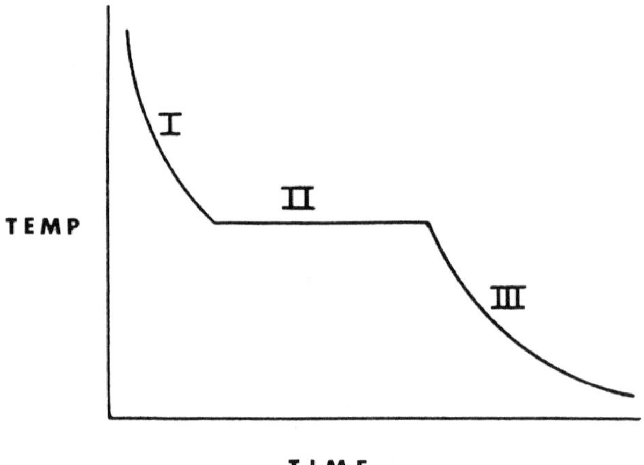

Fig. 9.2 Temperature-time curve for cooling of a molten metal. I, cooling of molten metal; II, solidification of the metal; III, cooling of solidified metal.

9.4 COOLING OF A MOLTEN METAL

9.4.1 Temperature—time curve

On cooling a pure molten metal, a temperature-time curve of the type shown in Figure 9.2 is obtained. This graph shows three portions: (I) for the cooling of the molten liquid; (II) a *plateau*—a horizontal portion—during this time the metal is solidifying, and there is evolution of latent heat of fusion which compensates for the heat loss to the surroundings; and (III) a portion for the cooling of the completely solidified metal.

9.4.2 Structure on solidification

Solidification starts at centres of crystallisation called *nuclei*.

Some of these nuclei may be impurities which exist even in a pure metal, scattered throughout the material. Growth of crystals from nuclei occurs in three dimensions, in the form of *dendrites* or

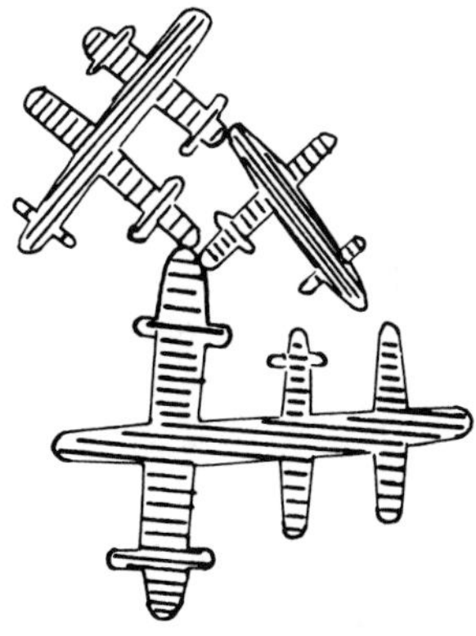

Fig. 9.3 Two dimensional representation of growth of dendrite.

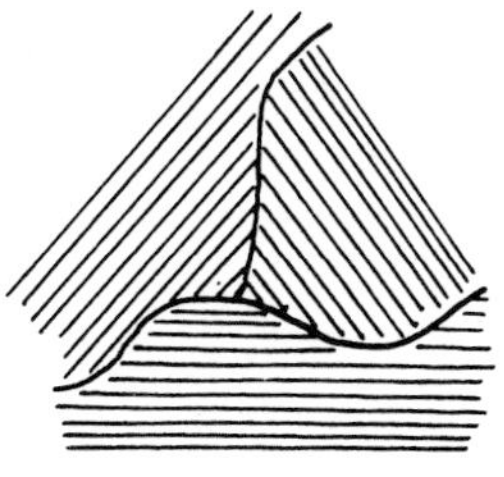

Fig. 9.4 Grain structure resulting from dendrite in Fig. 9.3

branched structures (Fig. 9.3). Growth continues until contact is made with adjacent growing crystals (Fig. 9.4), and solidification is complete when the pools of liquid between the dendrite arms have crystallised. Each nucleus gives rise via dendrites to one crystal or grain.

9.4.3 The grain structure of the solidified material

Each crystal of a metal is termed a *grain*. Each grain has grown from a nucleus. Within each grain, the orientation of the crystal lattice and the crystal plances is uniform. Adjacent grains have different orientations, because the initial nuclei acted independently from each other (See Fig. 9.5). Thus at the *grain boundary*—a narrow region 2 to 3 atomic diameters wide, the atoms take up positions intermediate between those of the atoms in the adjacent space lattices.

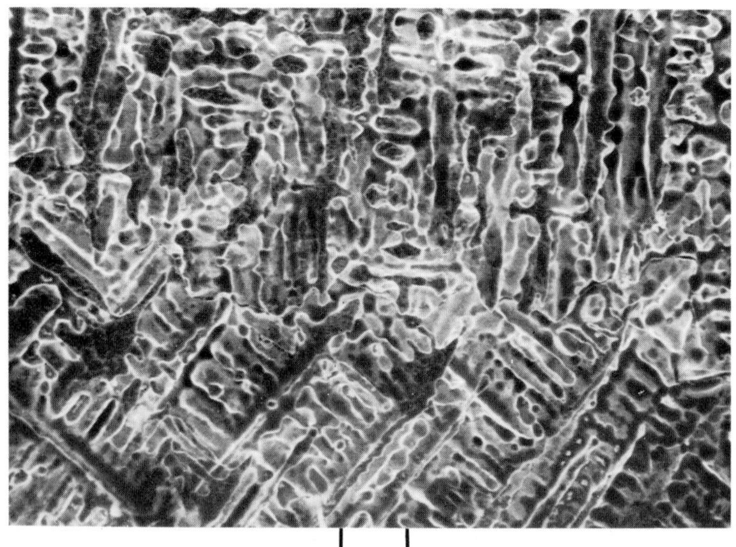

Fig. 9.5 SEM photograph showing different orientations of adjacent grains (Ni-Cr alloy). The distance between the markers represents 100 microns.

9.5 EXAMINATION OF GRAIN STRUCTURE

A surface of the metal is flattened, using emery or silicon carbide, then it is abraded and polished on a rotating disc, covered with chamois or other soft material which holds the polishing medium. The metal polish is removed by washing with water or alcohol.

The polished surface is then *etched*—treated with chemical agents, which attack the grain boundaries of the metal more than the grains themselves. This is because the atoms at the grain boundaries are more reactive, since they are not surrounded symmetrically by other atoms, as are the ones in the centre of the grain. Either acids or alkalies are used as etching agents—these may be in aqueous or alcoholic solution.

Etching of the prepared metal specimen produces grooves at the grain boundaries. On observing an etched metal microscopically, these grooves reflect light away from the observer more than the surface of the grain, so appear as black lines (Fig. 9.4).

9.6 RELATIONSHIP OF MICROSTRUCTURE TO MECHANICAL PROPERTIES

(a) *Elastic strain* in a metal is mainly due to a stretching of the inter-atomic bonds. The modulus of elasticity is determined by the chemical composition, and is scarcely affected by microstructure.
(b) *Plastic deformation* involves the *slip* of layers of atoms over each other. Slip does not occur by the movement (or shear) of an entire plane of atoms over the next layer in a single movement—this would require an enormous stress. Instead, the slip occurs by a localised region of shear, which passes progressively through the length of the slip plane. This localised shear zone is called a *dislocation* (Fig. 2.8).

In general, pure metals are very ductile, because each grain has many different slip planes in various directions. Dislocation movement is easy in metals because of the nature of metallic bonding. In contrast to this, dislocations are much less mobile in non-metallic crystals.

The proportional limit, or yield stress, is a measure of the ease with which dislocations can move in a metal. The yield stress of a pure single crystal of a metal is low, but may be raised by obstructing the movement of dislocations. This may be achieved by:
(a) Grain boundaries—a polycrystalline metal will have a higher yield stress than a single crystal. The yield stress is higher for a material of finer grain size, which has more grain boundaries.
(b) Other dislocations—if a metal is cold worked, large numbers of

dislocations accumulate internally. As a result, there is an increase in hardness and yield stress—hence *work hardening*.

(c) Alloying—see Chapter 10.

In general, obstruction of the movement of dislocations results not only in an increase in yield stress and hardness, but also in a lowering of ductility and impact resistance.

9.7 FACTORS AFFECTING GRAIN SIZE AND STRUCTURE

9.7.1 Rate of cooling

Slow cooling results in the formation of a *coarse grain structure*, whereas rapid cooling usually give a *fine structure* (Fig. 9.6). Rapid cooling produces more nuclei of crystallisation, thus more grains in a given volume of material, so that each grain is smaller. The structures in Figure 9.6 and both *equiaxed*—that is, the grains are not elongated (compare Fig. 9.7).

Rapid cooling of a molten metal is obtained in the following cases:

(a) when a mould of high thermal conductivity is used.

(b) if the bulk of the casting is small, and

(c) if the metal has been heated to only just above its fusion temperature.

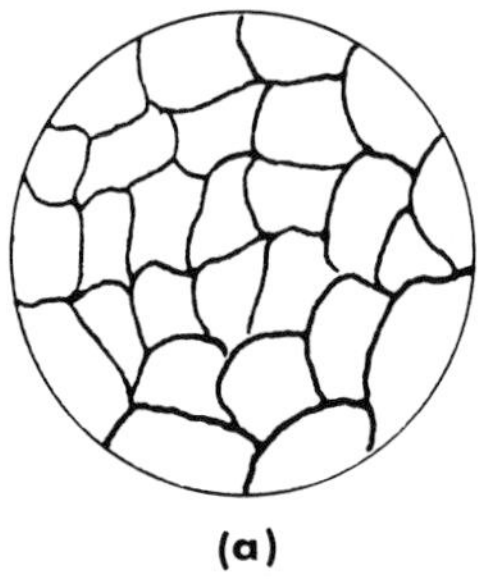

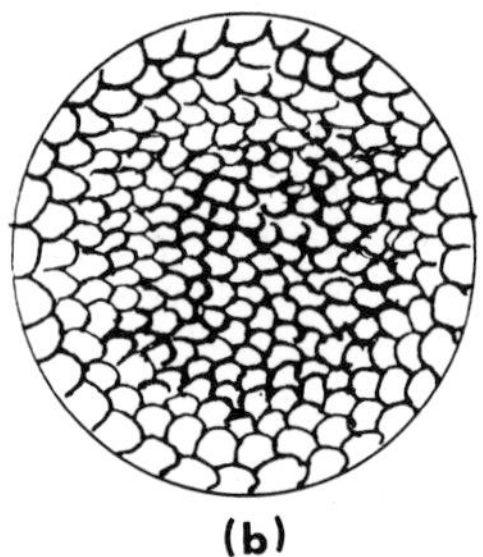

Fig. 9.6 Grain structures: (a) coarse equiaxed structure, (b) fine equiaxed structure.

After solidification the metal can then be cooled either slowly, or rapidly by *quenching* it in a cooling liquid such as water or oil.

9.7.2 Nucleating agents

Either impurities or additives can act as nucleating agents, so *refining* the grain structure.

9.7.3 Cold working

Hammering, rolling or drawing into a wire transforms the equiaxed structure into a *fibrous structure* (Fig. 9.7).

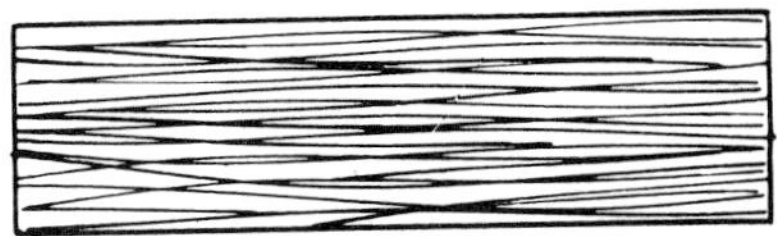

Fig. 9.7 A length of wire with a fibrous grain structure.

9.7.4 Stress relief anneal (recovery)

After cold working, there are internal stresses in a metal—these can cause cracking or distortion. A stress relief anneal can overcome these—it is a low temperature heat treatment which has little effect on the fibrous grain structure.

9.7.5 Recrystallisation

Further heating of a cold worked material can alter its grain structure, the new structure consisting of small equiaxed grains. In this case the metal is said to have been *recrystallised*.

The *recrystallisation temperature* is that temperature at or above which a metal will recrystallise rapidly. *Cold working* (as in Section 9.7.3) is defined as working below this temperature.

9.7.6 Grain growth

If a metal is overheated, or heated for too long, during recrystallisation, *grain growth* occurs. This results in a material of coarser grain structure.

Both grain growth and recrystallisation occur by means of *diffusion* or movement of the metal atoms across grain boundaries.

9.8 PRACTICAL POINTS

The following general practical points are important:

(a) Cooling a molten metal should be done rapidly, to get a fine grain structure, if strength and hardness are important.

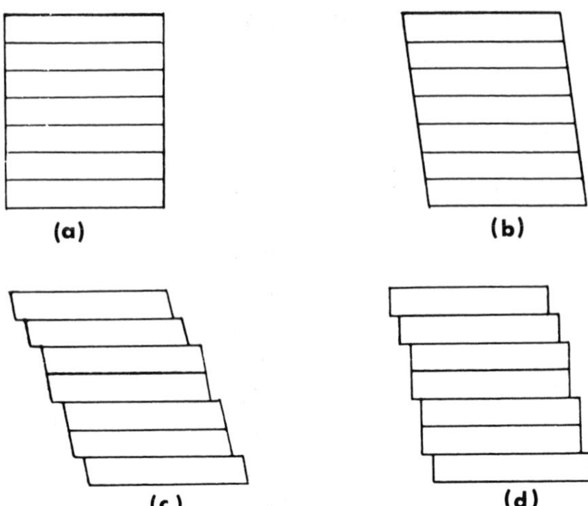

Fig. 9.8 Slip planes: (a) horizontal lines represent slip planes; (b) elastic deformation when material stressed; (c) under greater stress, slip and plastic deformation occur; (d) stress removed, permanent deformation.

(b) Cold working increases hardness and strength—this is known as *work-hardening*. However, this reduces the percentage elongation, so the material becomes more brittle. It becomes liable to fracture if further cold work is carried out, because the potential for further slip has been lost.
(c) The internal stresses of a cold worked metal can be removed by a heat treatment at a temperature well below the recrystallisation temperature.
(d) Recrystallisation gives a fine grain structure. Sometimes cold working followed by heat treatment is used to obtain a fine structure, to improve the properties of the material.
(e) Overheating, causing grain growth, must be avoided if properties such as high yield stress and hardness are desired.

9.9 METALS IN DENTISTRY

Pure metals are very seldom used in dentistry (exceptions—gold foil, Chapter 23, and platinum in laboratory procedures with dental porcelain, Section 28.3.1). Generally pure metals are too soft and ductile to make them suitable for dental applications. Mechanical properties can often be improved by using mixtures of metals. These are called *alloys* (Ch. 10).

READING REFERENCES

These are given at the end of Chapter 10.

10. Alloys

10.1 INTRODUCTION

An *alloy* is a mixture of two or more metallic elements; sometimes an important constituent may be a metalloid, or even a non-metal (example, carbon in steel, Section 10.6), provided the mixture of elements displays metallic properties. Many of the principles discussed in Chapter 9 for pure metals also apply to alloys—e.g. Sections 9.3 to 9.7, though the temperature-time curves are often different. (Compare Fig. 10.4 with Fig. 9.2).

In the previous chapter it has been shown that the properties of a metal depend on its thermal and mechanical treatments. The properties of an alloy depend not only on these factors, but also on its composition. The mechanical properties of an alloy can be very different from those of the component metals or metalloids. For example, an alloy of 50% gold and 50% copper has an ultimate tensile strength greater than that of either gold or copper.

Alloys may be classified as *binary* (2 constituents), *ternary* (3 constituents), *quaternary* (4 constituents), etc. The greater the number of constituents, the more complex becomes the structure of the alloy. For simplicity, binary alloy *systems* will be considered (Sections 10.2 to 10.4).

A *system* refers to all possible percentage compositions of the alloy. For example, the gold-silver system refers to all combinations of the two from 100% gold to 100% silver.

The properties of alloys are illustrated by two examples of contrasting structure and properties—the gold alloys (Section 10.5) and steel (Section 10.6). Section 10.7 lists the uses of alloys in dentistry, with references to future chapers, where the composition and properties of other alloy systems can be found.

10.2 BINARY ALLOYS

10.2.1 Introduction

When two molten metals are mixed, they usually form a solution. A *solution* is defined as a perfectly homogeneous mixture.

On cooling such a solution, one of three things may happen:

(a) A solid solution can be formed (Section 10.2.2);

(b) The two metals may be completely insoluble in the solid state, though this is rare (Section 10.2.3), or,

(c) There may be partial solid solubility (Section 10.2.4).

Additionally, or alternatively intermetallic compounds may be formed (Section 10.2.5).

10.2.2 Solid solutions

In a solid solution there is only one *phase* present. A *phase* is defined as any physically distinct, homogeneous, mechanically separable part of a system. Solid solutions may be of two types:

(a) Substitutional solid solutions. These are formed where two different types of atoms occur in different positions in the same crystal lattice (Figs. 10.1 and 10.2). This type of solid solution is likely to be formed between two metals if:

- (i) their atomic sizes differ by less than about 15%,
- (ii) they have the same type of crystal lattice, for example, face centered cubic, body centered cubic or hexagonal close packed (Section 2.4.1),
- (iii) they have the same chemical valency, and,
- (iv) they do not react to form intermetallic compounds (Section 10.2.5).

In Table 10.1 are data for gold, and some metals which form substitutional solid solutions with gold (see Section 10.5.2).

Table 10.1 Properties of some metals

Metal	Atomic diameter (Å)	Approximate percentage difference in size from gold	Crystal lattice	Usual valencies
Gold	2.88	—	f.c.c.	1.3
Copper	2.55	11.5	f.c.c.	1.2
Silver	2.92	1.4	f.c.c.	1.2
Platinum	2.77	3.8	f.c.c.	2.4
Palladium	2.74	4.9	f.c.c.	2.4

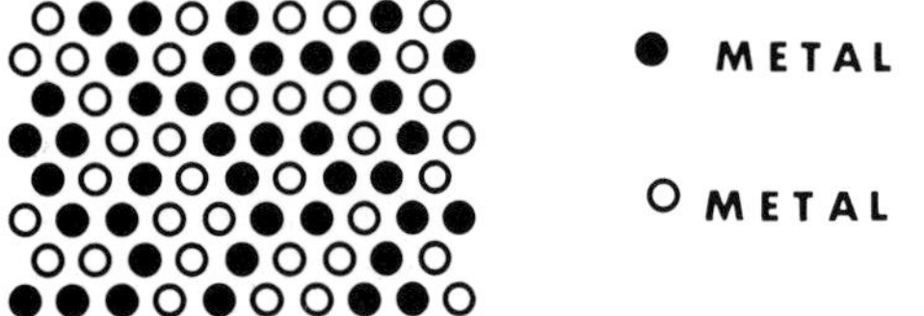

Fig. 10.1 Random or disordered substitutional solid solution.

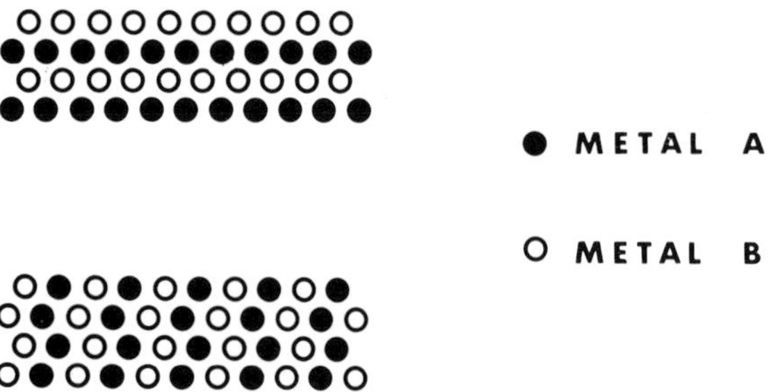

Fig. 10.2 Two examples of ordered substitutional solid solutions.

Substitutional solid solutions may be either *disordered* (Fig. 10.1) with a random distribution of the atoms of the two metals, or *ordered* (Fig. 10.2). (See Section 10.4.3.)

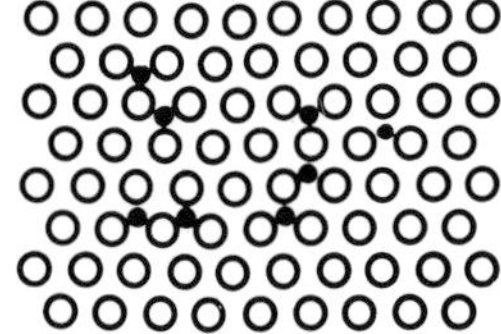

Fig. 10.3 Interstitial solid solution.

(b) Interstitial solid solutions (Fig. 10.3), where very small atoms can be accommodated in the interstices or spaces between larger atoms, for example, carbon in iron (Section 10.6).

10.2.3 Insolubility in the solid state

When this occurs, as in the bismuth—tin system, the solid alloy is heterogeneous, containing two phases. Even in the example quoted, complete solid insolubility is never obtained.

10.2.4 Partial solid solubility

This occurs, for example, in the silver-copper and lead-tin systems.

10.2.5 Intermetallic compounds

Metals with chemical affinity for each other can form intermetallic compounds. For example, the compound Ag_3Sn can be formed between silver and tin—this is an essential constituent of dental amalgam alloys (Ch. 22). In the formation of these compounds the normal chemical valency of the metals does not always apply.

10.3 PHASE DIAGRAMS (or thermal equilibrium diagrams)

10.3.1 Derivation

These diagrams are composition-temperature graphs. They are derived principally from cooling curve data. Figure 10.4 is the cooling curve of a binary alloy—it has no horizontal plateau like that of a pure metal (though, for one exception to this see Section 10.3.3), but two points X_L and X_S, where there are observed changes in the rate of cooling. Above temperature T_L the alloy is completely molten; between T_L and T_S the material is solidifying; at temperatures below T_S the alloy is completely solid.

To obtain the phase diagram for an alloy system (metals A and B), mixtures of different known compositions are prepared (e.g. 90% A and 10% B; 80% A and 20% B, etc.) and values of T_L and T_S determined for each. For the pure metals A and B, since the cooling curve has a horizontal plateau (Fig. 9.2), $T_L = T_S$.

All the results are plotted on a graph such as Figure 10.5, which is the *phase diagram*. There are two lines on this diagram:

(a) The upper line is obtained by joining up the plotted points of T_L values for the various compositions. It is called the *liquidus*; for any composition and temperature above this line, the alloy is completely molten.

(b) Similarly the lower line is obtained by joining up the plotted points of T_S. This line is called the *solidus*; below this the material is completely solidified.

The area between the two lines represents the range of temperature and composition for the partially solidified alloy.

Note: Phase diagrams are obtained when there are equilibrium conditions in a system; this does not apply if an alloy is cooled rapidly.

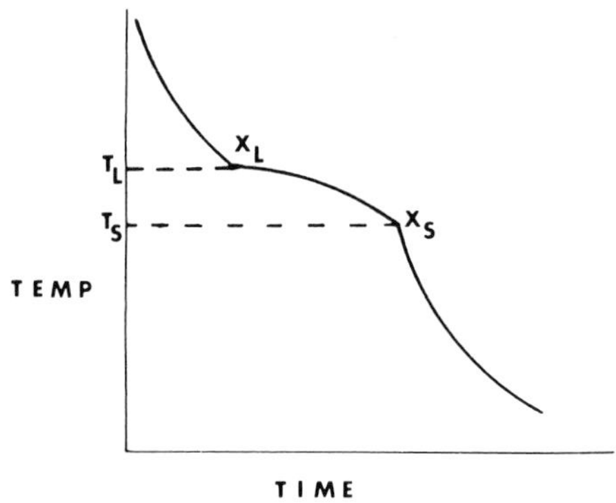

Fig. 10.4 Cooling curve of an alloy. Above temperature T_L the alloy is completely molten; below temperature T_S the alloy is completely solid.

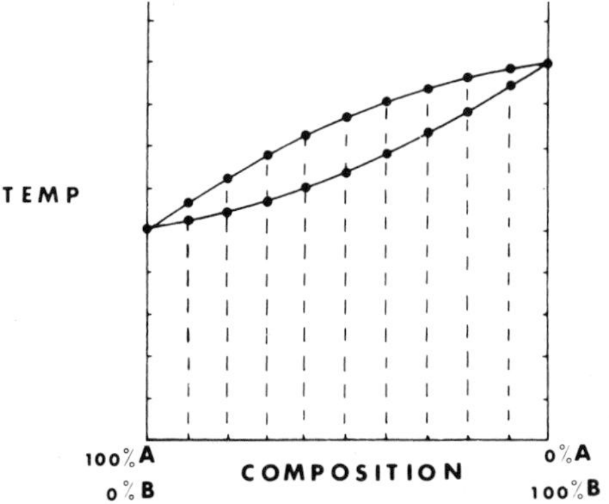

Fig. 10.5 Phase diagram for a binary solid solution.

10.3.2 Binary solid solutions

Figures 10.5, 10.6 and 10.9 are examples of phase diagrams for solid solutions. Consider in Figure 10.6, an alloy of 70% A and 30% B, at

900°C (point 0)—it is completely molten. On cooling to 800°C (point L_1) it begins to solidify. With a solid solution alloy the composition of the solid which forms is not the same as that of the liquid from which it forms. The composition of the solid which does form can be found by drawing a horizontal line through L_1 to the point where it interests the solidus at S_1. In this instance, the solid forming will have a composition of 30% A and 70% B, in distinction to the liquid from which it formed, which had a composition of 70% A and 30% B.

As soon as any solid is formed, this means that the composition of the liquid remaining will be different from that prior to the onset of solidification. At any temperature below L_1, but above the solidus, the composition of the liquid remaining, and of the solid formed, will be found by drawing a horizontal line at that temperature to intersect the liquidus and solidus. For example, at 750°C (Fig. 10.6), the composition of the total solid which has formed is S_2 and that of the liquid remaining is L_2. The solid forming becomes progressively richer in A as solidification proceeds as does the composition of the remaining liquid. The material completely solidifies at S_3.

The consequence of this is that provided the alloy is rapidly cooled after solidfying (see below) the composition of each grain of the alloy is not uniform—this is called *coring*. In the example above, the first material to solidify (that is, in the centre of the dendrites) is richer in B than the rest of the alloy, whereas the last material will be richer in metal A. Such a *cored structure* can be undesirable, particularly in relation to the corrosion resistance of the alloy (Section 11.3.1).

If the alloy had been cooled slowly, or reheated then cooled slowly, there would have been little or no coring—the latter process is called *homogenisation.*

Homogenisation depends on the movement, or *diffusion* of metal atoms. The greater the temperature, the greater is the thermal energy of the atoms, so they can diffuse more readily. At room temperature, the rate of diffusion in metallic materials is negligible, so no homogenisation can occur. Thus rapid cooling to room temperature does not permit much diffusion to occur.

The phenomenon of *order hardening* can occur in substitutional solid solutions—this is discussed in Section 10.4.3.

10.3.3 Binary eutectics

A phase diagram for a binary system where there is complete solid

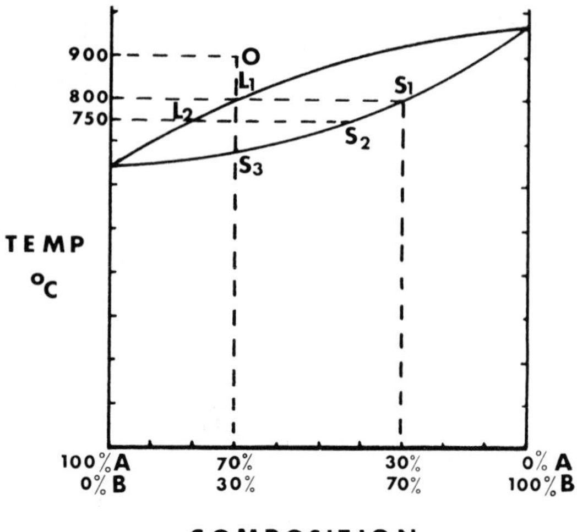

Fig. 10.6 Phase diagram for a binary solid solution.

insolubility (if this were possible in practice) is shown in Fig. 10.7. CEF is the liquidus, and CDEGF is the solidus. At E the liquidus and solidus coincide. A material of this composition is called a *eutectic alloy*. There are two features of interest here:

(a) The eutectic alloy is the lowest melting alloy of the system.

(b) The temperature-time curve for this alloy has a horizontal plateau (like that of a pure metal, Fig. 9.2).

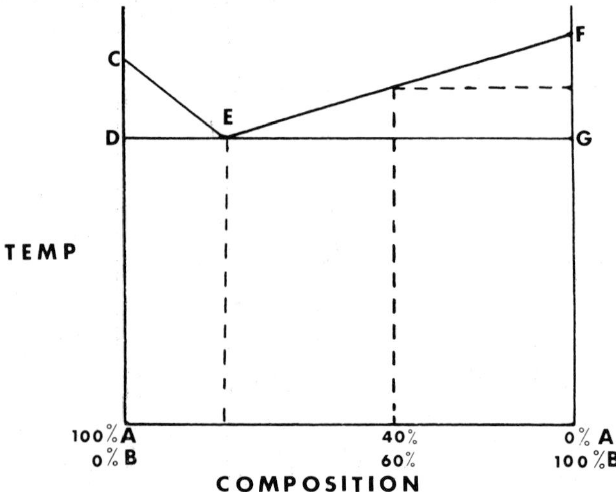

Fig. 10.7 Phase diagram for a binary system where there is complete solid insolubility.

On solidifying an alloy of composition E, there is simultaneous crystallisation of metals A and B, side by side, to form two phases. On cooling an alloy of composition 40% A and 60% B (Fig. 10.7), with more of metal B than the eutectic composition, pure B crystallises until the remaining molten liquid has the same composition as E, at which point A and B crystallise together.

Similarly on cooling an alloy of composition 80% A and 20% B, with more of metal A than the eutectic composition, pure A crystallises until the remaining liquid has the composition at E, when A and B crystallise together.

10.3.4 Partial solid solubility

Figure 10.8 is a phase diagram that occurs in a binary alloy system with partial solid solubility (as in Ag—Cu and Pb—Sn systems). CEF is the liquidus and CDEGF the solidus, as before. Below this latter line, the material is completely solid. Two lines are drawn in this area, namely, AD and BG. These represent the limits of the solubilities of B in A and A in B respectively at various temperatures. From the form of these lines it will be apparent that as temperature falls the solubility of B in A and A in B also falls. To the left of AD, B is soluble in A (called the α-solid solution) and to the right of BG, A is soluble in B (called the β-solid solution). The structure of the alloy under the line ADEGB is a mixture of α- and β-solid solutions.

If a molten alloy of composition I in Figure 10.8 is solidified (the eutectic mixture), the α- and β-solid solutions crystallise independently, similar to 10.3.3, where the pure metals behave in a similar manner. For alloy II in Figure 10.8 the β-solid solution crystallises first, followed by a mixture of α and β. Alloy III forms the α-solid solution when it solidifies, but on further cooling can exceed the solid solubility of metal B in A.

One of two things can happen in this case:

(a) On slow cooling, some of the β-solid solution may precipitate from the solid solution—this is the basis of *precipitation hardening*, discussed in Section 10.4.4.

(b) With rapid cooling, the alloy may not be at an elevated temperature for sufficient time to allow precipitation, which requires diffusion of metal atoms. Thus a *supersaturated solid solution* is the result.

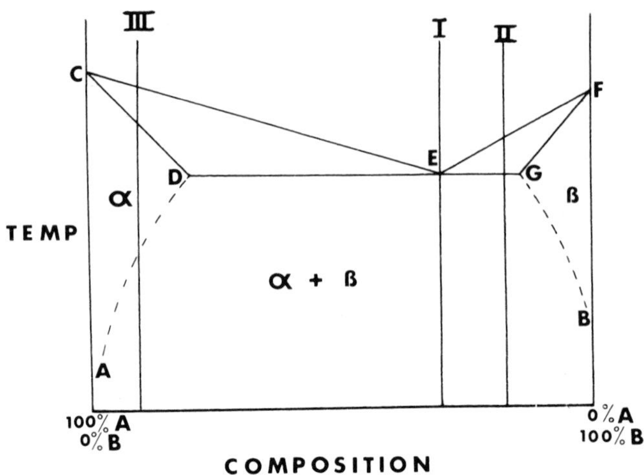

Fig. 10.8 Phase diagram for a binary system where there is partial solubility in the solid state.

10.4 MECHANICAL PROPERTIES

10.4.1 Work hardening

The properties of an alloy can be altered by cold working, as for a metal (Sections 9.6 and 9.7.3)—the consequences of work hardening, or *strain hardening* are:
(a) an increase in hardness,
(b) greater yield stress and ultimate tensile strength, and
(c) less ductility.

10.4.2 Solution hardening

In a binary substitutional solid solution, the atoms of two constituent metals are of different sizes (examples—Table 10.1), though the size difference is usually less than 15% (Section 10.2.2) Consequently the crystal lattice of such as alloy is distorted by the presence of either smaller or larger atoms. These distortions hinder the movement of dislocations, so raising the yield stress. Thus, for example, gold alloys containing copper, silver, etc. are harder, stronger and less ductile than pure gold.

10.4.3 Order hardening

This is best illustrated by the gold-copper system, for which

Figure 10.9 is a simplified phase diagram. Below the solidus, there are two areas designated (1) and (2). These represent conditions of temperature and composition where reactions can occur in the solid state, provided that the alloy is maintained at an elevated temperature for sufficient time to permit diffusion of atoms.

The reaction occurring in this system is called *ordering*. If an alloy of say 50% gold and 50% copper is cooled rapidly from 450°C, the lattice structure is *random* or *disordered* (Fig. 10.1). But slow cooling permits the formation of an ordered substitutional solid solution (Fig. 10.2). In area (1) of Figure 10.9, the ordered lattice has three copper atoms to each gold atom (Cu_3Au), and in area (2) there are equal numbers of atoms of the two metals in the lattice (CuAu).

Such an ordered structure is termed a *superlattice*. The unit cell of the CuAu superlattice is face-centered *tetragonal*—this differs from a face-centered cubic structure in that only two of the three axes of the unit cell are equal in length.

The formation of a certain volume of a tetragonal lattice within a cubic structure involves contraction on one of the crystal axes; this sets up strains which interfere with the movement of dislocations. Hence the yield stress, ultimate tensile strength and hardness are raised, and this is termed *order hardening*.

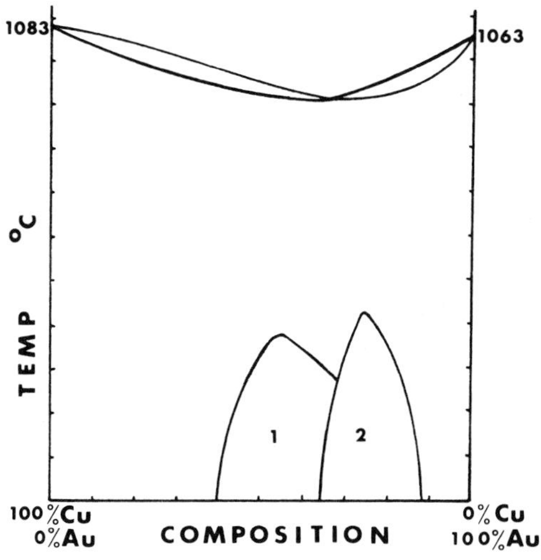

Fig. 10.9 Simplified diagram of the gold-copper system. Area 1—formation of Cu_3Au superlattice. Area 2—formation of CuAu superlattice.

10.4.4 Precipitation hardening

When precipitation occurs (Section 10.3.4, Fig. 10.8), as in the Cu—Ag system, the precipitated phase reduces the mobility of dislocations, thus increasing strength and hardness, and reducing the ductility.

10.4.5 Eutectic alloys

The general properties of eutectics are:
(a) they are hard but brittle,
(b) they have low melting points, and can be useful as solders (Ch. 44),
(c) their resistance to corrosion may be poor (Section 11.3.1).

10.5 GOLD ALLOYS

10.5.1 Pure gold

Pure gold is soft and ductile, so it is not used for cast dental restorations and appliances, but only where it can be substantially work hardened (Ch. 23). Thus casting golds for inlays, crowns, bridges and partial dentures contain alloying elements, the most common being copper, silver, platinum, palladium, nickel and zinc.

10.5.2 Effect of alloying elements

(a) Copper. From Figure 10.9 the following observations can be made:

- (i) Gold and copper form a solid solution in all proportions.
- (ii) The liquidus and solidus are close together, and coincide at one point; such an alloy shows little tendency to form a cored structure.
- (iii) When copper is alloyed with gold, the melting point of the alloy is less than that of gold.
- (iv) Solution hardening occurs, and order hardening can occur for alloys containing approximately 40 to 88 per cent gold, if the correct heat treatment is given.

Copper also has the following effects:

- (i) It imparts a red colour, if present in sufficient quantity.
- (ii) It reduces the density of the alloy—its density is about half that of gold.

Only a limited amount of copper can be used in a dental alloy, since corrosion may result (Section 11.5.1). In general, a dental gold alloy should have at least 75% noble metals (gold, platinum and palladium) to ensure adequate corrosion resistance.

(b) Silver forms a solid solution with gold in all proportions, and there is partial solid solubility in the silver-copper system. Silver has the following effects on a dental gold alloy:

(i) It slightly increases the hardness and strength by solution hardening.
(ii) Precipitation hardening can occur with copper present in the alloy, and under the appropriate thermal conditions.
(iii) It can allow tarnishing to occur.
(iv) Molten silver can dissolve gases such as oxygen, leading to porosity in a casting.
(v) It tends to whiten the alloy, and overcome the reddening effect of copper.

(c) Platinum

(i) Platinium forms a solid solution with gold, but increases the tendency for coring to occur.
(ii) Precipitation hardening can occur by reaction with copper.
(iii) It increases the melting point of the alloy.
(iv) It helps the corrosion resistance of the alloy.

(d) Palladium is similar to platinum in its effects on dental gold alloys, and is a less expensive metal.

(e) Zinc is included as a *scavenger*. When the alloy is being melted prior to casting, oxidation of some of the constituents (e.g. copper) can occur. The presence of an oxide of copper in the casting is undesirable, since it embrittles the alloy. Zinc oxidises more readily than all the other constituents of a gold alloy. Zinc oxide can be removed as a slag from the molten alloy.

(f) Other constituents such as nickel and iridium may be present; the latter metal helps to refine the grain structure of the alloy.

10.5.3 Dental casting golds

These are discussed in Chapters 29 and 35.

10.6 STEEL AND STAINLESS STEEL

10.6.1 Steel—constituents and properties

Steel is an alloy of iron and carbon, with up to 2% carbon. Alloys with greater quantities of carbon are *cast iron* or *pig iron*.

Iron can exist in two forms; face-centered cubic above 910°C, and body-centered cubic below this temperature (Section 2.4.1). Carbon is practically insoluble in body-centered cubic iron (soluble up to

0.02%), but is more soluble in face-centred cubic iron; this interstitial solid solution (Section 10.2.2) is called *austenite*.

Part of the simplified phase diagram for the iron-carbon system is shown in Figure 10.10. It can be seen that on cooling austenite, transformations occur as the solubility of carbon reduces with decreasing temperature.

A mixture containing 99.2% iron and 0.8% carbon produces a structure similar to that of a eutectic, since after cooling austenite slowly below a well-defined temperature (723°C), the solid material may be observed metallographically to have transformed to an intimate mechanical mixture of two components. One of these components is *cementite*, an intermetallic compound, Fe_3C, which comes out of solution as the iron changes from face-centered cubic to body-centered cubic. The other component is *ferrite*, which is an extremely dilute solid solution of carbon in body-centered cubic iron. This mixture of constitutents is called *pearlite*.

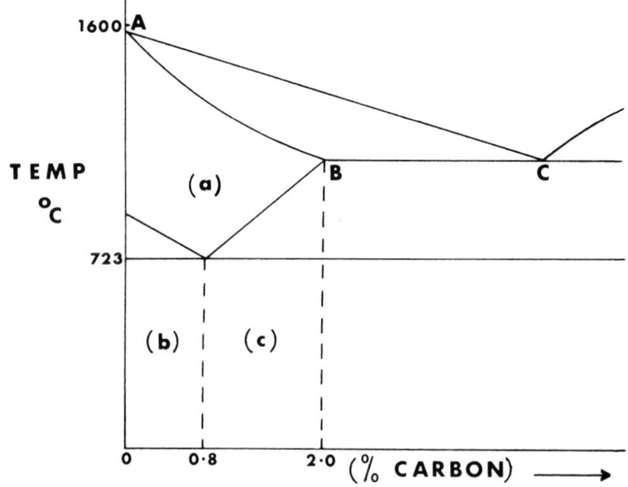

Fig. 10.10 Part of the simplified phase diagram for the iron-carbon system. AC, liquidus; ABC, solidus; (a) austenite (solid solution); (b) ferrite and pearlite; (c) pearlite and cementite.

This mixture (0.8% C, 99.2% Fe) is not a eutectic, since the transformations occur in the solid state. It is called a *eutectoid steel*, since the structure produced is similar to a eutectic.

Alloys with less than and greater than 0.8% carbon are called *hypo-eutectoid* and *hyper-eutectoid* steels respectively.

If austenite is cooled rapidly, there may not be sufficient time for the carbon to diffuse out of the solid solution to form cementite. In this case the alloy consists of a distorted b.c.c. lattice containing carbon; this material is called *martensite*. Because of the distortion of the lattice, martensite is an extremely hard and brittle material. (N.B. Contrast this to gold alloys, where rapid cooling produces a softened alloy—Section 10.5.)

A rapidly cooled steel would be too brittle for some applications, particularly for the cutting edge of burs (Ch. 46) or other dental instruments. Such materials can be *tempered*, that is, heated to between 200 to 450°C, held at a given temperature for a known length of time, and cooled rapidly—see Table 10.2. This procedure permits diffusion of carbon atoms from the crystal lattice to occur; in this way some cementite is formed.

In addition to iron and carbon, steels have small quantities of other constituents (stainless steel is a special case, and is discussed in Section 10.6.2), for example:

(a) Chromium may be added in small quantities to improve the tarnish resistance (stainless steel has much larger quantities of chromium, Section 10.6.2).

(b) Manganese may be used as a scavenger for sulphur, analogous to the effect of zinc on oxygen in gold alloys (Section 10.5.2).

(c) Molybdenum, silicon, nickel, cobalt, etc., may also be present.

Steel is discussed further in Chapter 46, in relation to its uses for dental instruments.

Table 10.2 Heat treatment of steels

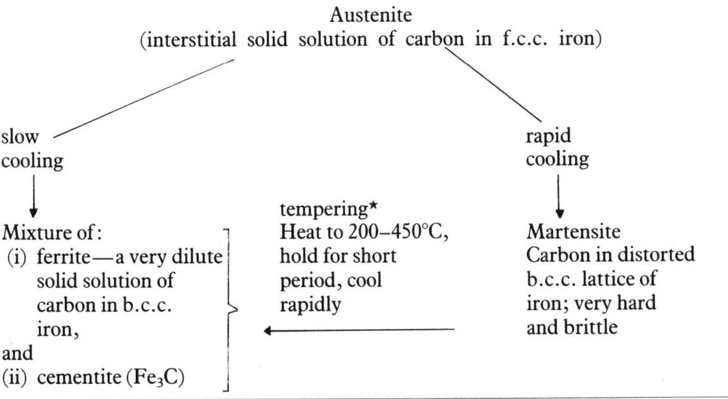

* The temperature and time of tempering a steel instrument must be carefully controlled, and depend on:
(i) the use to which the instrument will be put (Ch. 46), and
(ii) its composition.

10.6.2 Stainless steel

In addition to iron and carbon, stainless steel contains chromium, and often nickel. These have the following effects:
(a) Chromium, if present in sufficient quantities, renders the alloy resistant to corrosive attack. The mechanism of this is discussed in Section 11.2.
(b) Chromium and nickel both reduce the *critical temperature*—the temperature at which the austenitic structure breaks down on cooling.
(c) Nickel also helps the corrosion resistance and strength of the alloy.

Two types of stainless steel are of importance:
(a) Austenitic stainless steel which contains so much chromium and nickel that the austenitic structure—a solid solution (Table 10.2)—remains even on cooling to room temperature. Such alloys may have 18% chromium and 8% nickel (often called '18/8 stainless steel') or 12% of each of these constituents ('12/12 stanless steel'). These materials can be hardened by cold working, but not hardened by heat treatment, and so are not suitable for cutting instruments. 18/8 stainless steel can be used for denture base construction (Ch. 36), and for orthodontic wire (Ch. 38).
(b) Martensitic stainless steel, may contain 12 to 13% chromium, a small amount of carbon, but no other major constituents.

These alloys can be hardened by heat-treatment—contrast to the above.

10.7 ALLOYS IN DENTISTRY

(a) Steel is used for burs and dental instruments (Ch. 46).
(b) Dental amalgam is the most widely used filling material—an alloy of silver and tin, sometimes with smaller quantities of copper and zinc, when mixed with mercury, sets rapidly to give a hard strong material (Ch. 22).
(c) Gold alloys are used for inlays, crowns and bridges. Alternatives to gold include silver-palladium, nickel-chromium etc (Ch. 29).
(d) The following alloys can be, or have been, used for cast partial dentures: (Ch. 35)

- (i) gold alloys,
- (ii) cobalt-chromium alloys,
- (iii) silver-palladium alloys, and
- (iv) aluminium bronze.

(e) Stainless steel can be used as a denture base (Ch. 36).
(f) The following alloys are, or have been, used in the form of wires (Ch. 38):
   (i) stainless steel,
   (ii) gold alloys,
   (iii) cobalt-chromium alloys,
   (iv) nickel-chromium alloys,
   (v) nickel-titanium, and
   (vi) beta titanium.
(g) Some die materials consist of polymers with metallic fillers (Ch. 40). Also a bismuth-tin alloy can be sprayed into an inpression (Section 40.3.4).
(h) Dental solders (Ch. 44).

READING REFERENCES

Alexander W, Street A 1979 Metals in the service of man, 7th edn. Penguin, Harmondsworth, Middlesex

A very readable introductory book on metallurgy.

John V B 1974 Understanding phase diagrams. Macmillan, London

This is a concise introduction to phase diagrams. The following sections are of particular interest: 4.2 (Total Solid Insolubility), 4.3 (Interpretation), 4.4 (Solid Solubility), 4.5 (Phase Diagram for Total Solid Solubility), 4.6 (Partial Solid Solubility), 4.10 (Effects of Phase Diagram Type on the Properties of Alloys), Chapter 5 (Real Systems), including an extensive discussion of the iron-carbon system (5.4) and Chapter 6 (Experimental Determination of Phase Diagrams).

Bates J F, Knapton A G 1977 Metals and alloys in dentistry. International Metals Review 22: 19.

This extensively reviews the dental applications of metallic materials.

11. Corrosion and electrodeposition

11.1 INTRODUCTION

11.1.1 Definition and types of corrosion

Corrosion can be defined as a chemical reaction between a metal and its environment to form metal compounds. Many metals can react spontaneously with either a gaseous or aqueous environment. The compounds thus obtained are chemically more stable than the metals from which they have been formed.

The extraction of metals from compounds has been discussed in Section 9.2. Corrosion may be considered to be the reverse reaction to the extraction process. Corrosion is obviously undesirable, as it can spoil the aesthetics of an alloy, and in extreme cases can severely weaken the material, as in the rusting of iron. To avoid this in both dental and implant alloys only a few types of alloy can be used, and conditions that favour corrosion must be avoided as far as possible.

Corrosion reactions can be classified into two types:

(a) Non-aqueous corrosion, when metals can react to form compounds such as oxides and sulphides. Examples include:

(i) tarnishing of brass due to formation of sulphides.
(ii) discoloration of the surfaces of castings caused by oxidation,
(iii) oxidation of metal surfaces during soldering and heat treatment procedures.

(b) Aqueous corrosion can occur in the oral environment (Section 11.1.2) and this occurs by electrochemical reactions (Section 11.2).

11.1.2 The oral environment

In many respects the mouth is an ideal environment for aqueous corrosion of metals and alloys to occur. The presence of moisture, temperature fluctuations, and the changing pH caused by diet and the decomposition of foodstuffs, can all contribute to this phenomenon.

11.2 ELECTROCHEMISTRY

11.2.1 Conductors of electricity

Conductors of electricity are of two main types:
(a) *Electronic conductors*, such as metals, where the movement of electrons causes conduction.
(b) *Electrolytic conductors*, or *electrolytes*, for example, fused salts and aqueous solutions of acids, bases and salts, where conduction of electricity is accompanied by the movement of ions.

11.2.2 Current-consuming (electrolytic) cells

Consider an electrolyte containing cations M^+ and anions A^-. If two electronic conductors, or electrodes, are placed in this electrolyte and an electrical potential difference established between them by a battery, then movement of ions will occur. Cations, M^+, move to the negatively charged electrode or *cathode* and anions move to the *anode* or positively charged electrode (Fig 11.1). Such a process is called *electrolysis*.

For the above, the following reactions can be written:

At the cathode: $M^+ + \text{electron} \rightarrow M$
At the anode: $A^- \rightarrow A + \text{electron}$

An anodic reaction, then, is one that produces electrons, whereas a cathodic process consumes electrons.

11.2.3 Current-producing (galvanic) cells

Consider now two electrodes of different metals, e.g. copper and zinc, immersed in an electrolyte of sulphuric acid (Fig 11.2). When electrical contact is made between the electrodes, a current will flow.

The following reactions occur:

At the anode: $Zn \rightarrow Zn^{2+} + 2$ electrons
At the cathode: $2H^{+} + 2$ electrons $\rightarrow H_2$

As in the previous section, electrons are produced at the anode and consumed at the cathode. This is an example of a *galvanic* or corrosion cell. Zinc atoms are being converted to zinc ions (essentially an oxidation reaction), and passing into solution. Thus the zinc is being corroded.

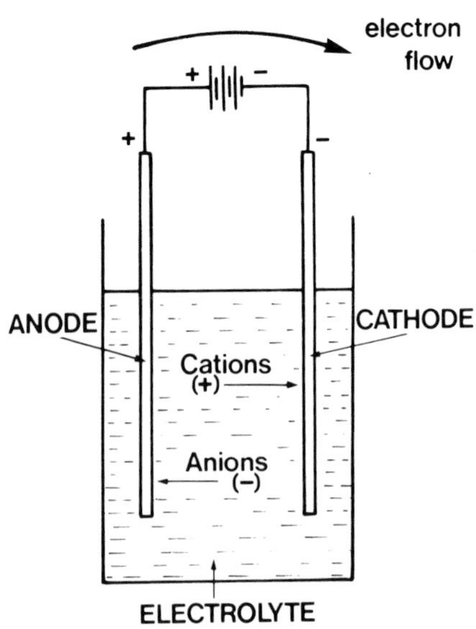

Fig. 11.1 Current-consuming (electrolytic) cell.

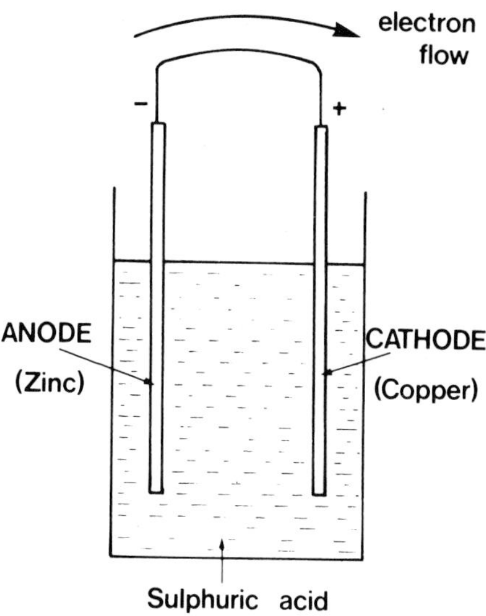

Fig. 11.2 Current-producing (galvanic) cell.

11.2.4 Electrode potential

Consider the reversible reaction:

$$M \rightleftharpoons M^{n+} + n \text{ electrons}$$

The forward reaction liberates electrons, and the reverse one consumes them. When electrons are produced this causes a potential on the electrode. This *electrode potential* is therefore a measure of the extent to which the above reaction proceeds from left to right, so indicating the tendency for the metal to corrode.

The standard potential of an electrode is usually expressed relative to that of the reaction:

$$H_2 \rightleftharpoons 2H^+ + 2 \text{ electrons}$$

which given the value zero. Some standard electrode potentials are given in Table 11.1.

Table 11.1 Electrode potentials of some metals*

Metal	Reaction	Electrode potential (volts)**
Gold	Au^{+} + electron → Au	+1.50
Platinum	Pt^{2+} + 2 electrons → Pt	+0.86
Palladium	Pd^{2+} + 2 electrons → Pd	+0.82
Silver	Ag^{+} + electron → Ag	+0.80
Mercury	Hg^{2+} + 2 electrons → Hg	+0.80
Copper	Cu^{+} + electron → Cu	+0.47
Copper	Cu^{2+} + 2 electrons → Cu	+0.34
Hydrogen	$2H^{+}$ + 2 electrons → H_2	0.00
Iron	Fe^{3+} + 3 electrons → Fe	−0.045
Lead	Pb^{2+} + 2 electrons → Pb	−0.12
Tin	Sn^{2+} + 2 electrons → Sn	−0.14
Iron	Fe^{2+} + 2 electrons → Fe	−0.44
Chromium	Cr^{2+} + 2 electrons → Cr	−0.56
Zinc	Zn^{2+} + 2 electrons → Zn	−0.76
Aluminium	Al^{3+} + 3 electrons → Al	−1.70
Sodium	Na^{+} + electron → Na	−2.71
Calcium	Ca^{2+} + 2 electrons → Ca	−2.90
Potassium	K^{+} + electron → K	−2.92

* These were measured at 25°C in a molar solution of the metal.

** Sometimes the opposite sign convention is used—e.g. the electrode potential of gold is −1.50 volts. The signs used here are those recommended by the International Union of Pure and Applied Chemistry.

Two things can be derived from this standard *electrochemical series:*
(a) A greater difference in electrode potential between two metals indicates a greater tendency for an electrochemical reaction to occur.
(b) The metal that is lower in the series (as written in Table 11.1) forms the anode. The anode is the metal which corrodes and goes into solution. It should be noted that different electrolytes can sometimes cause changes in the relative position of metals in the series.

11.2.5 Polarisation

The tendency of materials to corrode has been discussed above. Other factors must be considered, such as the extent to which corrosion proceeds in a given time. This depends mainly on a phenomenon called *polarisation*, which is a combination of at least three factors:

(a) Activation polarisation results from the potential difference needed to enable the electrode reactions to proceed at a finite rate.
(b) Concentration polarisation, due to the accumulation of reaction products, can occur. For example, around a zinc anode, there may

be a high concentration of zinc ions, which will reduce the current until they diffuse away from the anode. Evolution of hydrogen at a cathode can occur in some cells.
(c) Polarisation due to the formation of a film on the surface of the electrode can reduce the rate of an electrochemical reaction. This film may be composed of adsorbed gases or metallic oxides (see Section 11.2.7) on passivity).

In terms of production of an electric voltage by such cells, polarisation can be a problem. In contrast to this, polarisation is an advantage in the context of limiting corrosion.

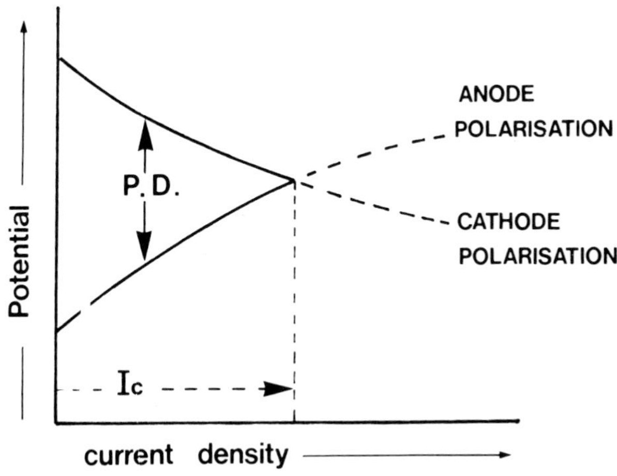

Fig. 11.3 Polarisation curves for a corrosion cell. P.D. marks the potential difference between anode and cathode. I_c is the maximum current density.

11.2.6 Anode and cathode polarisation

Figure 11.3 illustrates anode and cathode polarisation. Curves such as this are obtained by measuring the potential of each electrode for a given controlled current. As the current from the cell increases, the apparent electrode potential of the anode rises and that of the cathode decreases. The current at the point where these curves intersect, I_c, is called the *corrosion current*, and is a measure of the maximum current from the cell. Ideally, to reduce corrosion it is important to increase the polarisation of either or both electrodes to decrease the value of I_c. This may be achieved by metals which passivate (Section 11.2.7).

11.2.7 Passivity

For a metal capable of forming an oxide which is stable in the presence of an electrolyte, a curve such as Figure 11.4 is obtained. At point X there is a discontinuity in the curve and the potential suddenly increases from X to Y. The metal is said to be *passivated*, or rendered *passive*, at potentials above X, when it is covered by an oxide film.

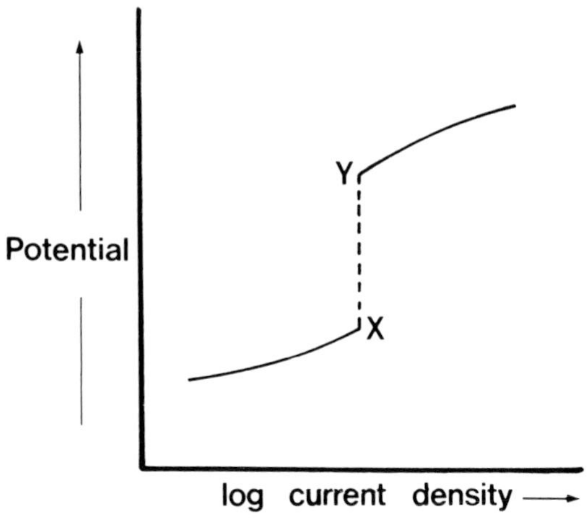

Fig. 11.4 Anodic polarisation curve for a metal, showing passivity at potentials between X and Y.

11.2.8 Potentiostatic measurements

To obtain experimental data on passivity, potentiostatic techniques are used which can yield data on the behaviour of the metal in the region of the discontinuity X...Y in Figure 11.4. Instead of measuring potential for a given controlled current as above, the potential is controlled and the current to maintain a given potential is measured. A curve such as Figure 11.5. is obtained for a passive metal. The point F is the *Flade potential*—the potential for which the minimum current density is obtained.

Metals such as titanium and chromium are easily passivated, that is, they have a low Flade potential. Likewise, alloys containing chromium, such as stainless steel can form passive layers.

It should be noted that the establishment of passivity depends on

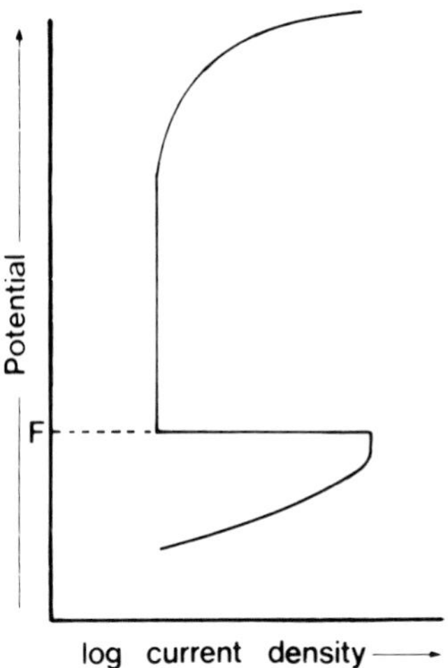

Fig. 11.5 Anodic polarisation curve for a metal, showing passivity at potentials between X and Y.

the nature of the electrolyte as well as the composition of the metal or alloy. For example, in the presence of chloride ions passivity is more difficult to achieve. The corrosion characteristics of dental alloys are often assessed in saline solutions (Fig. 11.6).

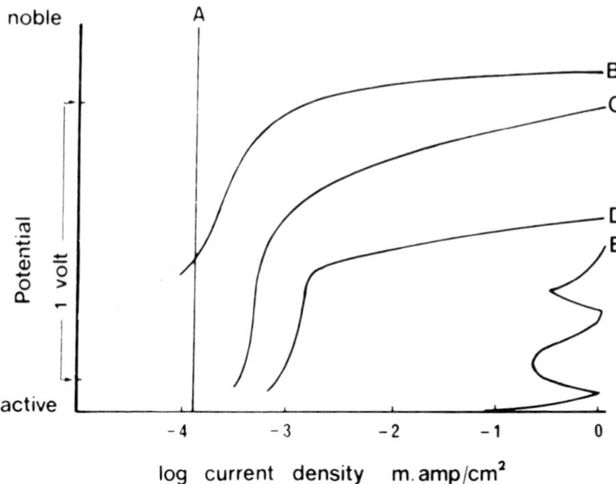

Fig. 11.6 Potentiostatically determined anodic polarisation curves of alloys in saline solution. A, titanium alloy; B, dental inlay gold alloy; C, cobalt chromium alloy; D, stainless steel; E, dental amalgam.

11.3 EXAMPLES OF ELECTROLYTIC CORROSION

11.3.1 Differences in composition of materials

Example 1. If a gold inlay comes into contact with an amalgam restoration, the amalgam can form the anode of an electrical cell, and so corrode.

Example 2. A soldered appliance or denture may corrode, since the composition of the solder differs from that of the alloys it joins.

Example 3. In a cored structure, differences in the composition within the alloy grains are found (Section 10.3.2). Thus part of a grain can be the anode, and part the cathode, in a galvanic cell. Consequently, homogenisation (Section 10.3.2) helps to improve the corrosion resistance of an alloy.

Example 4. Where there is solid insolubility (Section 10.3.3) or precipitation in an alloy with partial solid solubility (Section 10.3.4), different grains have different compositions. Again, this favours electrolytic corrosion.

11.3.2 Differences in composition of electrolyte

A homogeneous metal or alloy can undergo electrolytic corrosion where there is a difference in electrolyte concentration across the specimen.

Example 1. Consider the case of a metallic restoration which is partly covered by food debris. The composition of the electrolyte under this debris will differ from that of saliva, and this can contribute to the corrosion of the restoration.

Example 2. Where there are differences in the concentration of oxygen in an electrolyte, an *oxidation-type concentration cell* is formed. Corrosion is greater at portions of the metal or alloy with lower concentrations of oxygen. This can happen in an unpolished metallic restoration. The surface concavities become filled readily with food debris; this lowers the concentration of oxygen at those parts, which corrode, and lead to pitting of the filling.

Example 3. There can obviously be differences in the composition of the electrolyte in contact with different portions of a semi-buried dental implant.

11.3.3 Differences in stress

A metal which has been stressed by cold working, becomes more reactive at the site of maximum stress.

If stressed and unstressed metals are in contact in an electrolyte, the former will become the anode of a galvanic cell, and will corrode.

Example. In orthopaedic surgery, stainless steel plates and screws are frequently embedded in tissues. Any differences in the extent of cold working between screw and plate must be avoided. Similarly, different portions of the same piece of steel may be stressed to different extents, so favouring corrosion.

11.3.4 Stress corrosion

A combination of corrosion and stress conditions can cause failures of a metal by *stress corrosion.* At an anodic portion of a surface, electrolytic action can form a minute crack. This can increase in size as a result of stress concentration. More corrosion can occur in the enlarged crack, and so on, until eventual failure occurs.

11.4 CORROSION AND GALVANIC PAIN

In addition to corrosive attack on dental alloys, electrolytic corrosion can cause galvanic pain. Many people have experienced this when a piece of metal foil wrapping has inadvertently been taken into the mouth. If the foil contacts an amalgam restoration, an electric circuit is set up, usually completed by the tongue. The current causes painful stimulation of the tooth pulp.

Galvanic pain is occasionally encountered in the mouth, when dissimilar metal restorations come into intermittent contact. Long-term contact is unlikely to give severe galvanic pain, because polarisation can occur (Section 11.2.5).

One of the functions of a cement lining under a metal is to give electrical insulation of the pulp (Section 16.4.)

11.5 PREVENTION OF CORROSION

11.5.1 Choice of alloy

Alloys for long-term use in the mouth must be either (a) noble or (b) passive.

(a) Noble metals are those such as gold, platinum and palladium (Table 11.1). Dental gold alloys contain some copper, which has poorer corrosion resistance; however, such alloys must contain at least 70–75% noble metals.

(b) Passive alloys, such as those containing chromium, are widely used dentally.

Examples: stainless steel, cobalt-chromium and nickel-chromium.

11.5.2 Use of alloy

In addition to choosing the best materials, alloys must be used correctly, and situations which are likely to lead to corrosion, as in Section 11.3, must be avoided as far as possible.

11.6 ELECTRODEPOSITION

According to *Faraday's first law of electrolysis*, in an electrolytic cell, the amount of chemical decomposition is proportional to the quantity of electricity passed.

In *electrodeposition*, or *electroplating*, a material to be coated is made the cathode of an electrolytic cell (Fig 11.1). The anode is composed of the metal to be deposited on to the cathode surface. The electrolyte contains cations of the metal to be deposited. When current is passed through such a cell the anode dissolves, supplying cations, which are transported through the electrolyte to the cathode. Such copper and silver plating techniques are used in dental laboratories (Section 40.3.5).

Electropolishing is the reverse procedure, whereby a metal can be polished by making it the anode of an electrolytic cell (Sections 35.3.4).

READING REFERENCE

Cottrell A 1975 An introduction to metallurgy, 2nd edn. Arnold, London.

Chapter 23 includes an account of oxidation, corrosion in acids and alkalis, electro-chemical corrosion, and methods of prevention or control of corrosion.

12. Ceramics

12.1 INTRODUCTION

12.1.1 Definition and applications

Ceramic substances are composed of simple compounds of metallic and non-metallic elements. Examples include oxides, nitrides and silicates. Ceramics are used for pottery and porcelain, and as glasses, cements, refractories (heat-resistant materials) and abrasives. The dental applications are discussed in Section 12.12. A dental porcelain is essentially a glass prepared from a high purity feldspar (see below); it sometimes contains a crystalline phase (for example, to give increased strength). A pottery porcelain composition also contains feldspar, but with clay and quartz; firing produces a virteous body with a high proportion of filler.

12.1.2 History

The forming and burning of clay suspensions has been carried out since about 5000 B.C. Today, many new types of material are becoming available and ceramics are finding new uses—e.g. uranium dioxide as a nuclear fuel, metal-ceramic composites, glass-ceramics, etc.

12.2 CERAMIC RAW MATERIALS

The following types of materials are used in dental applications:
(a) Alumina (Al_2O_3) is a very strong hard oxide. It is prepared from alumina trihydrate by calcination, and the resulting form of alumina depends on the temperature used:

$$\text{alumina trihydrate} \xrightarrow{600°C} \gamma\text{-alumina} \xrightarrow{1250°C} \alpha\text{-alumina}$$

Alumina is a starting material in the preparation of aluminosilicate ion-leachable glasses (Section 12.8, Ch. 18) and is a constituent of some dental porcelains (Section 28.2.3).
(b) Boric oxide (B_2O_3) is a *ceramic flux*. A flux is included in glass formulations to lower the softening temperature of the glass. Boric oxide is also a glass former.
(c) Calcium oxide (CaO), potassium oxide (K_2O) and sodium oxide (Na_2O) act as fluxes.
(d) Feldspars are naturally occurring minerals, which are anhydrous aluminosilicates. The forms of feldspar include:

(i) potash feldspar ($K_2O.Al_2O_3.6SiO_2$)
(ii) soda feldspar ($Na_2O.Al_2O_3.6SiO_2$)
(iii) lime feldspar ($CaO.2Al_2O_3.2SiO_2$)

These materials are useful as fluxes in traditional pottery bodies.
(e) Fluorspar (CaF_2) is also a flux.
(f) Kaolin (or china clay) is an example of a clay material. It consists essentially of the mineral kaolinite, a hydrous aluminosilicate of composition $Al_2O_3.2SiO_2.2H_2O$. The functions of kaolin in a ceramic material are:

(i) it can be made into a plastic mixture with water, which can be moulded to the required size and shape.
(ii) a clay-water suspension maintains its shape during firing in a furnace.
(iii) at high temperature it fuses and can react with other ceramic materials.

(g) Silica minerals—silica (SiO_2) occurs in various allotropic forms—for example, quartz, cristobalite and tridymite, though the last of these is not very important dentally. Silica is a major ingredient in glasses, dental porcelain (Ch. 28), investment materials

(Ch. 42), and abrasive materials (Ch. 45). It is very hard, comparably infusible and stable material. Further properties are discussed in Section 12.6.

(h) Silicon carbide (SiC) is an abrasive.

(i) Zinc oxide is a widely used constituent of dental cement (Section 12.7, Chapter 17).

12.3 FORMING OF CERAMICS

12.3.1 Clay-based suspensions

The plastic mass of the ceramic—water mixture is dried and fired to give a hard material, as in dental porcelain (Section 28.3). The following factors are important in this process:

(a) The suspension should be plastic enough to allow it to be shaped readily.

(b) The material should have a high 'green' strength (this is the strength of the material before firing) to reduce the risk of damage during handling.

(c) There should be a low shrinkage on drying.

(d) The firing shrinkage should be as low as possible, for greatest accuracy. However, firing shrinkage of these materials can be of the order of 30 to 40% by volume.

(e) During firing, there should be no warpage or cracking.

(f) The fired material should be free of air bubbles.

12.3.2 Ceramic coatings

(a) A *glaze* can be applied to the surface of a fired porcelain, to give a smooth glossy non-porous finish. This is a mixture of clay in suspension, and a powdered glass. The glaze is brushed or sprayed on to the surface, and fired in the normal way (Section 28.3.4). In some cases a dental porcelain is self-glazing, and a glaze develops at the end of the firing cycle.

(b) A ceramic coating can be fired on to a metallic (e.g. gold) surface (Ch. 30).

12.3.3 Glass forming

Molten glass can be shaped by blowing, casting, drawing, pressing or rolling.

12.3.4 Concrete-type materials

Hydraulic cements come under this category; they are not used dentally.

12.4 CRYSTALLINE CERAMICS

These may have ionic or covalent bonds:
(a) Ionic crystals—compounds of metals with oxygen usually come into this class.
(b) Covalent crystals—for example, silicon carbide (SiC) which is very hard and has a high melting point.

For the structure of such materials, see Section 2.4.

12.5 NON-CRYSTALLINE CERAMICS

A *glass* may be defined as a product of fusion which has cooled to a rigid condition without crystallising.

Glasses are composed of silica (SiO_2), with other oxides, such as those of sodium, potassium, calcium, barium, etc. The composition of a glass can be controlled to give specific properties in respect of refractive index, colour, viscosity of molten material, etc.

The *fictive temperature* is the temperature at which a glass is transformed from a supercooled liquid into a *vitreous* (i.e. non-crystalline) solid.

Crystallisation of a glass can sometimes occur—this is called *devitrification*. For this to happen, a *nucleating agent* is required; this is a material on which crystal growth can occur. To achieve this in practice, an agent such as titanium dioxide (TiO_2) is dissolved in the molten glass. On cooling, the TiO_2 precipitates, and crystals of glass grow on it on subsequent heat treatment. Such materials are *glass-ceramics*.

These *glass-ceramics* have some advantages over other materials:
(a) The ceramic article is the same size and shape as the original glass.
(b) The material has greater hardness and strength than the parent glass.

12.6 PROPERTIES OF SILICA

12.6.1 Polymorphism

Polymorphic materials are those that can exist with more than one crystal structure. Silica is an example of such material in which changes of structure can occur. There are two types of structural transformation:

(a) *Displacive transformations* can take place where atoms become displaced, but no interatomic bonds are broken, when there is a temperature change. The following factors are characteristic of such processes:

(i) They occur at specific temperatures.
(ii) The transformations are rapid.
(iii) The high-temperature form has a greater specific volume, thus the formation of the high-temperature material is accompanied by an expansion.

(b) *Reconstructive transformations* of silica involve the breaking and remaking of Si—O bonds. These processes need more energy than the preceding type, and so usually occur more slowly.

12.6.2 Forms of silica

(a) Quartz, with a hexagonal structure, is the most stable form of silica.
(b) When quartz is heated to 867°C, a reconstructive transformation to tridymite occurs.
(c) At 1470°C, another reconstructive transformation takes place, to form cristobalite.
(d) At over 1700°C, cristobalite melts, and fused quartz, which is amorphous is produced.

Quartz (hexagonal structure)	$\overset{867°C}{\rightleftharpoons}$	Tridymite (rhombohedral structure)	$\overset{1470°C}{\rightleftharpoons}$	Cristobalite (cubic structure)	$\xrightarrow{1713°C}$	Fused quartz (amorphous)

Note: if fused quartz, cristobalite or tridymite are cooled rapidly, there is not sufficient time for the comparatively slow transformations to take place; so all four forms can exist at room temperature.

12.6.3 Displacive transformations

These can occur for quartz, tridymite and cristobalite, as follows:

(a) low quartz (or α-quartz) $\overset{573°C}{\rightleftharpoons}$ high quartz (or β-quartz)

(b) low tridymite $\xrightleftharpoons{105°C}$ middle tridymite $\xrightarrow{160°C}$ high tridymite
(or α -tridymite) (or β -tridymite)

(c) low cristobalite $\xrightleftharpoons{200–270°C}$ high cristobalite
(or α -cristobalite) (or β -cristobalite)

12.6.4 Dimensional changes

During displacive transformations, dimensional changes occur (Fi.g 12.1). Cristobalite and quartz both expand more than tridymite; this expansion is an important property of dental investment materials (Ch. 42). Fused quartz undergoes no such transformations, and has little thermal expansion.

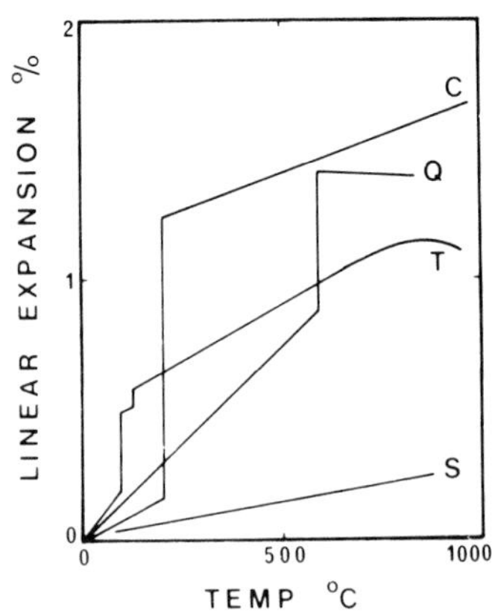

Fig. 12.1 Thermal expansion of the allotropes of silica. C, cristobalite; Q, quartz; T, tridymite; S, fused silica.

12.7 ZINC OXIDE

12.7.1 Sources

(a) Zinc oxide occurs as the mineral *zincite*.
(b) Zinc oxide can be prepared by the direct oxidation of zinc:

$$2Zn + O_2 \rightarrow 2ZnO$$

(c) Zinc oxide can be prepared by the decomposition of the

sulphate, nitrate, hydroxide or carbonate, e.g.,

$$ZnCO_3 \rightarrow ZnO + CO_2$$

12.7.2 Chemical reactions

The following reactions of zinc oxide are of dental interest:
(a) Reaction with phosphoric acid: zinc oxide can react with phosphoric acid to give zinc phosphate. This reaction is the basis of the zinc phosphate cements (Section 17.2).
(b) Reaction with eugenol: under certain conditions, particularly in the presence of moisture, zinc oxide can react with eugenol to give a chelate, zinc eugenolate:

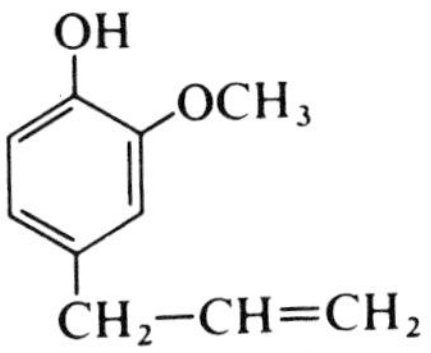

OH
OCH_3
$CH_2{-}CH{=}CH_2$

(eugenol)

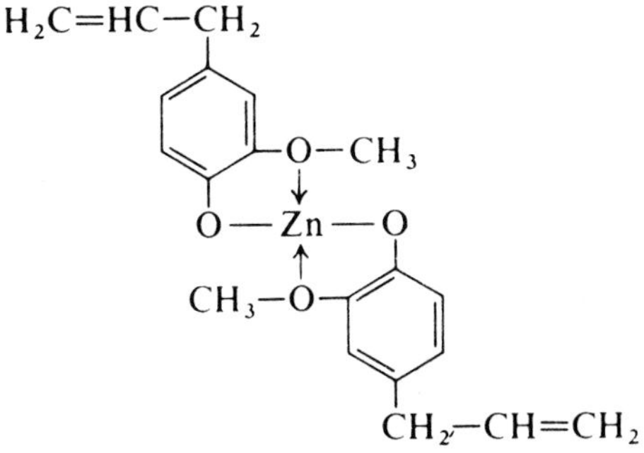

$H_2C{=}HC{-}CH_2$
$O{-}CH_3$
$O{-}Zn{-}O$
$CH_3{-}O$
$CH_2{-}CH{=}CH_2$

(zinc eugenolate)

This reaction is important in zinc oxide eugenol cements (Section 17.1) and impression materials (Section 25.3).
(c) Reaction with other *ortho*-substituted phenols: similar to the above, zinc oxide can react with, for example, guaiacol (2-methoxyphenol), 4-methylguaiacol, etc.
(d) Reaction with *ortho*-ethoxybenzoic acid (EBA): this reaction is

similar to the above, and is important in the EBA cements (Section 17.1.7).

(e) Reaction with aqueous polyacrylic acid: in this reaction, zinc polyacrylate is believed to be the main product; this reaction is employed in the polycarboxylate (polyacrylate) cements (Section 17.3).

12.8 ION-LEACHABLE GLASSES

Fluorine-containing aluminosilicate glasses are of particular interest. The chief constituents are SiO_2, Al_2O_3; CaO, Na_2O and fluorides. The detailed composition of such materials is given in Section 18.1.2.

The constituents of these glasses are fused together at temperatures up to 1400°C, the fluorides acting as fluxes (Section 12.2). The fused material is plunged into cold water which cracks it (this process is termed *fritting*) and makes easier the subsequent grinding to a find powder.

The aluminosilicate glass contains approximately equal numbers of Al and Si atoms, arranged as:

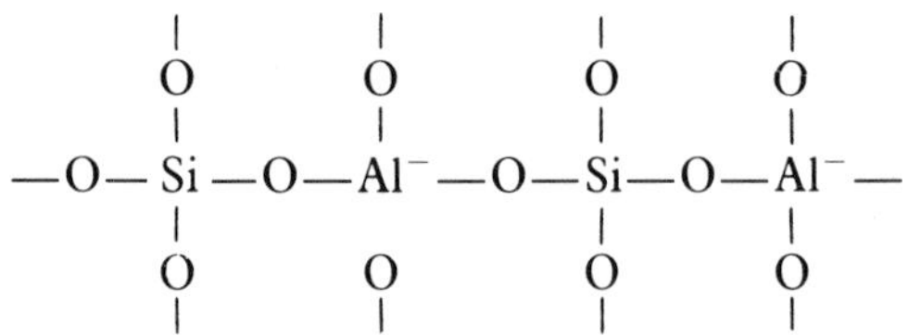

The aluminium has negative charges; these are balanced by Na^+ and Ca^{2+} which are present.

These glasses can react with, for example, phosphoric acid. Hydrated protons ($H_3O,^+$) from the liquid attack the aluminium sites with a negative charge, so decompose the surface of the glass. Forms of aluminosilicate glass can also react with weaker acids, such as aqueous solutions of polyacrylic acid. Further details of the dental applications of these reactions is given in Chapter 18.

12.9 GENERAL PROPERTIES

12.9.1 Chemical properties

Ceramics in general are extremely resistant to attack by chemicals (though note the exception in Section 12.8) a property that is of great advantage in dental applications. To dissolve a ceramic, strong chemicals such as hydrofluoric acid (HF) are required.

12.9.2 Mechanical properties

One of the problems associated with ceramics is their liability to fracture in tension. They exhibit little plastic deformation, and the impact resistance of many ceramics is low. Stresses within the material can cause internal cracks, which can propagate rapidly through a material until fracture occurs. Several factors can cause stresses:

(a) Dislocations in crystals (Fig. 2.8).

(b) Cooling of the sample from its firing temperature, due to differences in the coefficient of thermal expansion between different phases in the material.

(c) Abrasion of the surface can cause *stress concentration* to occur—the stress is concentrated where there is any irregularity of contour.

(d) Porosity within a material.

12.9.3 Thermal properties

The thermal conductivity of these materials is very low (Appendix-II, Table II.3). This is because there are no free electrons, as in metals (Section 2.2.3).

The coefficient of thermal expansion is also low; for example, the figure for porcelain is closer to that of enamel and dentine than other restorative materials (Appendix II, Table II.3).

12.9.4 Optical properties

From the dental viewpoint, these are excellent; dental porcelains are translucent, and can be coloured to match the shade of teeth.

12.10 COMPARISON OF CERAMIC WITH METALLIC MATERIALS

It is not always possible to make a sharp distinction between these two classes of materials. For example compounds between metals and metalloids, such as carbides, may be considered to be considered to be either ceramics, or intermetallic compounds. Nevertheless, it is useful to compare and contrast typical metals and ceramics:

(a) Chemical properties. Many metals and alloys can corrode (Ch. 11) whereas ceramics are very resistant to chemical attack (Section 12.9.1).
(b) Mechanical properties. Metals have values for tensile and compressive strength which are of a comparable order of magnitude. On the other hand, ceramics are considerably stronger in compression than in tension. They are also usually much more brittle than metals, and have low impact strengths.
(c) Thermal and electrical properties—metals are good conductors, ceramics are good insulators.

12.11 COMPARISON OF CERAMIC WITH POLYMERIC MATERIALS

(a) The stability of polymers at high temperature is usually less than that of ceramic materials.
(b) Mechanical properties. Generally polymers are less rigid and more easily capable of plastic deformation than ceramics.
(c) Crystallisation. Polymers and ceramics in general crystallise less readily, and have more complex structures than metals and alloys.

12.12 DENTAL APPLICATIONS

This list deals with the applications of ceramics in the order in which they will be discussed in the other sections of this book, and not necessarily in order of importance.
(a) The powder of cements (Ch. 17) and silicate filling materials (Ch. 18).
(b) Constituents of composite filling materials (Ch. 19).
(c) Dental porcelain, porcelain-fused-to-gold, and aluminous porcelain (Ch. 28 and 30).
(d) Some artificial teeth (Ch. 37).
(e) Constituents of dental investment materials (Ch. 42)
(f) Abrasive and polishing agents (Ch. 45).

READING REFERENCE

Van Vlack L H 1985 Elements of materials science and engineering, 5th edn. Addison-Wesley, Reading, Massachusetts

Chapter 7 gives an extensive account of the structure, properties and processing of ceramic materials.

13. Composite materials—theory

13.1 INTRODUCTION

Composite materials occur widely in nature. Bone and dentine, for example, contain a protein constituent, collagen, and a mineral material, apatite (see Ch. 14). Wood consists of strong and flexible cellulose fibres held together by lignin, which makes the material stiff.

It is not surprising that man has imitated nature by combining two materials to produce a composite, either to improve the properties of one constituent, or to yield a material with properties that are different from either constituent.

Neither is it surprising that composites are beginning to find applications as dental materials, due to the limitations of existing materials and the very exacting conditions of the oral environment.

13.2 METHODS OF COMBINING MATERIALS

13.2.1 Alloying

Any two-phase alloy system can be considered to be a composite, for example, eutectic alloys (Section 10.4.5)

13.2.2 Powder compacting

Reference has already been made to powder metallurgy (Section 9.3.3). The fabrication of tungsten carbide burs is an interesting example of the use of this method of compacting materials. Such burs (Section 46.3) consist of fine particles of the very hard tungsten carbide embedded in a softer matrix of cobalt.

13.2.3 Coating and bonding

One important example of this is the technique of fusing porcelain to a gold alloy. This technique, when used dentally, aims to obtain both the excellent mechanical properties of the gold alloys, and the good aesthetics of the ceramic constituent (Chapter 30.)

13.2.4 Fibre reinforcement

Perhaps the best known industrial example of this is the use of glass fibres to reinforce polymers. Such fibres have not frequently been used dentally, though one silicate filling material contains glass fibres (Section 18.1.2). Nevertheless, the theory of fibre reinforcement will be dealt with more fully in a subsequent section (13.3.1), as many important advances in materials science are being made in this direction.

13.2.5 Dispersion of a filler in a matrix

This is of great importance in composite filling materials (Ch. 19) which are becoming of increasing importance. This is discussed in Section 13.3.2.

13.3 REINFORCED POLYMERS

13.3.1 Fibres and whiskers

(a) Fibres. The following are currently used industrially—glass fibres (in polyester resin), silicon carbide and nitride, boron, and recently, carbon fibres (in epoxy resin).
(b) Whiskers. Ceramics can have poor mechanical properties, due to crystalline imperfections and surface irregularities (Section 12.9.2). If, however, single crystal filaments of a material (either metallic or ceramic) are grown under carefully controlled conditions, with few flaws and dislocations in their lattices (Section 2.4.2), tensile strengths much greater than 7 GN/m^2 may be achieved. Such *whiskers* (e.g. Al_2O_3) can be used to impart great strength to a composite.
(c) Principles of fibre reinforcement.

- (i) The polymer (the matrix) to be reinforced should be a material capable of plastic deformation (not brittle). It should also adhere to the fibre. Thus it can act as the medium which transmits stresses to the fibres.

(ii) Ceramic fibres should not be marred by surface cracks which will weaken them.
(iii) The principle of combined action—when a composite structure is under stress, there is an associated strain; the components of the material act together to equalise their strains.
(iv) Consider a reinforced structure with fibres aligned parallel to one another. If a tensile load is applied, parallel to the fibres, the matrix can flow plastically, and both the matrix and fibre will have equal strains. But if the fibre is stiffer (higher modulus of elasticity, Section 4.3.2) for a given strain it will take a higher stress than the matrix. In this way the fibres can significantly contribute to the strength of the composite.
(v) In practice, it is quite common to have random orientation of fibres in a matrix (e.g. fibre glass in polyester) so that the mechanical properties of the composite are *isotropic*—the same in all directions.

13.3.2 Particulate ceramic fillers

Ceramic-filled acrylics and other polymers are used dentally as restorative materials. The main functions of the particulate fillers are:
(a) to improve the mechanical properties such as compressive strength and modulus of elasticity,
(b) to reduce the coefficient of thermal expansion (see Appendix II, Table II.3),
(c) to reduce the shrinkage on setting of the material, and
(d) to contribute to the aesthetics.

The following points should be noted:
(a) The ceramic particles do not normally increase the tensile strength.
(b) The ceramic particles only increase the compressive strength if there is bonding between the two phases; special coupling agents are needed.
(c) The mechanism of particulate reinforcement of polymers is more complex than that of fibre reinforcement discussed above, but, as in the case of fibres, the load on the composite is shared between both polymer and ceramic phases.
(d) As a general principle smaller size particles give a greater improvement in mechanical properties.

13.4 REINFORCED CERAMICS

The propagation of a crack through a ceramic, such as dental porcelain, can lead to its fracture. However, if a stronger constituent, such as alumina (Al_2O_3) is present, it may hinder the progress of cracks and so strengthen the material. This principle has been used in aluminous porcelain (Section 28.2.3).

READING REFERENCE

Gordon J E 1976 The new science of strong materials, 2nd edn. Penguin, Harmondsworth. Middlesex.

This book gives an excellent account of the mechanical properties of solids in relation to their structure. Chapter 8 deals specifically with composite materials.

14. Enamel and dentine

14.1 INTRODUCTION

The purpose of this chapter is to consider briefly some important aspects of tooth tissue. Three reasons can be cited for the need for such information:

(a) In relation to biocompatibility, it is important to know the effects of chemical components of synthetic materials on human tissue.

(b) The properties of tooth substance should be known, because ideally a synthetic material should be similar (e.g. in terms of mechanical and thermal properties) to the material it replaces.

(c) It is very important to develop materials and techniques which are capable of durable bonding to tooth substances (Ch. 15).

This chapter is not a complete account of the structure and properties of enamel and dentine; only those aspects of the subject of relevance to dental materials science have been briefly considered. Further information can be obtained from standard works on dental anatomy (see reference at end of chapter).

14.2 THE STRUCTURE OF TEETH

Figure 14.1 shows a diagrammatic representation of a mid-plane section of an anterior tooth. The following features are noted:

(a) Enamel, a highly calcified substance, covers that part of the tooth which is visible. It is the hardest tissue in the body.

(b) The bulk of the tooth substance is dentine, which resembles bone in many respects.

(c) The root of the tooth is covered by cementum, a bone-like connective tissue.
(d) To the cementum is attached the periodontal membrane, which binds the tooth to its socket.
(e) The pulp of the tooth is soft tissue, containing nerves and blood vessels. The pulp is very sensitive to chemical, thermal and tactile stimulation.
(f) The diagram shows the dentinal tubules, which extend from the pulp to the interface with enamel or cementum.

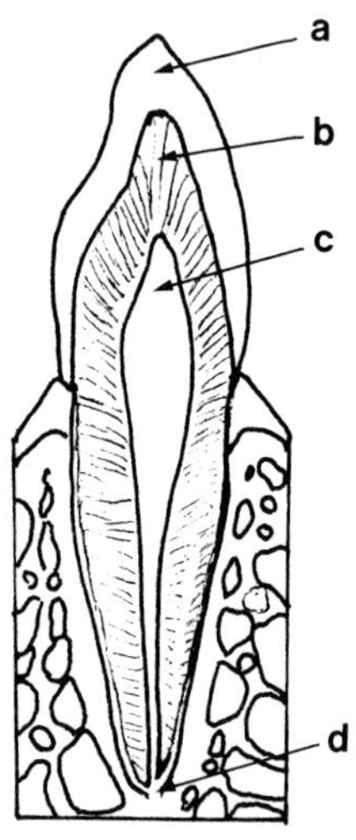

Fig. 14.1 Mid-plane section through an anterior tooth a. enamel b. dentine c. pulp d. apex

14.3 CHEMICAL COMPOSITION

Table 14.1 shows the approximate chemical composition of enamel and dentine.

Table 14.1 Approximate composition of enamel and dentine.

	Mineral vol%	phase (wt %)	Organic vol%	phase (wt %)	Water vol%	(wt %)
Enamel	92	(97)	2	(1)	6	(2)
Dentine	48	(69)	29	(20)	23	(11)

14.3.1 Enamel

The small quantities of organic matter consist of soluble proteins, peptides, insoluble protein and citric acid.

The mineral phase has an apatite structure, being principally hydroxyapatite, of empirical formula $Ca_{10}(PO_4)_6(OH)_2$.

14.3.2 Dentine

The organic matter, about 20% by weight, is mostly collagen (~18%) and small quantities of citric acid, insoluble protein, mucopolysaccharide and lipid.

As with enamel, the mineral component is hydroxyapatite.

14.4 ASPECTS OF STRUCTURE

14.4.1 Enamel

In enamel the hydroxyapaptite is in the form of rod-shaped units, termed enamel prisms. These are approximately 4–5 μm in diameter, and run from the interface with dentine to the enamel surface. In the inner enamel the prisms follow an undulating course. In the outer enamel the prisms are more regular and approach the enamel surface almost at right angles.

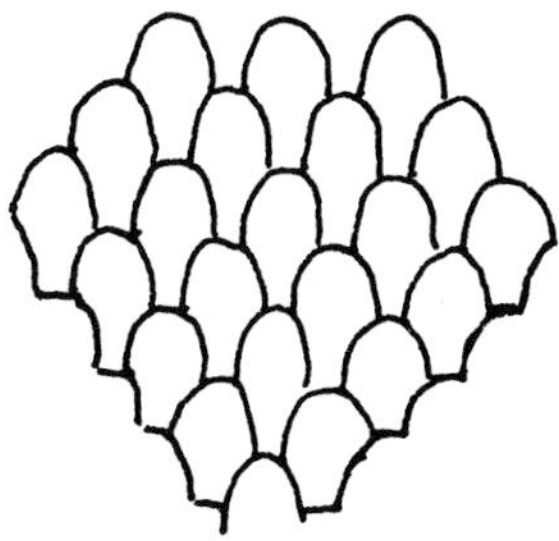

Fig. 14.2 Key-hole pattern for the interlocking of enamel prisms

There is no interprismatic substance, as was once believed. The prism boundaries appear to be almost horse-shoe shaped. It is thought that the prisms interlock according to a key-hole pattern (Fig. 14.2).

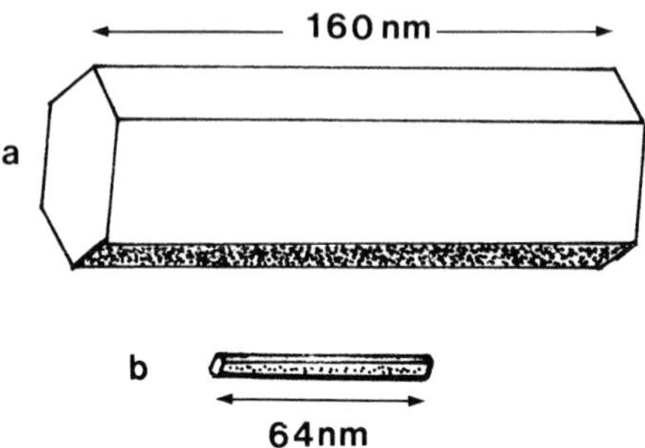

Fig. 14.3 Dimensions of hydroxyapatite crystallites in (a) enamel (b) dentine and bone

Within the prisms there are hydroxyapatite crystallites, which are slightly flattened hexagonal rods. Figure 14.3 gives the approximate dimensions of these, showing that the hydroxyapatite crystals in bone and dentine are much smaller than in enamel.

The surface of enamel has a greater organic content than deeper layers; organic material usually covers the surface.

14.4.2 Dentine

Figure 14.4 shows a diagrammatic representation of the cross-section of dentine, cut perpendicular to the tubules. The tubules contain slender prolongations or processes of the connective tissue cells, the odontoblasts, which line the pulp cavity. The tubules have an approximate diameter of 4 μm at the outer surface. There are also lateral branches, and some inter-branching also occurs. Peri-tubular dentine is a highly calcified annular layer within each tubule, which surrounds the odontoblastic process. In the tubules the space is filled with dentinal fluid, which is similar to tissue fluid in its composition. Fluid flows from the tubules of freshly cut dentine.

Between the tubules, the intercellular substance is composed of dense bundles of fibrils of collagen, embedded in a calcified substance.

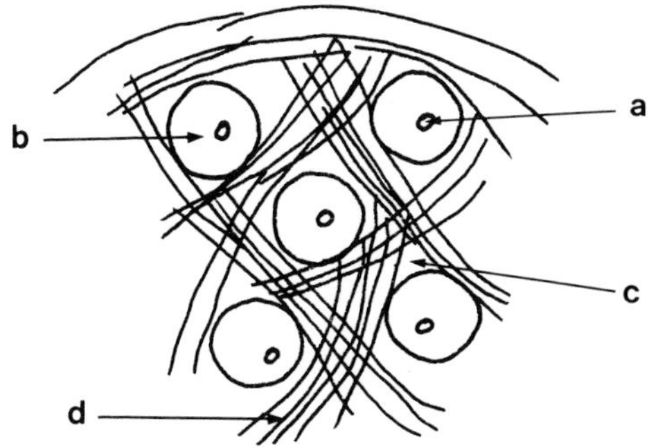

Fig. 14.4 Section of dentine, cut perpendicular to the dentinal tubules a. dentinal tubule b. peritubular dentine c. intertubular dentine d. collagen fibres

Secondary dentine can be found in response to stimuli due to, e.g. abrasion, erosion and the approach of caries.

14.5 PROPERTIES

Table 14.2 lists some of the more important properties of enamel and dentine. Ideally, these properties should be matched by any material designed to replace tooth tissue.

Table 14.2 Typical properties of enamel and dentine*

	Enamel	Dentine
Compressive properties		
Proportional limit (MN/m^2)	70–350**	160–175
Compressive strength (MN/m^2)	100–380**	250–350
Modulus of elasticity (GN/m^2)	10–80	11–12
Tensile properties		
Tensile strength (MN/m^2) —measured in tension	10	20–50
Tensile strength (MN/m^2) —diametral compression	30	30–65
Hardness		
Knoop hardness (KHN)	360–390	75
Thermal properties		
Thermal conductivity (W/mk)	0.88	0.59
Coefficient of thermal expansion (ppm/°C)	11.4	8.3

* Ranges of values taken from the literature
** Selected few data available; great variability in results which appear to depend on the orientation of the specimen

In some instances great variability in properties is seen, owing to the following difficulties in measurement:

(a) Teeth may be damaged by trauma, by caries, or during the extraction procedure.
(b) Storage of extracted teeth is difficult; pulp tissue may putrefy, and fungal growth can occur. Formalin as a storage medium will cause dehydration. Storage in water or solution of salts may cause changes in water content.
(c) Orientation of specimens is important, particularly in relation to enamel.

14.6 THE EFFECT OF CHEMICALS

14.6.1 The effect of fluoride on enamel

Fluoride ions can be substituted for hydroxy groups of hydroxyapatite, leading to the formation of fluorapatite. This latter substance is less soluble than hydroxyapatite; this may account for the observed fact that fluorised teeth are more resistant to dental caries.

14.6.2 Acid etching of enamel

Some current dental procedures use *acid etching* techniques to aid bonding of polymer-containing materials to enamel. The mechanism of this is given in Section 15.4.1, and practical details of the procedure in Section 20.4.

14.6.3 The effect of chemical agents on dentine

(a) Irritation can be caused when a substance passes through the dentinal tubules to the pulp. However, pulpal irritation is a complex phenomenon, and may also be related to the cavity preparation procedures, and to changes caused by dental decay.
(b) In attempts to aid bonding to dentine, remineralising solutions have been applied. Typically these contain calcium and phosphate ions.

14.7 RESUMÉ

Knowledge of the nature of tooth substances is important, since this relates to:
(a) techniques of bonding to enamel and dentine (Ch. 15).
(b) aspects of biocompatibility (Section 3.3).
(c) the properties of materials for the replacement of enamel and dentine (Section 19.2).

READING REFERENCE

Scott J H Symons N B B 1982 Introduction to dental anatomy, 9th edition. Churchill Livingstone, Edinburgh.

Section III of this book is recommended for detailed study of the structure and properties of the dental tissues.

15. Surface properties and adhesion

15.1 DEFINITIONS

Adhesion occurs when two unlike substances join together on being brought into contact, because of forces of attraction between them. *Cohesion* results from attraction between like molecules.

An *adhesive* is a material used to produce adhesion; the *adherend* is the substance to which the adhesive is applied.

Under certain circumstances, bonding can occur when a liquid flows into pores or crevices in the surface of the material. Because of the mechanical interlocking which occurs when the fluid material sets, a strong bond can be formed. This phenomenon is referred to as *attachment*. However, it is often called adhesion, or mechanical adhesion, in the dental literature. Dental techniques involving adhesion and attachment are often referred to as 'adhesive dentistry'.

15.2 PRINCIPLES OF ADHESION

15.2.1 Surface properties and bonding

The great majority of surfaces to which adhesive bonding is required are microscopically or macroscopically rough. There is a consequent danger of pockets of air being trapped between an adhesive and the surface, thus reducing the area of contact between the two (Fig. 15.1). However, if the rough surface is adequately wetted by an adhesive then this may increase the effective area of contact and hence improve the bond strength. For good adhesive bonding, surfaces should be cleaned to remove debris and weakly-bound deposits from them.

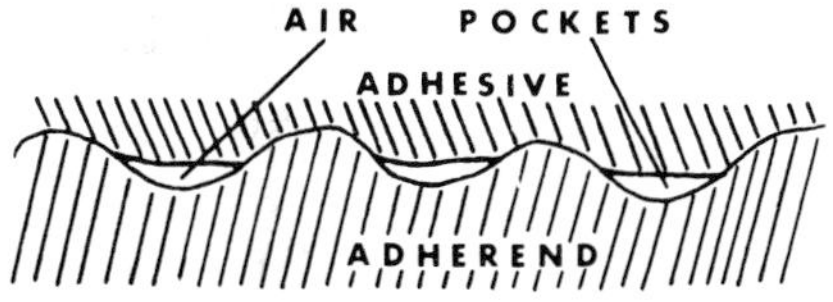

Fig. 15.1 Air trapped between adhesive and adherend.

Surface forces, such as van der Waals forces, are quite appreciable in magnitude, although weaker than primary chemical (covalent and ionic) bonds. However, van der Waals forces between material bodies fall off rapidly in magnitude with increasing distance of separation. In consequence of this factor and also that of surface roughness it is essential to apply a liquid adhesive to the surfaces to be joined. The adhesive must flow across the surfaces and fill any microscopic irregularities so that wetting of both the adherends is achieved. Subsequently the adhesive must be converted from a liquid to a solid form, to achieve mechanical strength and reasonably high rigidity in the adhesive. Solidification may be achieved by various means such as polymerisation of monomer liquid or evaporation of solvent from a resin.

15.2.2 Surface wetting

The ability of an adhesive to wet the surface of the adherend can be measured by the contact angle of a drop of liquid on the surface (Fig. 15.2). Materials of low *free surface energy* (or *critical surface tension*) will not be easily wetted e.g. waxes, and poly(tetrafluoro-

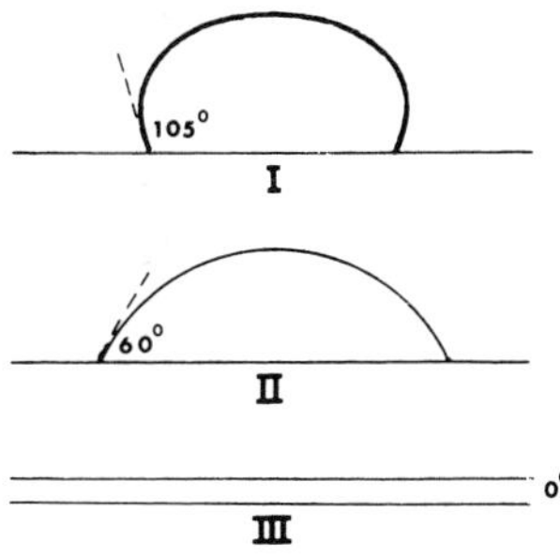

Fig. 15.2 Surface wetting. I, contact angle 105°; II, contact angle 60°; III, contact angle 0°.

ethylene)—PTFE—used in 'non-stick' cooking utensils. The surface energies of many surfaces may be increased by treatment in various ways. For example, dental enamel surfaces are treated by acid-etching which increases the surface energy (Section 15.4.1).

The contact angle of a liquid on a reasonably smooth surface is an inverse measure of the degree of surface wetting of the surface (Fig. 15.2). The contact angle depends on the surface energy of the solid and also on the *surface tension* of the liquid. (Surface tension effects arise from the different balance of inter-molecular attractions of molecules at a surface from those in the bulk of a material.)

For low contact-angle values to be achieved and surface tension of the fluid adhesive should ideally be lower than the critical surface tension of the solid. However, for *rapid* capillary penetration of a porous surface a reasonably high surface tension may be advantageous.

15.2.3 Requirements for setting adhesive systems

(a) The adhesive must give good wetting of the adherend.
(b) The adhesive should have a suitable viscosity to enable it to flow readily over the surface of adherend.
(c) The setting of the adhesive should occur without excessive dimensional changes—that is, little expansion or contraction.
(d) The thickness of the adhesive layer is important; too great a thickness can lead to poor bond strength (Fig. 15.3).
(e) The strength of the set adhesive must be taken into consideration.

Cohesive failure of a bond occurs if the adhesive fails; *adhesive failure* occurs where the adhesive and adherend part.

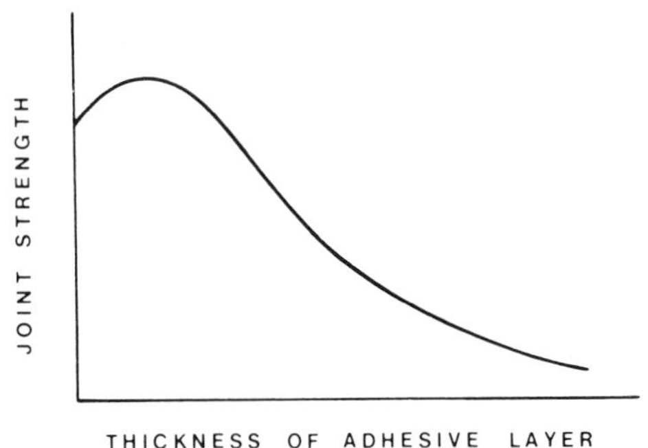

Fig. 15.3 The effect of thickness of adhesive layer on bond strength.

Consider, for example, an adhesive bond being tested in tension (Fig. 15.4a). One of three things may happen.

(i) failure of the adhesive bond (Fig. 15.4b).
(ii) tensile failure of the adhesive (Fig. 15.4c), or,
(iii) tensile failure of either adherend (Fig. 15.4d).

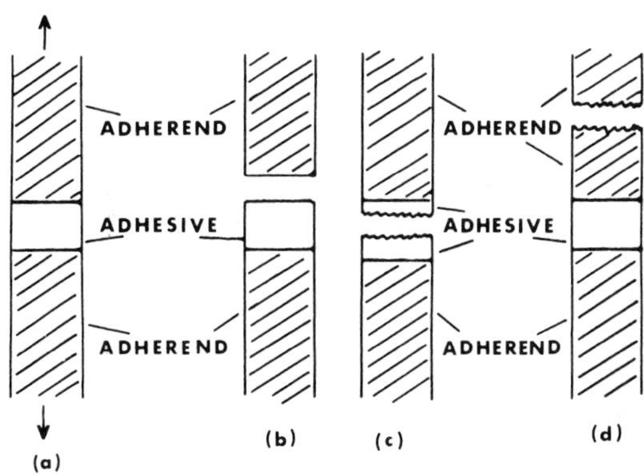

Fig. 15.4 Adhesive bonding. (a) Adhesive bond in tension. (b) Failure of adhesive bond. (c) Tensile failure of adhesive. (d) Tensile failure of adherend.

15.3 DENTAL CONSIDERATIONS

For adhesion to enamel and dentine, the following factors must be taken into account:
(a) The composition of the tissues—an adhesive should ideally react with both the organic and inorganic constituents (see Chapter 14).
(b) Ideally the adhesive should be *hydrophilic*—not repelled by water, which is present in enamel and dentine.
(c) The stability of the set adhesive in the oral environment is important.
(d) In a prepared tooth cavity, there may be considerable microscopic debris. Enamel surfaces may have deposits such as calculus on them.

15.4 METHODS OF OBTAINING BONDING TO ENAMEL AND DENTINE

15.4.1 Modification of enamel and dentine

Many types of surface treatments have been tried experimentally, in order to enhance bonding of materials to enamel and dentine. These include the use of enzymes, chelating agents, acids and alkalis.

The *acid-etch techniques* for modification of enamel are of great current importance. Phosphoric and citric acids of appropriate concentration, can within 1 to 2 minutes, remove about 5 μm of the surface enamel, and also selectively decalcify the enamel to a depth of from 15 to 120 μm. Stronger acids do not give selective decalcification. Weaker acids react too slowly with enamel. Currently available *acid etchants* are usually 30 to 50% solutions of phosphoric acid, some containing 7% zinc oxide.

Acid etching may aid bonding to enamel by:

(a) removal of surface debris.

(b) producing pores in the surface into which resin penetrates to form tag-like extensions, giving mechanical interlocking,

(c) increasing the free surface energy (critical surface tension) of the enamel so that it exceeds the surface tension of the resin, and consequently produces wetting, and,

(d) causing exposure of a greater surface area of enamel to the material.

Citric acid cavity cleansers also supplied, in attempts to improve bonding to dentine.

15.4.2 Potential adhesive systems

The following materials are of current interest:

(a) Polymers prepared from aromatic dimethacrylates (Chapter 19 and Section 20.4), in conjunction with acid-etch techniques.

(b) Cements containing poly(acrylic acid) solutions, such as zinc polycarboxylate cements (Section 17.3) and glass—ionomer cements (Section 18.3).

(c) Cyanoacrylates (Section 8.4.1 and 20.3).

15.5 DENTAL APPLICATIONS

Bonding to tooth substance is important in the following applications:

(a) The cementation of inlays, crowns and bridges (Ch. 16).

(b) Adhesive filling materials would not permit marginal leakage (Section 19.2).

(c) The prevention of dental decay, by sealing pits and fissures of teeth (Section 20.3.1)

(d) The direct bonding of bridges to etched enamel (Ch. 31).
(e) The direct cementation of orthodontic applicances to teeth (Section 38.6).

READING REFERENCES

Retief D H 1970 The principles of adhesion. Journal of the Dental Association of South Africa 25: 285.

This paper stresses the dental need for adhesion, the nature of adhesion and surface phenomena, and concludes with a summary of 15 points of importance.

Brauer G M 1975 Adhesion and adhesives. In: von Fraunhofer JA (ed) Scientific aspects of dental materials. Butterworth, London, Ch 2.

The main sections of this chapter deal with the reactivity of tooth surfaces, surface treatments to enhance adhesion, potential adhesive systems and adhesive test methods.

SECTION II

Cements, adhesives and non-metallic filling materials

16. Cements: classification, applications and requirements

16.1 APPLICATIONS

In this section of the book, a wide range of non-metallic materials is discussed, including dental cements, polymer based filling materials, and substances capable of bonding to tooth structure. Table 16.1 lists the dental applications of such materials. It should be noted that mention of a product in this table for a specific application does not imply endorsement of such technique; this table is a list of most of the materials that are or have been used, or have been suggested for specific applications.

16.2 CLASSIFICATION OF MATERIALS

The materials may be classified as follows:

(a) acid-base reaction cements—further classified in Section 16.3, and discussed in chapters 17 and 18.

(b) polymerising materials:
- (i) cyanoacrylates (Section 21.3)
- (ii) dimethacrylate polymers (Ch. 19 and 20)
- (iii) polymer-ceramic composites (Ch. 19)

(c) other materials:
- (i) calcium hydroxide (Section 21.1)
- (ii) gutta percha (Section 21.5)
- (iii) varnishes (Section 21.2)

16.3 ACID-BASE REACTION CEMENTS

16.3.1 Chief constituents

Dental cements are formulated as powders and liquids. The powders are amphoteric or basic (proton acceptors) and the liquids are acids or proton donors. On mixing the two together a viscous paste is

Table 16.1 Applications of materials

Dental application	Materials	Section
Cavity lining	Zinc oxide-eugenol	17.1
	EBA cements	17.1.7
	Zinc phosphate	17.2
	Calcium hydroxide	21.1
	Zinc polycarboxylate (polyacrylate)	17.3
Temporary restorations	Zinc oxide-eugenol	17.1
	EBA cements	17.1.7
	Copper cements	17.2.6
	Silver cements	17.2.7
	Gutta percha	21.5
	Silicophosphate cement	18.2
Restorations of deciduous teeth	Zinc phosphate	17.2
	Silicophosphate	18.2
	Glass-ionomer cement	18.3
Anterior restorative materials	Silicate cements	18.1
	Polymer-ceramic composites	19.3
	Glass-ionomer cements	18.3
Pulp capping	Zinc oxide-eugenol	17.1
	Calcium hydroxide	21.1
Root canal filling materials	Zinc oxide-eugenol and related materials	17.1, 21.6
	Gutta percha	21.5
	(Also, chloropercha, composite resin materials, epoxy resins)	21.5
Cementing agents, for inlays, crowns and bridges	EBA cements	17.1.7
	Zinc phosphate	17.2
	Zinc polycarboxylate (polyacrylate)	17.3
	Silicophosphate cement	18.2
	Glass-ionomer cement	18.3
Cementing agents for splints, and orthodontic appliances	Zinc phosphate	17.2
	Copper cements	17.2.6
	Zinc polycarboxylate (polyacrylate)	17.3
Agents for direct cementation of orthodontic appliances	Acrylic polymers; dimethacrylates	20.3.2
	Zinc polycarboxylate (polyacrylate)	17.3
Soft tissue adhesives	Adhesive bandage	21.7
	Cyanoacrylates	21.3
Periodontal dressings	Zinc oxide-eugenol, etc	21.4
	Zinc polycarboxylate (polyacrylate)	21.3
	Cyanoacrylates	21.3
Pit and fissure sealants	Dimethacrylate polymers	20.3.1
	Cyanoacrylates	20.3.1
	Glass-ionomer cements	20.3.1

formed, which subsequently hardens to a solid mass. The cements can be classified by the nature of the cement powder.

(a) Zinc oxide. This can react with a range of liquids, as detailed in Section 12.7. These cements are discussed in Chapter 17.

(b) Ion-leachable glasses, particularly fluorine containing aluminosilicates (Section 12.8—see Ch. 18).

Table 16.2 lists the chief components of acid-base reaction cements, and Figure 16.1 illustrates the five principal types of cement.

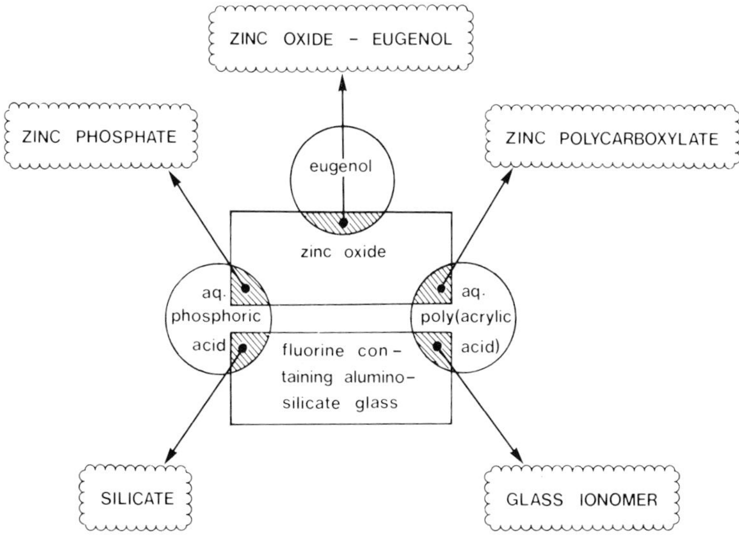

Fig. 16.1 The five principal types of dental acid-base reaction cements.

16.3.2 General reactions

A cement forming reaction is the interaction between an acid and a base, the product of which is a gel-salt. Equations for such reactions can be written in a simplified general form:

Table 16.2 Chief constituents of acid-base reaction cements

Cement powder (proton acceptor)	Cement liquid (proton donor)	Type of cement	Section	Related materials
Zinc oxide	eugenol	zinc oxide-eugenol (ZOE)	17.1	EBA cements (Section 17.1.7)
Zinc oxide	aqueous solution of phosphoric acid	zinc phosphate	17.2	Copper and silver cements (Sections 17.2.6 and 17.2.7)
Zinc oxide	aqueous solution of poly(acrylic acid)	zinc polycarboxylate or polyacrylate	17.3	Poly(acrylic acid) may be in solid form as a powder component
Fluorine containing aluminosilicate glass	aqueous solution of phosphoric acid	silicate cements	18.1	Silicophosphate cements (Section 18.2)
Fluroine containing aluminosilicate glass	aqueous solution of poly(acrylic acid) or copolymer	glass-ionomer	18.3	

MO	+ H_2A	$\rightarrow MA$	+ H_2O
proton acceptor	proton donor	gel-salt	

$MO \times SiO_2$	+ H_2A	$\rightarrow MA + \times SiO_2 + H_2O$
proton acceptor	proton donor	gel-salt

16.3.3 General structure

Set cements are heterogeneous; only part of the powder reacts with the liquids, and the final set material is composed of a core of unreacted powder surrounded by a matrix of reaction products, i.e. the gel-salt.

16.4 REQUIREMENTS OF CEMENTS

(a) They should be non-toxic, and non-irritant to the pulp and other tissues.
(b) Insoluble in saliva and liquids taken into the mouth.
(c) Mechanical properties—these must meet the requirements for their particular applications, for example, for a cavity lining, a cement should develop sufficient strength rapidly to enable a filling material to be packed on it.
(d) Protection of the pulp from effects of other restorative materials:
- (i) Thermal insulation—a cement is used under a large metallic restoration (e.g. amalgam) to protect the pulp from temperature changes.
- (ii) Chemical protection—a cement should be able to prevent penetration into the pulp of harmful chemicals from the restorative material.
- (iii) Electrical insulation under a metallic restoration to minimise galvanic effects (Section 11.4).

(e) Optical properties—for cementation of a translucent restoration (for example, a porcelain crown) the optical properties of the cement should parallel those of tooth substance.
(f) A cement should ideally be adhesive to enamel and dentine, and to gold alloys, porcelain and acrylics, but not to dental instruments.
(g) A cement should be bacteriostatic if inserted in a cavity with residual caries.
(h) Cements should have an obtundent effect on the pulp.
(i) Rheological properties are important: a luting cement should

have sufficiently low viscosity to give a low film thickness and should have adequate working time at mouth temperature to permit placement of the restoration.

READING REFERENCES

Smith D C 1971 Dental cements. Dental Clinics of North America 15 (1): 3

This review includes a discussion of the principal requirements for dental cements.

Wilson A D 1975 Dental cements-general. In: Von Fraunhofer (ed) Scientific aspects of dental materials. Butterworth, London, Ch 4

This chapter is an extensive discussion of the scope, applications, types, formation, structure and properties of dental cements.

Wilson A D 1978 The chemistry of dental cements. Chemical Society Reviews, 7: 265

This paper is a comprehensive review of the chemical composition and reactions of cements.

17. Cements based on zinc oxide

17.1 ZINC OXIDE–EUGENOL AND RELATED MATERIALS

17.1.1 Composition

(a) Powder
   (i) Zinc oxide (Section 12.7).
   (ii) Magnesium oxide may be present in small quantities; it reacts with eugenol in a similar manner to zinc oxide.
   (iii) Zinc acetate (or other salts), in quantities up to about 1%, are used as accelerators for the setting reaction.

(b) Liquid
   (i) Eugenol, the major constituent of oil of cloves.
   (ii) Olive oil, up to 15%.
   (iii) Sometimes acetic acid, to act as an accelerator.

17.1.2 Manipulation

These cements are mixed by adding the powder in small increments to the liquid, until a thick consistency is obtained. A powder/liquid ratio of between 4/1 and 6/1 by weight will give a material of the required properties; with experience, a suitable consistency can be recognised without weighing the materials. As a rule, a thin glass slab and stainless steel spatula are used.

17.1.3 Setting reaction

This is not yet fully understood. One or both of two things may occur on mixing the powder and liquid:
(a) Chemical reaction, to form a compound called zinc eugenolate (Section 12.7.2).
(b) Absorption of the eugenol by the zinc oxide may also occur.

Other factors to be noted are:
(a) The setting reaction between pure zinc oxide and pure eugenol will not occur in the absence of water. Thus, a mixture of zinc oxide and eugenol, without added accelerators, can be kept in a desiccator for several days without undergoing much change.
(b) The set materials contains both some unreacted zinc oxide and eugenol.

17.1.4 Setting time

This depends on:
(a) The powder:
  (i) Its method of preparation.
  (ii) The particle size—a finer powder will have a greater surface area exposed to the eugenol, so can react more quickly.
(b) The accelerating additives (Section 17.1.1).
(c) The powder/liquid ratio—a thicker mix gives a faster setting material.
(d) Exposure to moisture on mixing or the addition of water will accelerate the reaction.
(e) An increase in temperature also causes faster setting.

17.1.5 Properties

(a) Effect on the pulp—this is small, thus the material has been recommended for use in deep cavities near the pulp.
(b) Chemical properties—the solubility of the set cement in water is high—by far the highest of all dental cements—mainly due to the elution of eugenol.
(c) Mechanical properties—these are the weakest of all the cements (except calcium hydroxide, Section 21.1). See data in Appendix II.
(d) Protection of the pulp:
  (i) These cements have low thermal diffusivity—(Appendix II).

(ii) They can protect the pulp from the phosphoric acid of phosphate or silicate cements.
(iii) They can provide electrical insulation.

(e) Optical properties—the set cement is opaque.

(f) Adhesion—these cements do not adhere to enamel and dentine. This is one reason why they are not frequently used for the final cementation of dental restorations.

(g) These cements are *bacteriostatic* and *obtundent*.

17.1.6 Resin bonded cements

Zinc oxide—eugenol cements are available which contain either:
(a) hydrogenated rosin comprising about 10% of the powder, or
(b) polystyrene dissolved in eugenol, to give a 10% solution. The function of these additives is to increase the strength of the cement (Appendix II).

17.1.7 EBA cements

The letters EBA are an abbreviation for *ortho*-ethoxybenzoic acid, of formula:

$$C_6H_4(OC_2H_5)COOH$$

The formulation of cements containing EBA is in Table 17.1.

Table 17.1 Composition of EBA cements

Powder	Percentage by weight
Zinc oxide	60–74
Fused quartz or alumina	20–34
Hydrogenated rosin	6
Liquid	**Percentage by volume**
Eugenol	37.5
o-ethoxybenzoic acid	62.5

In comparing these cements with the unmodified accelerated zinc oxide–eugenol materials, two things should be noted:
(a) A higher powder/liquid ratio can be used for the EBA materials (7/1 or greater).
(b) The mechanical properties of EBA cements are considerably greater than those of unmodified zinc oxide–eugenol products (Appendix II).

17.1.8 Cements containing vanillate esters

Recently cements have been developed containing hexyl vanillate and *o*-ethoxybenzoic acid (HV-EBA), as a substitute for eugenol. This liquid is mixed with zinc oxide powder. It has been claimed that these cements have high strength and low solubility.

17.1.9 Special zinc oxide–eugenol products

Some zinc oxide–eugenol materials contain antibiotics such as tetracyclines, and steroids as anti-inflammatory agents. Their principal use is in pulp capping and root canal therapy. Another product also contains barium sulphate, which is radio-opaque.

17.2 ZINC PHOSPHATE AND RELATED MATERIALS

17.2.1 Composition

(a) Powder:
- (i) Zinc oxide is the principal constituent.
- (ii) Magnesium oxide may be present, up to about 10 per cent.
- (iii) Very small quantities of other oxides, or metallic salts (e.g. fluorides) may be present.

(b) Liquid. This is an aqueous solution of phosphoric acid, containing about 30 to 40% water. Zinc and/or aluminium phosphates are also present, formed by dissolving zinc oxide and/or aluminium hydroxide in the liquid.

17.2.2 Manipulation

(a) Consistency—the thicker the mix, the stronger is the set material. Thus for a cavity lining, a thick mix should be used. For cementation purposes a thinner mix is required, to permit the cement to flow as the restoration is being seated.
(b) Proportioning. It is not customary to measure the powder and

liquid but every effort to obtain consistent proportioning for the required consistency should be made. Too thin a mix should be avoided, because, in addition to affecting the strength, a thin mix has a lower pH and the set material is more soluble (Section 17.2.5).
(c) Mixing is carried out on a cool glass slab, adding the powder to the liquid in small increments to prolong the working time, and completing the procedure within 1 to 1½ minutes.
(d) The liquid should be kept in a stoppered bottle; loss of water from the liquid will lower its pH and slow down the setting (Section 17.2.4). A bottle of liquid which has become cloudy, due to loss of water, should be discarded.
(e) The powder is of similar composition to those of other cements (for example, zinc oxide–eugenol cements, Section 17.1.1), but each powder should only be used with the liquid supplied for it, to ensure the correct setting time and other properties.
(f) Cementing. Increase in temperature accelerates the rate of reaction of the cement (Section 17.2.4). Thus the cement sets faster at mouth temperature than at room temperature. The cement should be applied to the inlay (or crown, or bridge) before it is applied to the prepared cavity. If the opposite procedure were done, the cement in the tooth may begin to set before the restoration is seated.

17.2.3 Setting reaction

The surface of the particles of zinc oxide react with phosphoric acid, to give an insoluble phosphate, (Section 12.7.2). Magnesium oxide, if present, will react similarly. The final set material is heterogeneous, consisting in general of a core of unreacted zinc oxide particles in a matrix of zinc phosphate.

During setting:
(a) Heat is given out since the reaction is exothermic.
(b) Shrinkage occurs.

17.2.4 Setting time

This depends on:
(a) The powder. This is generally prepared commercially by heating the ingredients to above 1000°C, causing granulation, by a sintering process. Subsequently the solid is ground to a very fine powder. The rate of reaction of the powder with the liquid depends on:
- (i) The temperature to which it was heated; a higher temperature reduces the reactivity of the powder;

(ii) The particle size after grinding—a finer material reacts more quickly, since a greater surface area is exposed to the liquid.

(b) The liquid. The added buffering agents slow down the rate of reaction and improve the working time of the cement.

(c) The setting time also depends on manipulative variables. The following four factors will give acceleration of the setting reaction:

(i) A high powder/liquid ratio.
(ii) Fast rate of addition of powder to liquid.
(iii) The presence of moisture.
(iv) Higher temperature.

17.2.5 Properties

(a) Effect on the pulp. The pH of the freshly mixed cement may be between 1.6 and 3.6. The pH rises during setting, and approaches neutrality within one to two days. A thinner mix has a lower pH, and takes longer to reach neutrality. Pulpal reactions can occur. These can be minimised by protecting the pulp by one or more of the following:

(i) Zinc oxide–eugenol (Section 17.1).
(ii) Calcium hydroxide (Section 21.1).
(iii) A cavity varnish (Section 21.2).

(b) Chemical properties. The solubility of a set zinc phosphate cement depends on the powder/liquid ratio. A thinner mix gives a more soluble material. The solubility of the cement in distilled water is very low, but is higher in solutions of lower pH.

(c) Mechanical properties. These cements are stronger than zinc oxide–eugenol cement, but not as strong as silico–phosphate cements (Appendix II).

(d) Protection of the pulp. Phosphates are good thermal insulators (Appendix II), and may be effective in reducing galvanic effects.

(e) Optical properties. The set cement is opaque.

(f) Adhesion. These cements do not form chemical bonds with enamel or dentine. The retention of cemented restorations depends on the mechanical interlocking of the set material with surface roughnesses of the cavity and restoration.

(g) Rheological properties. The mixed unset cement appears to be near-Newtonian in behaviour (Fig. 17.1) with a viscosity of approximately 120 Nsm^{-2}. Viscosity-time curves do not show a horizontal plateau corresponding to a working time (Fig. 17.2).

(h) Film thickness. For most materials this is less than 40 μm and can be as low as 15 μm. Clearly this property depends on, among other things, the particle size of the powder, as supplied, and the extent to which this is changed during setting.

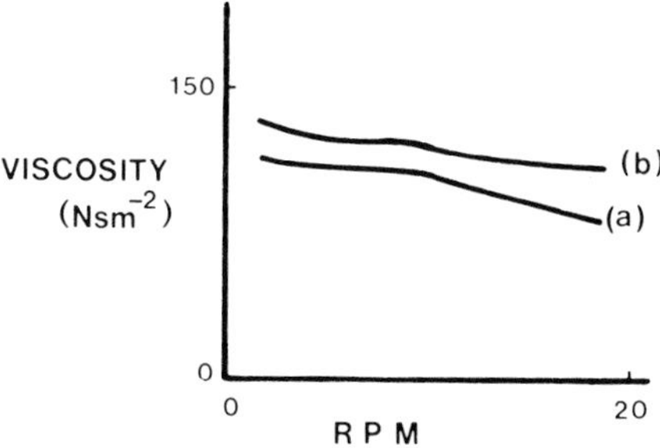

Fig. 17.1 Viscosity of (a) zinc phosphate, (b) zinc polycarboxylate cement as a function of rotation speed of a spindle viscometer. Viscosity measured at 25°C, 45 seconds after atart of mixing. (after Vermilyea et al 1977 J. Dent. Res., 56: 762.)

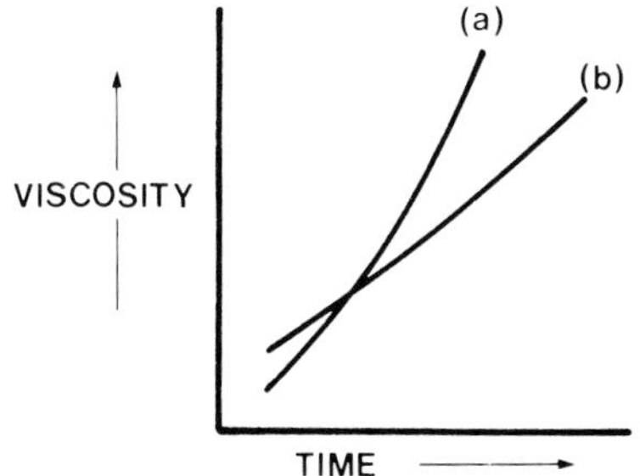

Fig. 17.2 Increase in viscosity with time of (a) zinc phosphate, (b) zinc polycarboxylate cement. (after Vermilyea et al 1977 J Dent. Res., 56: 762.)

17.2.6 Copper cements

These are similar to phosphate cements, except that the powder contains a copper compound in addition to zinc oxide. If copper(I) oxide (cuprous oxide) is used, the cement is red, while copper(II) oxide (cupric oxide) gives a black material.

The black copper cements have the following properties:

(a) Their effect on the pulp may be even greater than that of an unmodified phosphate cement.

(b) They are considered to be bactericidal, so have been used to prolong the life of deciduous teeth, if all the carious tooth substance cannot be removed.

They are sometimes used in the cementation of splints and fixed orthodontic appliances.

17.2.7 Silver cements

Some phosphate type cements contain silver salts in an endeavour to render them bactericidal.

17.3 ZINC POLYCARBOXYLATE CEMENTS

These cements, which are claimed to be adhesive to some dental tissues, have been developed in the last few years.

17.3.1 Composition

As originally formulated:
(a) The powder consists primarily of zinc oxide, though small quantities of magnesium oxide may also be present.
(b) The liquid is an approximately 40% aqueous solution of polyacrylic acid (Table 8.1), of average molecular weight between 20 000 and 50 000.

Recently developed commercial products have a number of variations:
(a) Some products are supplied with two liquids of different viscosities; the thinner liquid for cementing, and the more viscous one for cavity lining. The differences in viscosity are achieved by either:

- (i) differences in molecular weight; one manufacturer supplies two liquids, both containing 40–42% polyacrylic acid, but with molecular weights approximately 22 000 (lower viscosity) and 50 000 (higher viscosity) or:
- (ii) differences in concentration; for example, two solutions of polyacrylic acid, about 32% and 42% concentration, both polymers with molecular weight about 50 000.

(b) Many cements now contain the polyacrylic acid in the powder, around 15–18%. The liquids for these materials consist of about 95% water, pH 4.2–4.5 (compared to pH of 1.0–1.6 for polyacrylic acid solutions). One of the products is encapsulated for mechanical mixing.
(c) Another encapsulated materials contains about 43% alumina in the powder.
(d) One product contains a polymer with a structure slightly different from that of polyacrylic acid.
(e) Stannous fluoride is a constituent of one cement.

17.3.2 Manipulation

(a) Polyacrylic acid solutions are more viscous than the liquids of other cements, which affects the ease of mixing of the material.
(b) If the cement is being used to secure adhesion to enamel and dentine, it is important that the tooth surface should be clean and saliva-free (Section 17.3.5).
(c) The cement should be applied to the tooth as soon as possible after mixing, otherwise poor adhesion may result. If a cement mix begins to 'cobweb' on manipulation, it should be discarded. There is a continuous increase in cement viscosity during manipulation of the material (Fig. 17.2).
(d) Polycarboxylate cement will adhere to instruments, particularly those made of stainless steel. Thus:

- (i) It is useful to use alcohol as a release agent for the mixing spatula.
- (ii) Instruments should be cleaned before the cement sets on them.
- (iii) If cement does inadvertently adhere to a spatula, most of it can be chipped off quite easily. The remaining material can be removed in boiling sodium hydroxide solution.

17.3.3 Setting reaction

This may involve the formation of a salt, zinc polyacrylate. The set material is a cored structure containing a considerable quantity of unreacted zinc oxide.

17.3.4 Setting time

(a) This depends on the composition and method of manufacture of the powder and liquid.
(b) A faster setting time is achieved at higher temperatures.

17.3.5 Adhesive properties

The tensile bond strength of various cements are compared in Table 17.2. The following should be noted:
(a) Under ideal conditions of manipulation, the adhesion of a polycarboxylate to a clean dried surface of enamel is much greater than that of other cements. It has been found in some experiments to measure tensile bond strengths that the cement breaks in tension before the cement–enamel joint fails (as in Fig. 15.4c).

Table 17.2 Adhesion of cements

Cement	Adherend	Approximate tensile bond strength MN/m^2
Zinc polycarboxylate	Enamel, dry and polished	8.5
Zinc polycarboxylate	Enamel, wet with water	8.5
Zinc polycarboxylate	Enamel, wet with saliva	4.4
Zinc polycarboxylate	Dentine, dry	3.9
Zinc polycarboxylate	Dentine, wet with saliva	1.9
Zinc phosphate	Enamel, dry and polished	3.6
Zinc phosphate	Dentine, dry	1.7
Copper phosphate (black)	Enamel, dry and polished	2.9

(b) Wetting the enamel surface with distilled water has little effect on the bond strength. This is to be expected, since the liquid is an aqueous solution.
(c) The presence of saliva will reduce considerably the bond strength to enamel (Table 17.2).
(d) It appears that a polycarboxylate will adhere better to a smooth surface than to a rough one. This mode of action contrasts with zinc phosphate cements, where a rough surface helps mechanical interlocking (Section 17.2.5).
(e) The adhesive bond to dentine is not as good as that to enamel (Table 17.2).
(f) The bond between polycarboxylate and dentine is also affected by saliva (Table 17.2).
(g) The cement does not adhere well to gold or porcelain. Techniques of tin plating metallic restorations have been developed to improve bonding to such cements (Section 30.6).
(h) Adhesion to stainless steel is excellent. The cement has thus been used for the cementation of fixed orthodontic appliances.

17.3.6 Other properties

(a)The experiments so far carried out suggest that these cements have very little irritant effect on the pulp.
(b) Chemical properties—these cements are more soluble than zinc phosphate materials. Some products may also absorb water, which can cause the material to become soft and gel-like.
(c) Zinc polycarboxylate cements are almost as strong as phosphate materials in compression, and stronger in tension (Appendix II).

(d) From the nature of these cements, it is probable that they have good thermal insulation properties.
(e) The set cement is very opaque, because of the large quantity of unreacted zinc oxide that is present.
(f) Rheological properties are broadly similar to those of zinc phosphate cements (Section 17.2.5; Figs. 17.1 and 17.2).

18. Cements based on ion-leachable glasses

18.1 SILICATE CEMENTS

18.1.1 Introduction

These were introduced for anterior fillings around 1903. Since that date there have been considerable developments in these materials, though their properties still leave much to be desired. Although alternative materials are available for anterior restorations (Ch. 19) they also have some undersirable properties.

The requirements for anterior restorative materials are discussed in Section 19.2, and a comparison of silicates with some polymer-based restorative materials is given in Table 19.3.

18.1.2 Composition

(a) Powder

(i) An analysis of four modern materials gave the following results:

silica (SiO_2)	31.5–41.6%
alumina (Al_2O_3)	27.2–29.1%
lime (CaO)	7.7– 9.0%
sodium oxide (Na_2O)	7.7–11.2%
fluoride (F^-)	13.3–22.0%
phosphorous pentoxide (P_2O_5)	3.0– 5.3%
zinc oxide (ZnO)	0.1– 2.9%

(Date from: Wilson A D 1970 Chemistry and industry, 19 December, p 1613)

(ii) Fibreglass is present in at least one available material.
(iii) Arsenic is an impurity in some of the powder constituents; the material should contain less than 2 parts per million of arsenic, otherwise pulpal damage can occur.

(b) Liquid

The composition is similar to the liquid used for phosphates (Section 17.2.1). An analysis has given the following data:

phosphoric acid (H_3PO_4)	48.8–55.5%
aluminium (Al)	1.5– 2.0%
zinc (Zn)	4.2– 9.1%

(Data from: Wilson A D 1970 Chemistry and industry, 19 December p 1613)

The liquids for silicates and phosphates must not be used interchangeably, as each has been prepared to give the correct properties with its own powder.

18.1.3 Mixing

To obtain the optimum properties from a silicate restorative material, two things are important in the mixing procedure: the material should be mixed both quickly and as thickly as possible—the reasons for this are discussed in Section 18.1.7.

(a) Mixing by hand

(i) Use a thick glass slab; this should be cooled in order to allow more powder to be added to a given amount of liquid in the limited time available. The slab should not be cooled below the temperature at which the water vapour present in the air saturates the air and begins to condense (this is, the *dew point*), otherwise the condensed moisture will be incorporated in the material, and affect the setting time (Section 18.1.5), and possibly adversely affect the solubility and mechanical properties of the set cement.

(ii) Steel spatulas should not be used; they are liable to be abraded by silicate powder, leading to discoloration of the material. Agate or cobalt–chromium (stellite) spatulas are usually used, though plastic ones are also available.

(iii) The correct powder/liquid ratio is important. Too thick a mix will produce a crumbly mass, since all the powder particles will not be wetted by the liquid. A mix which has too much liquid will have a longer setting time and lower pH, and will produce a set material which is weaker, more soluble and more prone to staining. A typical powder/liquid ratio is 1.6 g/0.4 ml.

(iv) The powder should be incorporated into the liquid as quickly as possible, and mixing should be complete within one minute. It is usual to add half the total quantity of powder to the liquid initially, and smaller quantities as the mixing proceeds. The powder is folded into the liquid to ensure that all the particles are properly wetted. The mixed material should have a consistency like putty.

(b) Mechanical mixing

Measured quantities of powder and liquid can be mixed mechanically in a gelatin capsule. A number of materials are supplied in capsules which contain both the pre-proportioned powder and liquid; the latter is sealed in one section of the capsule. Prior to mixing the seal is broken by applying pressure to the capsule.

The advantages of such systems are:

(i) the material is not handled until after mixing, so there is less chance of contamination,
(ii) the correct powder/liquid ratio is obtained without guesswork or time-consuming weighing procedures, and
(iii) rapid mixing can be achieved, for example, in 10 to 15 seconds.

Evolution of heat occurs on mechanical mixing; this accelerates the setting, so may reduce the working time. This temperature rise is due:

(i) mainly to heat from the exothermic reaction between powder and liquid, and
(ii) also to heat from friction of the abrasive powder.

18.1.4 Setting reactions

The following processes are believed to occur during the setting reaction:

(a) The surface of the glass powder is decomposed by the liquid. Hydrated protons (H_3O^+) from the liquid disrupt the aluminosilicate network by attacking the aluminium sites which are negatively charged (Section 12.8). Other cations (Na^+, Ca^{2+}) are displaced by hydrated protons; as a result there is degradation of the glass network to form a hydrated siliceous gel.

(b) The powder is *amphoteric*, that is, it can react chemically as an acid in the presence of strong bases, and as a base towards strong acids. The reaction between the acid liquid and amphoteric powder is therefore an acid–base reaction, and as a consequence, the pH of the aqueous phase increases. The ions liberated from the surface of the glass particles migrate to the liquid phase (leaving a siliceous gel behind); they are subsequently precipitated as phosphates and fluorides as the pH rises. Hardening is complete within 24 hours when these precipitation processes have gone to completion. The principal binding agent is alumino–phosphate gel, which contains a little crystalline basic phosphate—$Al_2(OH)_3PO_4$.

(c) Only the surface of the powder particles is attacked by the phosphoric acid. In all, about 20% of the powder is consumed in the reaction. The set material has a cored structure consisting of:

(i) unreacted glass particles,
(ii) these are sheathed by a surface layer of siliceous gel, and
(iii) they are embedded in a largely amorphous gel, where aluminium phosphate is the essential binding agent.

18.1.5 Setting time

(a) This depends on the composition of the material, as supplied by the manufacturer. It is also influenced by the particle size of the powder—the finer the particles, the more rapid is the setting.

(b) In addition, the following factors give slower setting:

(i) longer mixing time,
(ii) lower temperature,
(iii) loss of water from the liquid, and
(iv) lower powder/liquid ratio.

18.1.6 Important practical points

(a) Care of the liquid—this can readily lose water in a warm atmosphere. The manufacturer usually supplies excess liquid in a bottle, so that the last portion can be discarded when the powder is finished. A liquid in which crystals have formed should also be discarded.

(b) The mixed material should be inserted into the cavity in one portion. If small increments are used complete bonding between the portions will not occur and the set material will be weaker.

(c) Immediately after filling the cavity the surface is covered with a strip of cellulose acetate or celluloid. Care should be taken to avoid movement of this strip until the material has set, otherwise the

forming gel structure will be broken and the restoration weakened.
(d) A lining is usually required. In shallower cavities a phosphate cement may be used. In very deep cavities, a liner is required to protect the pulp from the effects of phosphoric acid—for example, zinc oxide–eugenol, calcium hydroxide or a varnish. However a silicate material should not be placed directly on a slow-setting zinc oxide–eugenol base, as this leads to eventual discoloration of the restoration by unreacted eugenol. For this reason several linings may be used in deep cavities—for example, zinc oxide–eugenol followed by zinc phosphate.
(e) Protection from moisture contamination is most important:
- (i) The material should be inserted into a dry cavity; the use of a rubber dam can ensure that a dry field of operation is maintained.
- (ii) On removal of the cellulose acetate or celluloid strip, the surface of the restoration should be painted with a varnish to protect it from saliva for a few hours.
- (iii) Failure to observe these precautions will permit the gel that forms to absorb moisture and swell; also dissolution of some of the cement constituents may occur.

(f) The cellulose acetate or celluloid leaves a smooth surface on the restoration. Ideally, this should not be disturbed as subsequent polishing will not produce as good a surface.
(g) Crazing, or surface cracking, can occur if premature drying out of the silicate is allowed to occur.

18.1.7 Properties of the set material

(a) Effects on dental tissues:
- (i) As already mentioned, pulpal reactions can occur due to the chemical constituents of this material.
- (ii) Silicate restorative materials have anticariogenic properties. It is believed that this is related to their fluoride content. In other words, fluoride uptake by the enamel adjacent to the restoration can occur. This reduces the enamel solubility, similar to the effect of topically applied fluoride solutions.

(b) One of the chief criticisms of silicate cement restorations is that they erode in oral fluids. It is believed that two things can occur in this process:
- (i) Some of the constituents of the gel matrix dissolve.
- (ii) Particles of unreacted silicate powder are then washed away.

In the laboratory, the 'solubility' of a silicate is measured by exposing discs of the material in distilled water at 37°C for 24 hours. In such experiments it has been found that:

(i) the solubility of a silicate is greater for a lower powder/liquid ratio.
(ii) the solubility decreases after two or three days, and
(iii) the solubility is also greater at lower pH values, and even in neutral citrate solutions.

This last finding can be explained in terms of the structure of the set material (Section 18.1.4), since citrates can attack the precipitated phosphates.

(c) Mechanical properties
From Appendix II it can be seen that these materials are stronger in compression than other cements, though not as strong as dental amalgam. Their hardness is about the same as dentine (Appendix II).

(d) Thermal properties

(i) Coefficient of thermal expansion—this is lower than that of any other restorative material, and is close to that of enamel and dentine (Appendix II).
(ii) Thermal conductivity—this is also low (Appendix II).

(e) Aesthetics—Initially silicate restorations have excellent aesthetic properties, and can match tooth colour well if the correct shade of material is chosen. The index of refraction of a silicate is not dissimilar from that of enamel and dentine. The materials are translucent, due to the gel-like nature of the matrix and the fact that the core is a glass.

Over a period of time, silicates can become stained, particularly if the surface has been roughened by abrasion or erosion.

If a silicate restoration is allowed to dry out, the surface may become powdery and more opaque. This is particularly likely to happen in patients who are mouth-breathers.

A gap may form between the restoration and cavity margin, due to dissolution. This crevice may stain and appear as a black line.

(f) Adhesion—no adhesive bond is formed between a silicate cement and enamel and dentine.

(g) Dimensional changes on setting—a slight contraction occurs.

(h) The surface of a silicate restoration is difficult to polish satisfactorily.

(i) Comparative properties—in Chapter 19 a comparison of the available types of anterior restorative materials is given (Section 19.9).

18.2 SILICOPHOSPHATES

(a) The liquid of these cements is similar to that supplied for zinc phosphate and silicates.

(b) The powder is a mixture of:

(i) silicate powder and

(ii) zinc oxide, as for the zinc phosphate cement powder.

Some materials are simple mixtures of the two powders; in others the two types of powder are partially fused together.

(c) The object of combining these two types of cement is:

(i) to obtain the good aesthetics of the silicate materials, and

(ii) to obtain the somewhat lower initial solubility of the phosphate cements.

(d) The properties of silicophosphates are intermediate between those of silicates of phosphates; the properties of an individual material will depend on whether it more closely resembles a silicate or a phosphate.

(e) The manipulation and factors influencing setting time are similar to those of silicate cements.

(f) The setting reaction is the same as for silicate cements, except that the formation of zinc phosphate must also be taken into account. The set material is again a cored structure.

(g) These materials are or have been used:

(i) for fillings in deciduous teeth, and temporary restorations,

(ii) as semi-translucent cements for porcelain jacket crowns, and

(iii) as die materials (Section 40.3.1).

18.3 GLASS-IONOMER CEMENTS

18.3.1 Introduction

These experimental cements are related both to dental silicate cements (Section 18.1) and polycarboxylate (or polyacrylate) cements (Section 17.3), combining certain properties of both. The name 'ASPA' by which they are sometimes known is derived from Alumino Silicate PolyAcrylic acid.

18.3.2 Composition

(a) Polymer: As originally formulated, a 45–50% aqueous solution

of acrylic acid/itaconic acid co-polymer (Appendix III, no. 21) stabilised with 5% tartaric acid to prevent thickening and gelling on storage (see Fig. 18.1). As with polycarboxylates, many products now contain the polymer in solid form. The supplied material is a mixture of ceramic (see below) and polymer particles. Some products contain poly (maleic acid) instead of acrylic acid co-polymers.
(b) Ceramic powder: this is related to that of dental silicate cements. It is prepared by fusing a mixture of quartz and alumina in a fluorite/cryolite/aluminium phosphate flux at 1000–1300°C, and quenching the melt to form an opal glass. However, dental silicate glasses are only suitable for reaction with strong acids such as phosphoric acid.

To obtain a suitable rate of reaction with weaker acids such as polyacrylic acid, the glass is made more basic by increasing the ratio of Al_2O_3/SiO_2 in the fusion mixture.

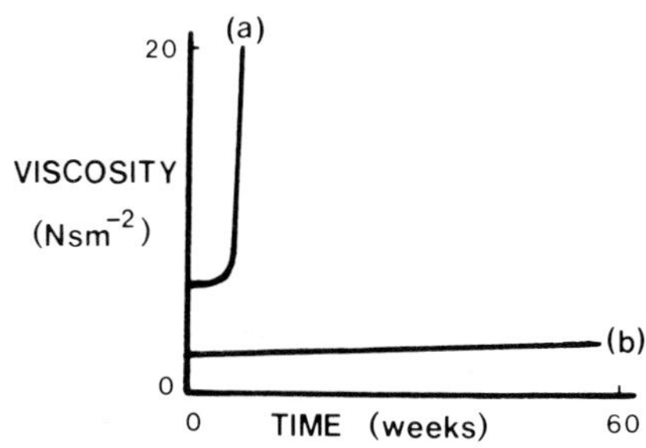

Fig. 18.1 Viscosity of cement liquids, as determined by a falling sphere viscometer. (a) 50% poly (acrylic acid) solution shows gelling after about 4 weeks (b) acrylic acid/itaconic acid co-polymer, stabilised with tartaric acid. (after Crisp et al., J. Dent. Res., 54, 1173, 1975.)

18.3.3 Setting

(a) On mixing powder and liquid, calcium and aluminium ions are extracted from the surface of the powder particles.
(b) Ca^{2+} and Al^{3+} ionically cross-link the polyacrylate chains, causing the cement to gel, set and harden. (see Fig. 18.2)

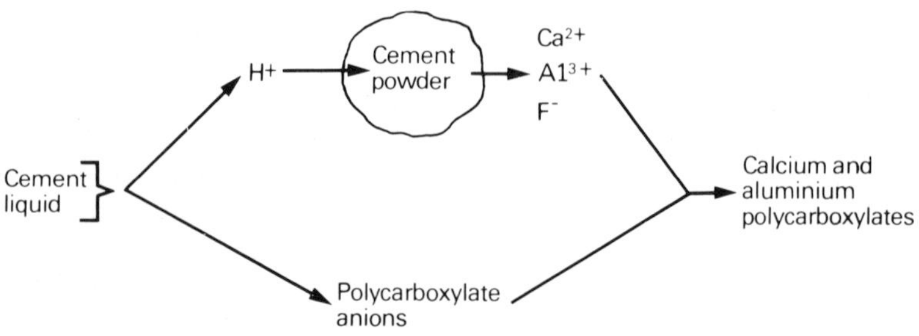

Fig. 18.2 Reactions in glass–ionomer cements

18.3.4 Structure of set material

The set material contains opal glass particles, sheathed in a siliceous gel, embedded in a metal polyacrylate matrix.

18.3.5 Properties

(a) These cements have some of the merits of silicate, particularly in terms of strength, translucency and fluoride content; in these respects they are superior to the zinc oxide-based materials.
(b) Glass-ionomer cements also have the adhesive properties of zinc polycarboxylate cements.

18.3.6 Applications

These cements are used for (i) erosion and abrasion cavities (without cavity preparation), (ii) as fissure fillings, (iii) as lining cements—e.g. glass-ionomer cement can be etched by phosphoric acid (Fig. 18.3). This etched cement can bond composite resins to dentine, since micromechanical attachment between composite and cement is achieved, (iv) for the restoration of deciduous teeth, (v) as repair materials around the margins of old restorations and (vi) as luting cements, particularly for use with tin-plated restorations (Section 30.6).

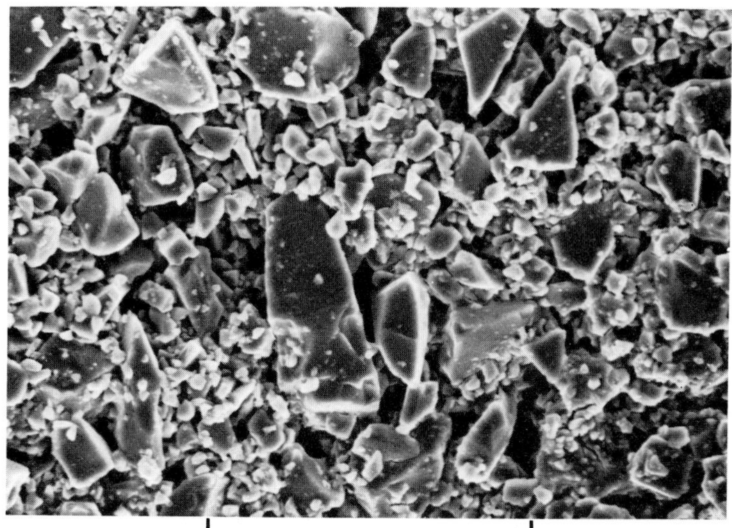

Fig. 18.3 SEM photograph of etched glass–ionomer cement. The distance between the marks represents 100 μm

18.4 CERMETS

(a) Composition

Cermet cements contain an ion–leachable glass fused with a fine silver powder, which can react with a polymeric acid to form a set cement.

(b) Properties

(i) Good biocompatibility
(ii) Cariostatic
(iii) Tougher and better wear resistance than glass ionomers
(iv) Adhesive

(c) Applications

(i) Core build-up materials
(ii) They are being used experimentally as posterior filling materials.

READING REFERENCE

Wilson A D Kent B E Clinton D Miller R P 1972 The formation and micro-structure of dental silicate cements Journal of Materials Science 7: 220

This is an extensive review of recent research on silicates

Dubert L W Jenkins C B G 1972 Tooth coloured filling materials in clinical practice. Wright, Bristol

Included in this book are details of the manipulation of silicates (and other restorative materials).

Wilson A D Kent B E 1972 A new translucent cement for dentistry. Bristish Dental Journal 132: 133

Kent B E Lewis B G Wilson A D 1973 The properties of a glass-ionomer cement. British Dental Journal 135: 322

Crisp S Ferner A J Lewis B G Wilson A D 1975 Properties of improved glass-ionomer cement formulations. Journal of Dentistry 3: 125

These three papers describe the development, properties and composition of glass-ionomer cements.

Wilson A D 1975 Dental cements based on ion-leachable glasses. In: von Fraunhofer J A (ed) Scientific aspects of dental materials Butterworth, London, Ch 6

Contains detailed information about the chemistry and structure of silicate, silico–phosphate and glass–ionomer cements.

McLean J W 1984 Alternatives to amalgam alloys. British Dental Journal 157: 432

This paper includes brief information on cermets, which have just recently become commercially available.

McLean J W Powis D R Prosser H J Wilson A D 1985 The use of glass–ionomer cement in bonding composite resin to dentine. British Dental Journal 158: 410

The technique of using acid etched glass–ionomer cement to bond composite resin to dentine. This paper gives research data and clinical technique.

19. Polymer-ceramic composite filling materials

19.1 HISTORICAL PERSPECTIVE

In the previous chapter, the limitations of silicate filling materials have been noted. To avoid the problems associated with silicates, polymeric filling materials were developed. These are essentially autopolymerising acrylics, the chemistry of which is discussed in Section 8.3. Acrylic filling materials fall far short of the ideal requirements (as detailed below), and are not considered in detail. Particular problems that arise with these materials include high water absorption, high coefficient of thermal expansion, large shrinkage on polymerisation and low strength. Comparative properties are given in Table 19.3.

To overcome some of the above problems, ceramic-filled polymers were developed. Some early materials were based on acrylic resin, but subsequently, dimethacrylate polymers were proposed. Modern composite materials are ceramic filled dimethacrylates. Considerable development has taken place over the last 20 years. Such materials are very widely used and are beginning to find application for posterior restorations.

19.2 REQUIREMENTS FOR TOOTH FILLING MATERIALS

(a) Biological considerations:

(i) Not irritant to the pulp or to the gingiva.
(ii) Low systemic toxicity.
(iii) Cariostatic.

(b) They should not dissolve or erode in saliva or in fluids taken into the mouth. Low water absorption is also important.

(c) Mechanical properties should be adequate to withstand the forces of mastication, and should be similar to those of enamel and dentine in respect of modulus of elasticity and strength. Good abrasion resistance to dentifrices and constituents of food is also important. Posterior restorations are particularly subjected to conditions of abrasive wear.

(d) Thermal properties:
(i) The coefficient of thermal expansion should be similar to that of enamel and dentine.
(ii) They should have a low thermal diffusivity.

(e) Good aesthetic properties are required, particularly for fillings in anterior teeth. Thus the restoration should initially match the tooth in colour, translucency and refractive index. Over a period of time there should be no staining or discolouration.

(f) Ideally, adhesion between the filling and enamel and dentine should occur.

(g) There should be minimal dimensional changes on setting of these materials.

(h) The material should readily take and retain a smooth surface finish.

(i) Radio-opacity of the material would enable:
(i) detection of secondary caries.
(ii) indentification of overhanging ledges, and
(iii) detection of incompletely filled cavities due to trapped air.

(j) Rheological considerations: the material should have an adequate working time during which there is little or no viscosity change, followed by rapid hardening.

19.3 CONSTITUENTS OF COMPOSITES

The components of modern composites may be listed as (i) principal (higher molecular weight) monomers, (ii) diluent (lower molecular weight) monomers, (iii) inorganic fillers, (iv) silane coupling agents, (v) polymerisation inhibitors, (vi) initiator/activator components and (vii) u.v. stabilisers.

19.3.1 Principal (higher molecular weight) monomers

Many composites are based on an aromatic dimethacrylate system, the monomer being the reaction product of bisphenol-A and glycidyl methacrylate, often called BIS-GMA or Bowen's resin (formula in Appendix III no. 7). This highly viscous monomer can undergo free radical addition polymerisation to give a rigid cross-linked polymer (Section 8.6). A monomer similar to BIS-GMA, but without hydroxy groups, has also been used (Appendix III, no. 7).

Some products use alternative monomers which are described as urethane dimethacrylates (Appendix III, no. 49). The properties of composites based on these latter monomers are in general similar to those of materials containing Bowen's resin.

19.3.2 Diluent (lower molecular weight) monomers

Other monomers are included in composite formulations to reduce the viscosity of the material to enable proper blending with the inorganic constituents, and to facilitate clinical manipulation. The monomer of choice may be:

(i) monofunctional, such as methyl methacrylate.
(ii) difunctional monomers are usually preferred (see below). e.g. ethylene glycol dimethacrylate (Section 8.5) or triethylene glycol dimethacrylate (Appendix III, no. 48).

Greater quantities of diluent monomer give composite materials of lower viscosity, but also with greater shrinkage on polymerisation.

Note: Difunctional monomers are usually preferred to monofunctional ones because:

(i) they have less shrinkage on polymerisation
(ii) they give a more cross-linked structure, which is harder and stronger, and has a lower coefficient of thermal expansion
(iii) they are less volatile
(iv) they give polymers with lower water absorption.

19.3.3 Inorganic fillers

(a) Types of fillers

A wide variety of fillers has been used:

(i) Early composites contained glass fibres and beads, synthetic calcium phosphates and fused silica.
(ii) Current materials may contain lithium aluminosilicates, crys-

talline quartz, or barium aluminoborate silica glasses (see Fig. 19.1). This latter material has the following formulation (wt.%): SiO_2, 50; BaO, 33; B_2O_3, 9 and Al_2O_3, 8. Many composites contain a combination of a barium glass and another filler.

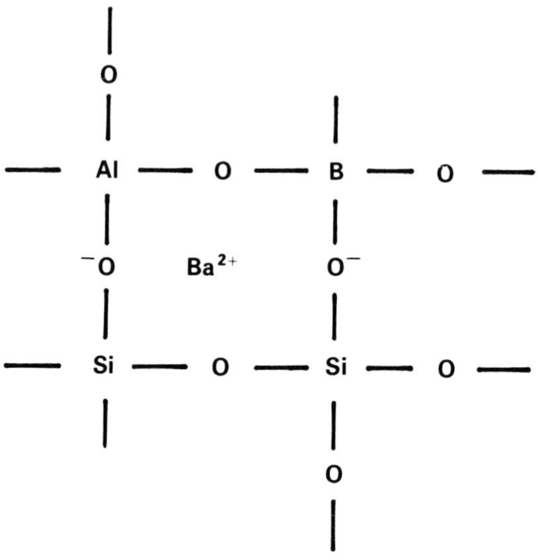

Fig. 19.1 Possible structure of barium aluminoborate silicate glass (after Bowen R L 1979 J. Dent. Res. 58: 1492)

(iii) A strontium glass is incorporated in one product; it is claimed that this softer material renders the composite easier to polish.

(iv) Recently a number of products have been developed which contain a filler of particle size about 0.05 μm, in contrast to the above fillers, which are typically 10–40 μm. This microfine filler consists of silica.

The quantity of filler is important. Composites with the larger size particles contain typically 78% (by weight) of filler. Some recent products for posterior restorations contain up to 87% filler. However, products with microfine silica contain less inorganic fillers. It is technically difficult to add large quantities of microfine silica to a fluid monomer, since it acts as a thickening agent and confers thixotropy. It is usual for the filler to be prepared in a matrix of cured resin, which is then ground, and incorporated in a difunctional monomer. Present day microfine composites contain from 25 to 63% SiO_2 (by weight). A British standard specification defines composites as containing 50% or more by weight of inorganic filler.

(b) Effects of fillers on properties

The incorporation of inorganic fillers has the following effects on a polymer:

(i) Improvement in mechanical properties such as compressive strength, modulus of elasticity and hardness.
(ii) Reduction in coefficient of thermal expansion.
(iii) Contribution to the aesthetics; glass is able to refect the colour of the surrounding tooth material.
(iv) Reduction in the contraction on setting.
(v) Less heat evolved in polymerisation.
(vi) The composite is radio-opaque if barium or strontium glasses are used.

(c) Classification of materials

Available products can be broadly classified into four groups, based on type and quantity of filler content; as in Table 19.1, which also gives some general comments on comparisons between the various materials.

19.3.4 Silane coupling agents

It is important, for reinforcement of the polymer by the filler to occur, that the two constituents should be bonded together. To achieve this, the filler is usually treated with a vinyl silane compound (Appendix III, no. 50).

19.3.5 Polymerisation inhibitors

Since dimethacrylate monomers will polymerise on storage, an inhibitor is necessary. Hydroquinone has been widely used, but was responsible for causing discolouration of the material. The monomethyl ether of hydroquinone is now used (Appendix III, no. 18). Only a few parts per million of this compound are required.

Table 19.1 Classification of composites according to filler type

Type	Typical Particle size (μm)	% (by weight) of filler	General comments
Large particle	15–35	78	Difficult to polish; surface roughens on abrasion of resin matrix; surface may attract plaque. Good mechanical properties.
Fine particle	1–8	70–86	Good mechanical properties with superior finishing and polishing characteristics than the above.
Microfine filled	0.04	25–63	Easy to obtain and maintain smooth surface which does not attract plaque. However, mechanical properties are poorer; wear resistance may be poor; also greater shrinkage on setting and more absorption of water owing to lower filler content.
Blended filler	0.04 and 1–5	77–80	Developed in attempts to obtain the benefits of both types of filler.

19.3.6 Initiator/activator systems

(a) Chemical activation

Benzoyl peroxide initiator and tertiary amine activators, or sulphinic acid type initiators may be employed. Of the tertiary amines, N, N-dimentyl-*p*-toluidine was used as activator, but now N, N-dihydroxyethyl-*p*-toluidine is widely used (Appendix III, no. 12).

(b) u.v. Activation

Composites containing benzoin methyl ether (Appendix III, no. 5) have been developed. On application of u.v. light of appropriate wavelength, energy is absorbed and free radicals are generated to initiate polymerisation. This system has now been susperceded by visible light curing (see below) because of:

(i) limited depth of polymerisation,
(ii) layering techniques attempting to overcome this problem may cause faults within the material,
(iii) potential harmful effects such as skin cancer and eye damage.

(c) Visible light activation

Composites have been developed which contain an α-diketone and an amine. On application of visible light of wavelength 460–485 nm free radicals are generated (Appendix III, no. 51). Visible light cured materials are now very widely used (see Sections 19.4, 19.5(a) and 19.6.3).

19.3.7 u.v. stabilisers

To prevent discolouration with age of composites, compounds are incorporated which absorb electromagnetic radiation. Clinical evidence suggests that this improves colour stability. (Example: 2-hydroxy-4-methoxybenzophenone, Appendix III, no. 20).

19.4 LIGHT SOURCES

The available lights for curing composites may be classified as in Table 19.2. The light output will have a spectral distribution similar to that in Figure 7.3.

Table 19.2 Classification of light sources

Mode of transmission of light	General comments
Fibre optic system	Fibre optic system needs to be handled with care to avoid fracture of some of the glass rods
Fluid-filled hose	Avoids above problem but fluid may deteriorate over a period of time
Pistol grip	These lights are generally more compact and lightweight than the above.

The following components will be included in most systems:

(i) a quartz-halogen bulb;
(ii) appropriate light filters;
(iii) a switch;
(iv) a timing device;
(v) a curing tip; this may vary from around 5 mm in diameter up to 7 mm or more for curing larger surfaces as in posterior composites.

19.5 SELECTION OF MATERIALS

(a) Chemical *versus* visible light-curing.

Advantage of chemical activation: no elaborate equipment needed.

Advantages of visible light activation: command setting—no increase in viscosity until application of light; also they require no mixing, so problems of air incorporation are avoided (see Figs. 19.2 and 19.3).

(b) Microfine *versus* conventional fillers.

Advantage of microfine filled material: can take and retain good surface finish.

Advantages of conventional materials: better mechanical properties, lower coefficient of thermal expansion.

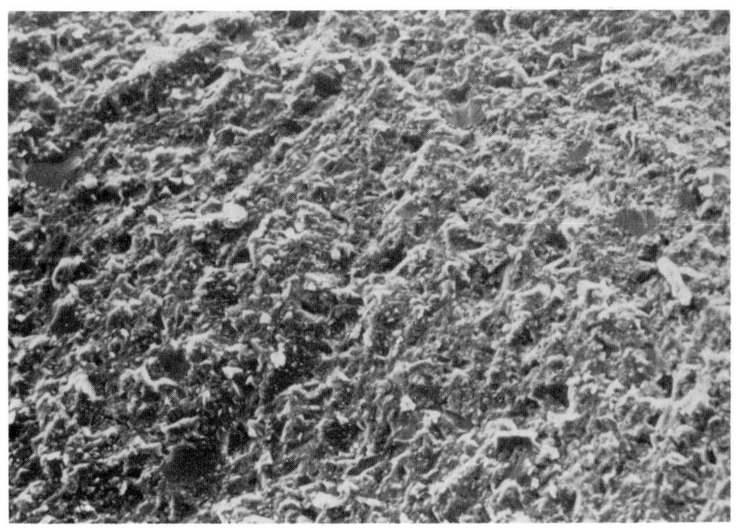

Fig. 19.2 SEM photograph of a light cured microfine composite.

(c) Difference between microfine materials: at least three different formulation types are available:

(i) A two paste system: the base paste contains monomer and filler prepared in a matrix of cured resin; the 'catalyst' paste contains benzoyl peroxide dispersed in a phthalate ester. The total inorganic filler content may be well below 50%.

(ii) Some products are based on Bowen's resin with difunctional diluent (Section 19.3.2) and contain 50 to 60% inorganic filler and 16 to 20% organic filler.
(iii) A light activated microfine composite is available, with around 63% silica.

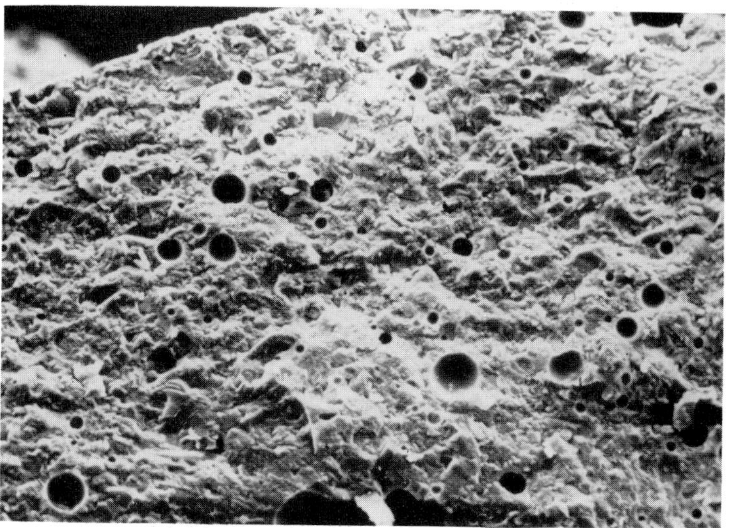

Fig. 19.3 SEM photograph of a chemically activated microfine composite (same magnification as Fig. 19.2). Note the presence of porosity.

19.6 MANIPULATION

19.6.1 General factors

(a) It has often been recommended that enamel margins should be bevelled. However, some aspects of this are controversial, particularly in relation to bevelling in stress-bearing locations.
(b) A base is required to protect exposed dentine, to avoid the possibility of irritation from organic constituents of the restorative material. Calcium hydroxide cements are usually used (Section 21.1). Alternatively etched glass-ionomer cements have been recommended (Section 18.3.6). Eugenol-containing materials should be avoided, since eugenol can act as a plasticiser for the polymer.
(c) Bonding to enamel—all enamel surfaces contacted by resin should be etched (Section 20.4). It is wise to check that the calcium hydroxide base has not been disturbed by the etchant.

(d) Intermediate resins or bonding agents, if applied to the etched enamel, can improve retention and reduce marginal leakage of the restoration.
(e) Cellulose acetate matrix bonds should be used to give optimum surface finish.
(f) Contamination by blood or saliva should be avoided.
(g) Pressure should be applied during setting for better marginal adaptation.

19.6.2 Chemically activated materials

(a) The two pastes should be mixed thoroughly in the correct proportions (usually equal volumes).
(b) Stainless steel spatulas should not be used for mixing, as they are not sufficiently abrasion resistant.
(c) Avoid contamination of one paste by the other.
(d) As far as possible, avoid the incorporation of air during mixing.
(e) During mixing of some products, tints can be added to permit colour matching between composite and tooth.
(f) The mixed materials should be placed in the cavity without delay.

19.6.3 Light-cured materials

(a) In general, most commercially available light sources will polymerise most light-cured materials, though some systems are more efficient than others.
(b) Under-curing must be avoided at all costs. This gives a material with a hard outer 'skin' and soft material at the base of the cavity.
(c) Under-curing may result if the light source is not sufficiently close to the surface of the material being polymerised.
(d) Over-curing is not harmful. This may be a wise precaution if using a light with a material from a different manufacturer.
(e) Darker shades of material absorb more light, so require longer curing times.
(f) In some instances, material may begin to polymerise if exposed to strong ambient light.

19.6.4 Finishing procedures

(a) If surface finishing is required, this is probably best achieved by:

(i) abrading the material with a diamond stone or tungsten carbide bur.
(ii) polishing with a white stone.

(b) Surface glazes are supplied with some materials; these are essentially unfilled polymers. Though a glaze can give a smooth surface initially, it is unlikely that its benefit will last long.

19.7 APPLICATIONS

(a) Anterior restorations. Composites are now the most widely used materials for this application. Microfine filled materials may not be sufficiently durable for larger restorations.
(b) Posterior restorations (Fig. 19.4). There is great current interest in the application of composites as substitutes for dental amalgam. Long term clinical data are not yet available to assess the performance of the materials. They can be recommended for use where aesthetic considerations are of paramount importance. This type of material is much more sensitive to technique variations than amalgam.
(c) Laminate veneer systems are available to improve the aesthetics of stained and discoloured teeth. A thin polymeric or ceramic veneer

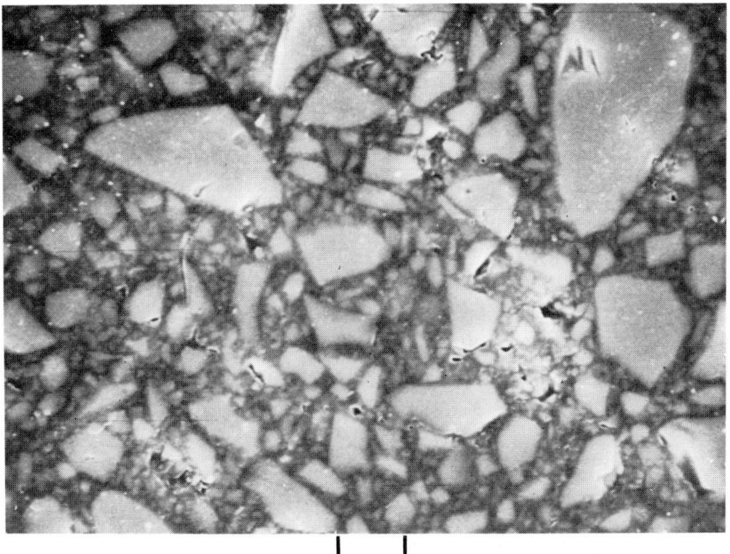

Fig. 19.4 SEM photograph of a posterior composite filling material, showing filler particle size distribution. The distance between the marks represents 10 μm.

is cemented to acid etched enamel by a resin.
(d) Composites have been recommended as core build up material, on to which a crown can be cemented.
(e) Composites are used for resin-bonded bridge systems (Ch. 31).

19.8 CRITIQUE OF COMPOSITES

(a) Biological considerations. In terms of pulpal irritation, composites appear to be superior to silicate cements and unfilled acrylics. However, plaque can accumulate on a rough composite surface.
(b) Composites have a very low solubility. The polymer component absorbs some water which may make the material swell to partially counteract polymerisation shrinkage.
(c) Mechanical properties are generally good (Table 19.3), though microfine materials are not usually as strong and rigid as the conventional composites.
(d) Thermal properties
 (i) Conventional composites have less thermal expansion than unfilled resins. Microfine filled materials with higher inorganic filler content have lower coefficients of thermal expansion (Table 19.3).
 (ii) Composites are good thermal insulators.
(e) Aesthetics. Though initial aesthetics of composites can be good, the resin may discolour over a period of time. Also, accumulation of plaque (see (a) above) can cause discolouration.
(f) Bonding. Composites are not adhesive to enamel and dentine, though bonding to enamel using acid etch techniques can be achieved. Coupling agents to secure adhesion to dentine are being developed and have recently become available (Ch. 20).
(g) Dimension change on setting—this is comparatively small for polymers prepared from difunctional monomers, and which are heavily filled.
(h) With many composites it is difficult to obtain a smooth surface finish by abrading and polishing techniques. Also, abrasive wear in service roughens the material, because the polymer phase wears more rapidly than the harder ceramic material. However, materials with microfine fillers can take and retain a smooth surface finish.
(i) Many composites are radio-opaque.
(j) Rheological properties. Unmixed composite pastes are usually Bingham bodies (Fig. 19.5). Chemically activated composites show a continued increase in viscosity from the conclusion of mixing (Fig. 19.6).

Table 19.3 Comparative properties of anterior restorative materials

	Silicate	Acrylic	Conventional composites	Microfine filled composites
Pulpal irritation	Yes	Yes	Yes	Yes
Anticariogenic properties	Yes	No	No	No
Resistance to oral fluids	Poor	Good	Good	—
Compressive strength (MN/m^2)	200	70	170–260	250
Tensile strength (MN/m^2)	15	30	35–55	30
Thermal properties				
expansion ($\times 10^{-6}$/°C)	8	81	20–35	50–77
diffusivity (10^{-3} cm^{-2} sec^{-1})	2.29–2.51	low 1.25	low 6.75	low
Aesthetics				
initially	Excellent	Excellent	Excellent	Excellent
long term	Staining	Discoloration at margins	Possible staining and rough surface	No surface roughening
Adhesion to enamel and dentine	Poor	Poor	Poor	Poor
Dimensional changes on setting	Slight contraction	Contraction considerable	Contraction (½–1% after 24h) less than acrylics	Contraction
Surface finish	Difficult to polish	Can be trimmed and polished easily	More difficult to finish than acrylics	Easy to trim and polish

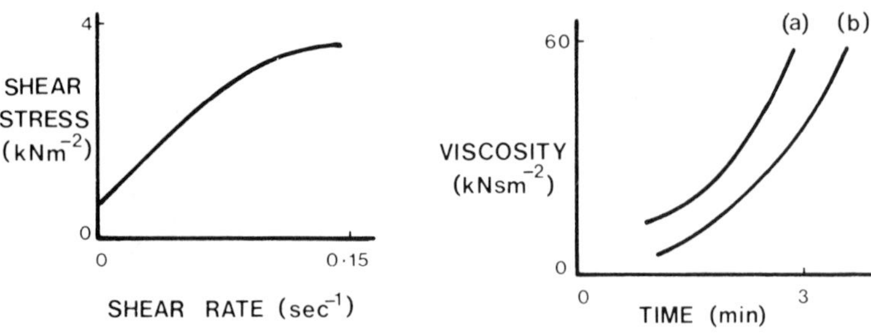

Fig. 19.5 Rheological characteristics of a composite paste (Compare with Fig. 5.3) (After Braden 1977 J. Dent. Res. 56: 627).

Fig. 19.6 Apparent viscosity at shear rate of 13 s^{-1} *versus* time, for setting composites. (After Watts D C et al 1980 J. Oral Rehab. 7: 478).

19.9 COMPARATIVE PROPERTIES OF ANTERIOR RESTORATIVE MATERIALS

These are listed in Table 19.3.

READING REFERENCES

Bowen R L 1979 The components in composite restorations. Journal of dental research 58: 1493

This article lists the basic components of composite restorative materials and is a useful source for further references.

Lutz F, Setcos J C, Phillips R W, Roulet J F 1983 Dental restorative resins. Dental clinics of North America 27: 697

This paper gives a classification of, and the clinical characteristics of, composites.

Combe E C 1985 Creating successful composite restorations. In: Derrick D D (ed) The dental annual Wright, Bristol, p 34–42

Factors influencing the choice and manipulation of contemporary materials.

Watts D C, Amer O, Combe E C 1984 Characteristics of visible-light-activated composite resins. British dental journal 156: 209

A comparative study of light curing systems.

20. Techniques and applications of bonding to enamel and dentine

20.1 INTRODUCTION

For a proper understanding of this chapter, the theory of adhesion and attachment (Ch. 15) should be understood. Also, the nature and properties of the various materials should be known; this includes adhesive cements (zinc polycarboxylate, Section 17.3; glass-ionomer cement, Section 18.3) and materials based on aromatic dimethacrylates (Ch. 19).

20.2 ADHESIVE SYSTEMS

(a) Bonding to enamel can be obtained by:
- (i) adhesion of a cement containing poly(acrylic acid) or related material,
- (ii) the attachment of a polymer to acid-etched enamel.

The two systems are compared and contrasted in Table 20.1.

(b) Bonding to dentine can be obtained by:
- (i) the adhesion of certain cements, as above; experimental mineralising solution, containing calcium and phosphate ions, have been developed in attempts to improve the bond,
- (ii) the bonding of a polymer-containing composite restorative material to dentine, by the use of a coupling agent, as detailed below.

20.3 PRACTICAL APPLICATIONS OF 'ADHESIVE DENTISTRY'

20.3.1 Fissure sealants

(a) Most current sealants are based on difunctional monomers, with diluent monomers to reduce the viscosity. In composition they are essentially similar to composites, but without added filler (Section 19.3). Similar to composites, some of these materials are chemically activated, while others require the application of ultraviolet or visible light (Section 19.3.6). Bonding to enamel is achieved by the acid etch technique (Section 20.4).

(b) Two sealants have been supplied, which gave disappointing results, are perhaps best considered as means of topical fluoride application. These are:

(i) a material described as an acrylic polymer containing an amine-fluoride, and

(ii) a polyurethane with sodium monofluorophosphate.

(c) Glass-ionomer cements are under investigation as fissure sealants and fillings.

(d) A sealant based on methyl-2-cyanoacrylate with silicate fillers gave disappointing results in clinical trials.

Table 20.1 Comparison of systems for bonding to enamel

	Acid etch systems	Direct adhesion systems
Materials	(i) Aromatic dimethacrylate polymers (ii) Other polymer-based materials	Cements containing polyacrylic acid or similar materials: (i) Zinc polycarboxylate (ii) Glass-ionomer cement
Composition, as supplied	(i) Contains monomers (ii) No aqueous phase	(i) No monomers present (ii) Water present
Setting reaction	Polymerisation Fillers, where present, do not take part	Salt formation involving fillers
Preparation of tooth surface	Enamel is etched (Sections 15.4.1 and 20.4)	Enamel is cleaned, not etched
Bonding mechanism	Attachment	Adhesion

20.3.2 Orthodontic attachments

As outlined in Section 38.6, the acid-etch technique is now being widely used for direct bonding of orthodontic appliances.

20.3.3 'Adhesive' restorations

(a) Dimethacrylate-based restorative materials are being used for

incisal edge restorations, and for aesthetic coatings for teeth, where the enamel is mottled or stained. Acid etch techniques are used to achieve bonding to enamel.
(b) Resin-dentine coupling or bonding agents are now being marketed. These usually contain phosphorus or halophosphorus esters of Bis-GMA resin. There is as yet no clinical evidence on the long-term efficacy of these products.
(c) In the case of abrasion cavities, acid etching is not very suitable because dentine is exposed. Glass-ionomer cements have become available for this type of restoration.
(d) The direct bonding of bridges to etched enamel can be achieved. (See Ch. 31).

20.4 PRACTICAL CONSIDERATIONS OF THE ACID ETCH TECHNIQUE

The following points should be noted for successful etching of enamel:
(a) The tooth surface should first be cleaned with a pumice slurry using a bristle brush, followed by washing with water. Prophylaxis pastes containing constituents which are immiscible with water should be avoided.
(b) The acid etchant (either liquid or gel) is placed on to the dry enamel surface with a cotton wool pledget held in tweezers, usually for 60 seconds.
(c) The etched surface must be copiously washed with water, for at least 15 seconds.
(d) The surface must be dried. Check that the drying air jet is not contaminated with oil or water.
(e) The etching procedure will have raised the free surface energy of the enamel, and so increased its wettability. Contamination with ionic material (e.g. saliva, blood, tissue exudate) will lower the free surface energy. Thus, between etching and application of the resin, the patient must not be permitted to rinse or otherwise contaminate the surface.
(f) Etched enamel has a characteristic white frosted appearance. The teeth of patients living in areas with fluoridated water supplies are more resistant to acid attack, and may need further acid etching.
(g) The rules can be summarised as follows: CLEAN, ETCH, WASH, DRY, APPLY.

20.5 SUMMARY OF CURRENT STATUS

(a) Acid etch techniques in conjunction with dimethacrylate resin can be very successful.
(b) The problem of bonding to enamel appears to have been largely solved; bonding to dentine is much more difficult.
(c) Cements containing polyacrylic acid, and similar polymers, are capable of considerable chemical development.
(d) For success, any bonding technique requires meticulous attention to manipulative detail.

READING REFERENCES

Ibsen R L, Neville K 1974 Adhesive restorative dentistry, Saunders, Philadelphia

This book gives information on many techniques of bonding to tooth substance. There is a discussion of some common causes of failure in adhesive procedures.

Silverstone L M 1976 Should I be using pit and fissure sealants or amalgam? International Dental Journal 26: 29

The author shows that fissure sealants can have a highly significant effect in the prevention of occlusal caries.

Council on Dental Materials, Instruments and Equipment 1984. Resin detine bonding systems. Journal of the American Dental Association 108: 240

This gives a brief review and status report on coupling agents for bonding resins to dentine.

21. Miscellaneous materials

21.1 CALCIUM HYDROXIDE

21.1.1 Composition

(a) The simplest products of this type contain only an aqueous suspension of calcium hydroxide. However, such materials are not sufficiently strong to withstand the forces of packing a filling material such as amalgam.
(b) Other products contain, in addition either aqueous methyl cellulose or a resin dissolved in a volatile solvent such as chloroform; these materials are more cohesive and stronger than the above.
(c) One product contains a phenolic compound, which reacts with calcium hydroxide to form a mass consisting of calcium phenolate in which there is an excess of unreacted calcium hydroxide.

21.1.2 Properties

(a) Calcium hydroxide can neutralise the free phosphoric acid of a phosphate cement; a thickness of about 0.25 mm is sufficient to serve as an effective barrier against the passage of acids.
(b) The pH of these materials is around 11 to 12; this degree of alkalinity is inimical to the survival of micro-organisms found in carious dentine.
(c) Mechanical properties: compressive strength after 24 hours is 6–10 MN/m^2; tensile strength 1–2 MN/m^2.
(d) Solubility is high—a value of 25–30% in water after 1 week has been quoted.

21.1.3 Uses

(a) Used under cements containing phosphoric acid, to protect the pulp from chemical damage.
(b) Often used as a lining material under polymer-ceramic restorations.
(c) Used for pulp capping.

21.2 VARNISHES

These consist of a resin such as copal or rosin, in a volatile organic solvent, e.g. acetone, ether or chloroform. When used under an amalgam restoration, these varnishes do not give a thick enough film to provide thermal insulation, even if several layers are applied.

A cavity varnish will reduce the penetration of fluids round the amalgam and into the dentinal tubules. Such varnishes can also reduce the diffusion of phosphoric acid from phosphate cements and silicate restorative materials.

Not all varnishes are suitable for use under acrylic fillings, as the solvent may dissolve or soften the acrylic.

21.3 CYANOACRYLATES

Cyanoacrylate monomers have the general formula:

$$\begin{array}{c} \quad\;\; CN \\ \quad\;\; | \\ CH_2{=}C{-}COOR \end{array}$$

where R may be, for example, a methyl, ethyl, propyl or butyl group.

These materials polymerise rapidly when spread into a thin film, and in the presence of moisture (Section 8.4.1). The outstanding property of such materials is their adhesion, even to moist tissues. Their suggested applications have included:
(a) use as pit and fissure sealants. (Section 20.3.1)
(b) use as tissue adhesives in place of suturing, and,
(c) use as haemostatic agents—aerosol sprays can be used to prevent haemorrhage.

The inflammatory response of cyanoacrylates is important; in general, the methyl cyanoacrylate has the greatest toxicity.

21.4 PERIODONTAL DRESSING MATERIALS

21.4.1 Introduction

A periodontal dressing is a material placed over the periodontal tissues, normally after surgery. The need for dressings after some types of surgery is currently a matter of debate.

21.4.2 Requirements

(a) Biological: ideally there should be no irritant, allergenic or other toxic effect. There should be no disturbance in the microbial balance of the mouth.
(b) Retentive properties: A dressing should remain securely in place over the tissues until the operator desires to remove it.
(c) Other properties: There should be no deleterious effects on adjacent restorative materials.

21.4.3 Materials

(a) Zinc oxide—eugenol formulations are widely used, but there is a possible sensitising effect in up to 5 per cent of patients.
(b) A zinc oxide—fatty acid formulation is widely used.
(c) A recently introduced material contains poly(acrylic acid) in addition to poly(ethyl methacrylate), zinc oxide, n-butyl phthalate and alcohol. This material is compatible with chlorhexidine, which is widely used for plaque control.
(d) Other materials which have been used include: a paste which sets by solvent loss, a non-setting hydrogenated fat incorporating the antibiotic bacitracin, and cyanoacrylates.

21.4.4 Hazards

(a) Proprietary materials containing asbestos are no longer available in some countries, because of possible serious hazards.
(b) Antibiotics can permit endogenous, potentially pathogenic organisms to proliferate in some cases.

21.5 GUTTA PERCHA

This compound is an isomer of rubber (Appendix III, no. 17) and can be used, with added zinc oxide or wax as a temporary filling material. This material is not considered satisfactory for this purpose

for the following reasons:
(a) It is softened by heat before insertion into the cavity—both the temperature and pressure of insertion may cause pulpal irritation.
(b) It does not adapt well to the cavity,
(c) Considerable marginal leakage can occur—perhaps more than with any other restorative material.

In one technique, gutta percha with a creosote disinfectant is used as a temporary dressing in endodontic treatment of deciduous teeth. It is claimed that the creosote dissolves the gutta percha and improves the adaptation.

Gutta percha is also used:
(a) As an impression material (Section 25.5.2).
(b) Occasionally it is heated to test the vitality of a pulp.

21.6 ROOT CANAL FILLING MATERIALS

A root filling is a permanent restoration intended to obturate the pulp space of a tooth. The object of this treatment is to promote long term retention of a sound dental support for a functional crown. Materials introduced into the root canal as medicaments are excluded from this discussion.

Root fillings may be classified as rigid (points or cones), plastic (pastes, cements or sealers) and combinations of the two.

(a) Rigid root fillings
   (i) Metallic: silver cones can be used, but are prone to corrosion by apical fluids. Titanium cones avoid this problem. Close adaptation of a rigid metal cone to the irregularities of the canal wall cannot be obtained.
   (ii) Polymeric: gutta percha (Section 21.5) cones are widely used.

(b) Plastic root fillings: These are usually zinc oxide—eugenol based materials, containing constituents such as bismuth trioxide or precipitated silver, thymol iodide, resins, etc. These materials are not used on their own because of:
   (i) difficulties in control of the material—e.g. extrusion through the apical foramina,
   (ii) periapical irritation, and,
   (iii) resorption.

(c) Combination of rigid and plastic materials: It is usual to use a filling cone in combination with a plastic material, to overcome the problems detailed above.

21.7 ADHESIVE BANDAGE

A hydrophilic bandage, which adheres to mouth tissues, has recently become available. It can be used as a protective covering for sutures and surgical wounds.

The manufacturers state that the bandage contains harmless food additives such as gelatin, pectin, sodium carboxymethylcellulose and polyisobutylene.

The material dissolves in the mouth in 24 to 48 hours.

SECTION III

Metallic filling materials

22. Amalgam

22.1 INTRODUCTION

Definition: an *amalgam* is an alloy of mercury with another metal or metals. Mercury is a liquid at room temperature; its freezing point is −39°C. It can readily undergo *amalgamation* reactions with metals such as silver, tin and copper to give a set material.

Dental amalgam is the most widely used filling material for posterior teeth. Mercury is mixed with an alloy powder to give a plastic material which is packed into the prepared cavity. The hardened or set amalgam is stronger than any dental cement or anterior filling material (Appendix II).

Alloys for use with mercury for dental applications are often referred to as dental amalgam alloys. Strictly speaking this is a misnomer; they are not amalgam alloys, but alloys from which an amalgam can be prepared.

22.2 COMPOSITION

Alloys for the preparation of dental amalgam may be broadly classified into two types: firstly, conventional alloys, containing less than 6% copper—the chemical formulation of these materials has been very little changed over the years; secondly, copper enriched alloys, which have become available during the last few years (sometimes referred to as 'higher copper' alloys).

22.2.1 Conventional alloys

Conventional alloys contain the following principal constituents:

silver	67–74%	copper	0–6%
tin	25–27%	zinc	0–2%

An important difference between alloys containing zinc and those which are zinc free, is discussed in Section 22.6.8.

Some alloys contain or have contained up to 2 to 3% mercury—such alloys amalgamate more rapidly.

The chief difference between many conventional alloys is their particle size and shape. Lathe cut alloys (Section 22.3) may be coarse or fine grain; the latter are to be preferred (Sections 22.4.4). Alloys are particle size blended—that is there is a distribution of sizes to give greater packing efficiency of the particles. As an alternative to lathe cut materials, spherical particle alloys are available. Some alloys contain a blend of lathe cut and spherical particles.

22.2.2 Copper enriched alloys

Copper enriched alloys are of the following types:

(a) Blended alloys, sometimes referred to as 'dispersion modified' alloys; these contain two parts by weight of conventional composition lathe cut particles plus one part by weight of spheres of a silver-copper eutectic alloy (70% Ag + 30% Cu, approximately). The overall composition is approximately:

silver	69%	copper	13%
tin	17%	zinc	1%

(b) Single composition alloys; a number of different types are available:

(i) ternary alloys in spherical form, either: silver 60%, tin 25%, copper 15%, or:
silver 40%, tin 30%, copper 30%.

(ii) an alloy similar to the first of those detailed in (i) above, but containing particles in spheroidal form—that is, that particles are not perfectly spherical.

(iii) quaternary alloys in spheroidal form, containing:

silver	59%	copper	13%
tin	24%	indium	4%

(c) Alloys which are the reverse of type (a) above are available in some countries. That is, they contain 2 parts by weight of spheres of 60% Ag, 25% Sn and 15% Cu, plus 1 part by weight of conventional alloy. This latter component may be present either as spherical or fine grain lathe cut particles.

(d) Experiments have been carried out on alloys which are mixtures of conventional alloys and copper amalgam (see Section 22.7).

22.3 MANUFACTURE OF ALLOY

Conventional alloys are prepared by fusing together the pure metals to form an ingot which is then *homogenised* (Section 10.3.2) and cut into filings. Homogenisation helps to ensure that each filing has similar composition and properties. The size and shape of the particles of cut alloy are of great importance (Sections 22.4.4 and 22.6.8).

A freshly cut alloy reacts very rapidly with mercury. This may be explained partly by the dislocations and imperfections in the alloy lattice, which can increase its chemical reactivity. If the alloy filings are stored at room temperature for a few months the reactivity gradually decreases—such alloys are said to have been *aged*. The same results can be achieved much more rapidly by boiling the filings in water for 30 minutes. This rapid method of aging the filings is usually carried out by the manufacturer, to give a product of stable properties.

Spherical particles are prepared by an *atomisation* process—that is—spraying the molten alloy into an inert atmosphere, when the droplets of alloy solidify as spheres. Spherical particles are easier than irregular shaped particles to grade with respect to their particle size. A blend of sizes from 10 to 37 μm has been suggested.

22.4 MANIPULATION

22.4.1 Proportioning

(a) Mercury—the required quantity can be obtained by weighing or by using a volume dispenser. Clearly the latter method is quicker. It is important to use pure clean mercury.

(b) Alloy—this can be proportioned by:

(i) weighing.

(ii) using tables of alloy, particularly with mechanical mixing (Section 22.4.2).

(iii) having envelopes with pre-weighed quantities, or,
(iv) using a volume dispenser.

Two disadvantages of a volume dispenser are:

(i) It is difficult to measure any powder accurately by volume, as the weight of material per volume depends on the efficiency with which the particles are packed together, and
(ii) alloy can cling to the walls of the dispenser.

(c) Alloy/mercury ratio, in the final set amalgam it is desirable to have less than 50% mercury (Section 22.6.4). Two techniques have been recommended:

(i) The use of an alloy/mercury ratio of 5/7 or 5/8. the excess mercury makes the trituration easier, giving a smooth plastic mix of material. Before insertion into the cavity, excess mercury is removed from the mix by squeezing it in a dental napkin.
(ii) Minimal mercury techniques (Eames technique), where about equal weights of alloy and mercury are used, and no mercury squeezed out of the mix before condensation. This method is used in conjunction with mechanical mixing (Section 22.4.2).

Regardless of which method is used, excess mercury which becomes apparent during packing should be removed (Section 22.4.3).

22.4.2 Trituration

(a) Hand mixing by mortar and pestle.

A glass mortar and pestle are used. The *mortar* has its inner surface roughened to increase the friction between the amalgam and the surface. A rough surface can be maintained by occasionally grinding with carborundum paste. The *pestle* is a glass rod with a rounded end.

This technique is not widely used today; mechanical methods (see below) are more rapid, and involve less risk of exposure to mercury vapour (Section 22.4.6).

(b) Mechanical mixing

The proportioned alloy and mercury can be mixed mechanically in a capsule, either with or without a stainless steel or plastic pestle. A pestle, which should be of considerably smaller diameter than the capsule, should be used with tablet alloys, to help break up the material. The mechanical amalgamators have time-switches to ensure a correct and reproducible mixing time. A number of these materials are available in an encapsulated form, each capsule containing a controlled weight of alloy, and having the right quantity of mercury sealed in its lid. The seal is broken before putting the capsule on to the mechanical amalgamator.

The choice of trituration time is important, and will depend both on the type of alloy and the speed of the mixer. In particular copper enriched alloys require precise control of trituration conditions. Some such products require high energy mixing to break up the oxide coating which forms on copper-rich particles.

22.4.3 Condensation

For full details of this, and other clinical procedures, a textbook on operative dental surgery should be consulted.

The mixed material is packed into the cavity in increments in such a way that:

(i) each portion is properly adapted by a condenser of suitable size.
(ii) a load of up to 4 to 5 kg is applied to each increment, and,
(iii) as the mix is condensed , some mercury-rich material rises to the surface. Some of this can be removed, to reduce the final mercury content, and improve the mechanical properties (Section 22.6.4). The remainder will assist bonding with the next increment, to avoid the production of a weak laminated restoration.

A material should be condensed as soon as possible after mixing. If it is left too long, and has begun to set,

(i) proper adaptation to the cavity will be impossible.
(ii) elimination of excess mercury will be difficult.
(iii) bonding between increments will be poor, and,
(iv) lower strength values will result.

Mechanical condensers are also available, which apply vibration to pack the amalgam.

Amalgams prepared from spherical alloys need less packing pressure than those prepared from lathe cut alloys. However, condensation can be more difficult for spherical alloys, as the condenser point tends to pass right through the material instead of developing pressure. Generally spheroidal particle amalgams condense with more resistance than spherical materials.

22.4.4 Trimming and carving

When the cavity is overfilled, the top mercury-rich layer can be trimmed away and the filling carved to the correct contours. The amalgam prepared from a coarser grain alloy may be more difficult to carve, as the instrument may pull out large pieces of alloy from the surface. Spherical alloys are used where ease of carving is desired.

22.4.5 Polishing

Conventional amalgams are polished not less than 24 hours after insertion—that is, when the material has gained considerable strength. Since amalgams from copper enriched alloys gain strength rapidly (Table 22.1), it is sometimes recommended that they can be polished shortly after insertion.

22.4.6 Some precautions

(a) Mercury is toxic, so free mercury should not be exposed to the atmosphere. This hazard can arise during trituration, and condensation and finishing of restoration, and also during the removal of old restorations at high speed.
(b) Skin contact with mercury should be avoided, as it can be absorbed by the skin.
(c) Any excess mercury should not be allowed to get into sinks, as it can react with some of the alloys used in plumbing.
(d) Contamination of an amalgam by moisture must be avoided (Section 22.6.8).

22.5 SETTING REACTIONS AND STRUCTURE

22.5.1 Conventional alloys

(a) Nature of the alloy: silver and tin can form an intermetallic compound (Section 10.2.5), of formula Ag_3Sn. This is called the gamma phase of the silver tin system. This contains 73.15% silver and 26.85% tin. An alloy for dental use should have silver and tin in very nearly these proportions, though copper may replace a small amount of the silver (see below). The silver contributes to the resistance to tarnish of the amalgam. Tin reacts very readily with mercury, and makes amalgamation of the alloy easier. If too much tin is present, contraction occurs on setting of the amalgam and the strength and hardness of the set material are reduced.

Copper may replace silver to some extent; it increases the hardness and strength of the amalgam. Zinc, if present, acts as a scavenger for oxygen in the fusion of the alloy, similar to its application in gold alloys (Section 10.5.2).

(b) Setting mechanism: The reaction between dental amalgam alloys and mercury is very complex. Considered here are a few facts related to the reaction between the intermetallic silver-tin compound (Ag_3Sn)—the γ —phase—and mercury:

(a) During and after mixing the γ-phase dissolves in the mercury.

(b) Reaction occurs to give formation and crystal growth of at least two phases:

(i) The compound Ag_2Hg_3, with a body-centered cubic structure, called the γ_1 phase.

(ii) A tin-mercury compound with a hexagonal structure of formula $Sn_{7-8}Hg$, called the γ_2 phase.

These reactions may be written as:

$$Ag_3Sn + Hg \rightarrow Ag_2Hg_3 + Sn_{7-8}Hg + Ag_3Sn \text{ (unreacted)}$$

$$\text{or,} \quad \gamma + Hg \rightarrow \underbrace{\gamma_1 + \gamma_2}_{\text{matrix}} + \underbrace{\gamma}_{\text{core}}$$

(c) Structure of the set material: This is a cored structure, with a core of unreacted γ and a matrix of the γ_1 and γ_2 compounds, the latter of which forms a continuous network.

(d) After setting, further reactions may occur by diffusion processes.

22.5.2 Copper enriched alloys

The main feature of these materials is that the set structure is essentially free of the γ_2 component.

(a) Blended alloys. The reaction is essentially that between a mixture of Ag_3Sn plus Ag-Cu spheres and Hg, and takes place in two stages:

Stage 1: As for the reaction of conventional alloys (see above); the Ag-Cu does not participate.

Stage 2: A reaction between the γ_2 component and Ag-Cu spheres, leading to the production of a copper-tin compound, and more γ_1, thus:

$$Sn_{7-8}Hg + Ag - Cu \rightarrow Cu_6Sn_5 + Ag_2Hg_3$$

$$\text{or,} \quad \gamma_2 + Ag - Cu \rightarrow Cu_6Sn_5 + \gamma_1$$

The Cu_6Sn_5 is present as a 'halo' surrounding the Ag-Cu particles. The final set material consists of a core of (i) Ag_3Sn and (ii) Ag-Cu surrounded by a halo of Cu_6Sn_5, and a matrix of γ_1.
(b) Single composition-alloys. The structure of the materials is similar to that given above, except that the Cu_6Sn_5 is present in the γ_1 matrix rather than as a halo.

Notes:

(a) Experiments have shown that alloys in which about 10% of gold is substituted for some of the silver also produce amalgams free of the γ_2 phase.
(b) The absence of the γ_2 phase has great significance in terms of (i) corrosion properties (Section 22.6.2), (ii) strength (Section 22.6.4), (iii) creep properties (Section 22.6.5) and (iv) durability of the margins of amalgam restorations (Section 22.6.6).

22.6 PROPERTIES

22.6.1 Toxicity

The toxicity of mercury has already been stressed (Section 22.4.6). It is logical to ask if there are any likely toxic effects for the patient who has amalgam restorations. It is known that mercury penetrates into the tooth structure, and can discolour that tooth; traces may even reach the pulp. It is believed, however, that there are no systemic toxic effects.

22.6.2 Corrosion reactions

(a) Tarnish: amalgam can tarnish in the presence of sulphur, to give a layer of sulphides on the surface of the restoration.
(b) Corrosion of conventional amalgams: the set material is heterogeneous, which can encourage corrosion. Of the three phases present, the γ_2 is the most active electrochemically, being anodic in relation to both the γ and γ_1 phases. As γ_2 corrodes, essentially two products result:

- (i) Sn^{2+} ions are formed: in the presence of saliva, corrosion products such as SnO_2 and $Sn(OH)_6Cl$ are found.
- (ii) Hg is produced, which can react with some of the remaining hitherto unreacted γ phase.

(c) Corrosion of copper enriched amalgam.

- (i) No γ_2 is present, and Cu_6Sn_5 is the phase most prone to corrosion.

(ii) However, the corrosion currents associated with these systems are considerably less than that with conventional amalgam.
(iii) The volume of corrosion products is less than with conventional amalgam.
(iv) No mercury is produced as a result of the corrosion.

(d) Practical considerations:
(i) Corrosion resistance is greatly improved if the amalgam is polished. This process removes pits and voids on the surface, which aid concentration cell corrosion (Section 11.3.2).
(ii) If amalgam comes in contact with a gold restoration, an electrolytic cell may be set up (Section 11.3.1) leading to corrosion of the amalgam and incorporation of mercury on the gold restoration.
(iii) Corrosion of conventional amalgam can have a significant effect on long term mechanical properties. It has been shown, for example, that tensile strength is reduced by 30% when the network of γ_2 has corroded.

22.6.3 Marginal leakage

The initial marginal leakage of an amalgam restoration according to *in vitro* tests, reduces with time, because of sealing of the micro-fissures by products of corrosion breakdown.

22.6.4 Strength

The following factors can lead to the production of a weak amalgam restoration:
(i) undertrituration.
(ii) too high a mercury content.
(iii) too low condensation pressure
(iv) a slow rate of packing.
(v) corrosion (Section 22.6.2).

The rate of development of strength of an amalgam is of importance (Fig. 22.1). With amalgams which develop strength slowly, there is danger of early fracture of such a restoration. Generally, spherical and copper enriched amalgams have high early strengths (Table 22.1). Of the phases present in conventional amalgams the γ_2 is the weakest and softest.

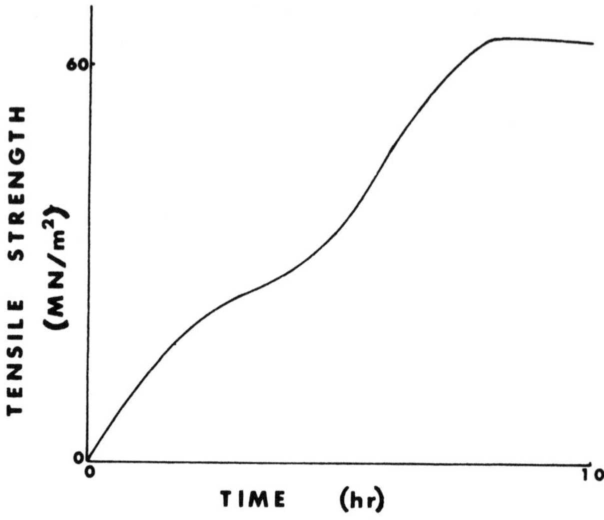

Fig. 22.1 The rate of increase of tensile strength of an amalgam with time.

Table 22.1 Typical properties of dental amalgam*

Amalgam type	Compressive strength (MN/m^2) 1 hour	Fully set	Static creep (%) after 7 days under pressure of 38 MN/m^2
Conventional, lathe cut	120–170	380–450	2.5–3.5
Conventional, spherical	140–180	380–450	0.3–1.5
Blended alloys	120–220	410–460	0.2–1.7
Single composition ternary alloys	230–320	460–540	0.02–0.3
Quarternary alloys (with indium)	210–240	430–480	0.06–0.1

* Range of values taken from research reports in the recent literature.

22.6.5 Creep

In general, set alloys with no γ_2 phase show less creep than conventional materials. (Table 22.1). In general:

creep of conventional alloys >> creep of blended alloys > Creep of single composition alloys

22.6.6 Marginal failure

'Ditching' of the margins of amalgam is a common occurrence.

Clinical trials have shown that new alloy formulations show much less marginal breakdown than conventional materials. The following observations are relevant:

(a) Poor technique can cause breakdown—e.g. an unsupported ledge of amalgam extending over the enamel may fracture during mastication.

(b) In general, materials with high creep values have been shown to have poorer durability of margins. This does not, however, necessarily prove that there is a cause and effect relationship between the two phenomena. In general:

integrity of blended alloys > integrity of single composition alloys > > integrity of conventional alloys

(c) A theory has been propounded which links marginal breakdown with corrosion characteristics. It has been suggested that the mercury corrosion product (from conventional materials) reacts to form more γ_1 and γ_2 material, with associated expansion, termed 'mercuroscopic expansion'. The expanded material, weakened by corrosion, protrudes away from the supporting tooth structure, and fractures.

22.6.7 Thermal diffusivity

From the data in Appendix II, it can be seen that dental amalgam is a conductor of heat, whereas the enamel and dentine it replaces is a thermal insulator. Consequently, large amalgam restorations are usually lined with a thermal insulating cement (Section 16.4) to protect the pulp from temperature changes in the mouth caused by hot and cold foods and liquids.

22.6.8 Dimensional changes

Ideally there should be little or no contraction on setting of a dental amalgam, otherwise a gap between filling and cavity walls may result, enhancing the possibility of further decay. Too great an expansion should also be avoided, as this will cause the filling to protrude from the cavity.

In laboratory experiments, where free expansion is measured, it has been shown that a greater expansion on setting will result if:

(a) a higher alloy mercury ratio is used;

(b) there is a shorter trituration time;
(c) lower pressure during condensation is used;
(d) the alloy has a larger particle size, and
(e) if there is contamination by water before setting if a zinc containing materials. This will result in:
  (i) an electrolytic reaction between zinc (the anode) and the other metals which are cathodic (see Table 11.1), and the water as an electrolyte:
  (ii) hydrogen is evolved as a result of this reaction;
  (iii) the pressure of the evolved hydrogen may cause the amalgam to flow and
  (iv) this causes an expansion, which may not appear within the first 24 hours, but may become evident some days after insertion of the restoration.

22.7 COPPER AMALGAM

These have been used for restorations of deciduous teeth, because of the antibacterial effect of the copper.

The material is supplied as an amalgam, in the form of pellets, containing about 60 to 70% mercury and 30 to 40% copper. They are heated until droplets of mercury appear, and then triturated as with other amalgams, and then condensed into a cavity.

These alloys cannot be recommended for use, because of poor mercury hygiene associated with their use.

22.8 THE SELECTION OF AN AMALGAM ALLOY

A number of questions must be asked in selecting an amalgam alloy.
(a) Conventional or copper enriched alloy?
  (i) High copper alloys appear to be superior in many of their properties. Their better strength is probably not very important; correctly manipulated conventional materials are sufficiently strong. The better marginal integrity of high copper amalgams is important.
  (ii) The conventional materials are still widely used in some countries, particularly because of their lower cost.
(b) Which type of conventional alloy?
  (i) Finer grain alloys are to be preferred in terms of ease of carving; however, amalgams produced from extremely fine particles have a greater γ_2 content.

(ii) There appears to be little advantage in using spherical alloys of the conventional type, except in terms of ease of carving.
(iii) Zinc-free alloys are preferred in situations where moisture control is difficult.

(c) Which type of copper enriched alloy?
(i) The dispersion modified alloys have produced excellent results in clinical trials.
(ii) Alloys containing spheroidal particles may be easier to manipulate than those which are all spherical.

READING REFERENCES

Wing G 1975 Dental amalgam. In: von Fraunhofer J A (ed) Scientific aspects of dental materials Butterworths, London, Ch 8

This chapter discusses the structure, manipulation and properties of amalgam, with data on the properties of new alloy formulations.

Brown D 1976 The clinical status of amalgam. British Dental Journal 141: 80

This review discusses potential sources of failure of amalgam restorations, and the structure and properties of new alloys, particularly the dispersion alloy discussed in Section 19.2.2(a).

Merfield D P, Taylor A, Gemmell D M, Parrish J A 1976 Mercury intoxication in a dental surgery following unreported spillage. British Dental Journal 141: 179

This important recent paper discusses a case of mercury intoxication, and stresses the need for a wider awareness of the hazards associated with poor mercury hygiene.

23. Direct filling gold

23.1 METALLURGICAL PRINCIPLES

23.1.1 Welding

Welding is the joining of two metals without the use of an intermediary alloy. A successful weld requires adhesion between the two pieces of metal to occur. Gold has an unusual property, in that it can be easily welded at room temperature. Pieces of pure gold can be welded together in a cavity to form a restoration.

23.1.2 Work hardening

Pure gold, in the as-cast condition, is very ductile and too soft for use in dental restorations. However, the process of condensing pure gold in order to effect welding at room temperature causes work hardening of the metal. This improves its hardness and strength and reduces the ductility (Section 9.6). Nevertheless, direct filling golds are usually utilised only in Class III and Class V cavities, and not for situations where they would be subjected to direct masticatory stress.

23.2 MATERIALS

23.2.1 Gold foil sheet

Gold foil is manufactured by rolling and beating the material to form the required thickness of foil. As this considerably work hardens the metal, it is heat treated (stress relief annealed, Section 9.7.4, and recrystallised, Section 9.7.5) to increase its ductility and malleability, so that it is supplied in the fully annealed condition. Gold is supplied in books of foil, each sheet being 101.6 mm (4 inches) square. Laminated foil, with sheets of platinum between sheets of gold, has also been used.

The thickness of the foil is designated by a number—for example, one sheet of number 4 foil weighs 4 grains. Each sheet is cut into portions of varying size for different applications—for example, ⅛, 1/16, 1/32, 1/64, 1/128 of a sheet, etc. Each piece is then generally formed into a cylinder or pellet of gold, ready for clinical use.

23.2.2 Mat gold

This is prepared by electrolytic precipitation of gold as a powder and compression and sintering of the power. It is supplied as thin strips of gold, which can be manipulated in a similar manner to the foil.

23.2.3 Powdered gold

Gold powder, prepared by atomisation of the molten metal, or by precipitation, is supplied as a pellet, sometimes wrapped in gold foil.

23.2.4 Non-cohesive gold

Non-cohesive gold foil, which has gases such as ammonia adsorbed on to its surface, is sometimes preferred for lining a cavity as it can be readily adapted to the cavity floor and walls. This is then covered with a veneer of cohesive gold.

23.2.5 Direct gold alloys

It has recently been suggested that small quantities of calcium, platinum or silver (from 0.1–5% by weight) included in direct filling gold, can increase the hardness and strength, with no adverse effect on the corrosion resistance.

23.3 MANIPULATION

23.3.1 Degassing

Before insertion of gold foil into a cavity, it is heated. This is often called annealing, though in fact the gold has already been annealed by the manufacturer. The purpose of the heating is to remove adsorbed gases, particularly oxygen, from the metal surface, in order to improve the weldability. Clearly, the foil should also not be contaminated by handling, or by moisture in the cavity.

Gold foil can be heated on a container, above a gas or alcohol flame, or in an electric furnace. Temperatures of 250 to 350°C are usually recommended. The time of heating depends on the individual material, and the degree of surface contamination.

23.3.2 Compaction

The clean and decontaminated gold is packed into the cavity in increments. Each piece is condensed or compacted by (i) a plugger and hand mallet, (ii) a pneumatic vibratory condenser, or (iii) an electrically driven condenser. The first of these methods usually requires the greatest time and may be the most traumatic for the patient.

The area of the condenser point is important. If this is too large there is less pressure applied to the gold for any given force, and welding may not be achieved. If too small, the condenser will punch a hole in the metal rather than weld it. The area of the condenser point should be between 0.3 to 1.0 mm^2,

The force of compaction should be applied perpendicular to the surface of the foil. Failure to do this will result in shear stresses, which may cause a piece of foil to become dislodged.

23.4 PROPERTIES

23.4.1 Density

The density of pure gold is 19.32 g/cm^3. A gold foil restoration has a density of only about 16 g/cm^3. This difference can be accounted for by the presence of porosity where there has not been complete contact between the pieces of foil. Clearly the degree of porosity depends on the compaction technique that is used. It is important to minimise the number of internal voids to obtain the greatest strength.

23.4.2 Mechanical properties

It has been shown that:

(a) Properly condensed gold foil is about as hard as the type I inlay golds.

(b) The use of foil that has been laminated with platinum gives an even harder restoration. However, it can be difficult to obtain adhesion between different layers of foil.

As has been mentioned, the strength and hardness of a foil restoration are not sufficient to withstand the direct forces of mastication.

23.4.3 Other properties

(a) These materials cause the least gingival irritation of any restorative material.
(b) The corrosion resistance of gold is excellent.
(c) There is very little marginal leakage round a gold foil filling.

23.5 CRITIQUE OF GOLD FOIL

With proper manipulation, and great attention to detail, gold fillings can be prepared that will last for many years. Nevertheless these materials can be criticised on at least two grounds:
(a) The time taken to insert a gold filling is much greater than is normally required for other materials.
(b) It is a point of dispute whether the trauma during compaction has a damaging effect on the pulp. Automatic mechanical condensing procedures are both quicker, and possibly less traumatic.

READING REFERENCE

Knight T J 1972 Cohesive golds—a review of the literature. Journal of the Dental Association of South Africa 27: 101

This review deals with developments in new materials over the last ten years, the principles of cavity design, new manipulative techniques and biological effects.

SECTION IV

Impression materials

24. Impression materials: requirements and classification; impression trays

24.1 INTRODUCTION

The construction of the majority of oral appliances (for example, dentures, crowns, inlays, bridges and orthodontic appliances) requires the preparation of a model of patients' oral tissues. One of the range of impression materials is used to obtain a reverse or negative form of the tissues. This is converted into a positive model, using one of the available model and die materials (Ch. 40).

Impression materials, in the fluid or plastic state, are carried to the mouth in a suitably sized tray; hardening of the material takes place either on cooling or through chemical reaction. Materials which are more fluid displace the tissues less; these are generally known as *mucostatic* impression materials. More viscous impression materials are designated *mucocompressive*.

24.2 REQUIREMENTS

An impression material should have the following properties:

(a) Accuracy

This is clearly important, since a restoration or appliance fabricated in the laboratory cannot be more accurate than the impression from which a working model is prepared.

For great accuracy, the following factors are important:

(i) Rheological properties; the material must be in a fluid or plastic state on insertion into the mouth; it must be sufficiently fluid to record fine detail; it must have sufficient working time during which there is no significant increase in viscosity.

(ii) There should be negligible dimensional changes associated with the setting reaction or process.

(iii) Ideally the material should be elastic on removal from the

mouth, so that undercuts can be recorded without distortion of the impression. It should also adhere to the tray.
- (iv) There should be negligible dimensional changes on storage of the impression in the dental laboratory.
- (v) It should be compatible with model and die materials.

(b) Other properties

In addition, an impression material should:

- (i) be non-toxic and non-irritant, with an acceptable odour and taste;
- (ii) have a suitable setting time—the impression should not need to be in the mouth for more than five minutes, to avoid fatigue to both operator and patient; and,
- (iii) be stable on storage over a period of time.

24.3 CLASSIFICATION

The materials in common use can be classified as non-elastic or elastic, according to the ability of the set material to be withdrawn over under-cuts.

24.3.1 **Rigid materials** (Ch. 25)

- (a) Plaster of Paris.
- (b) Impression composition (compound).
- (c) Zinc oxide–eugenol and similar pastes.
- (d) Impression waxes.

24.3.2 **Elastic materials**

- (a) Hydrocolloids: (Chapter 26).
  - (i) Reversible: agar.
  - (ii) Irreversible: alginates.
- (b) Elastomers: (Chapter 27).
  - (i) Polysulphides (Rubber-base, Mercaptan, Thiokol).
  - (ii) Silicones.
  - (iii) Polyethers.

24.4 IMPRESSION TRAYS

These may be classified as *stock trays*, which are obtained in standard sizes, or *special trays*, fabricated from a model of the mouth of the patient.

(a) Stock trays may be:
  (i) Reusable—made of metal, supplied either with or without perforations.
  (ii) Disposable—usually perforated, and made of a polymer such as nylon or polystyrene.

(b) Special trays are all disposable, and may be made of self-cured acrylic or shellac.

25. Non-elastic impression materials

25.1 PLASTER OF PARIS

25.1.1 Chemistry

The chief constituent of impression plaster is calcined calcium sulphate hemihydrate. On mixing with water this reacts to form a rigid mass of calcium sulphate dihydrate. The chemistry of this system is discussed in Section 40.2.

During the setting an expansion may be demonstrated (Section 40.2.4)—this is substantially reduced by the addition of potassium sulphate (Section 40.2.6). As this accelerates the setting too much, borax is added to slow down the process (Section 40.2.6). Another additive is alizarin red; this imparts a pink colour to the impression enabling it to be distinguished from the model that is cast on it. A flavouring agent may also be present.

The additives may be blended with the plaster powder, or may be supplied as an aqueous solution to be mixed with plaster. In the latter case a suitable solution contains: 4% potassium sulphate, 0.4 to 1% borax (the precise value being chosen to give a desirable setting time; this may vary for different batches of plaster) and 0.04% alizarin red. This solution is called 'A.E' or 'anti-expansion' solution.

Some impression plasters may also contain:
(a) additives such as gum tragacanth, to improve the cohesive properties of the mixed plaster, and
(b) starch, incorporated so that the set plaster will disintegrate due to the swelling of the starch when boiling water is poured over

it—this facilitates removal of the impression from the cast model. Materials containing starch are called *soluble plasters*.

25.1.2 Manipulation

The plaster should be mixed with water or an A.E. solution in the ratio of 100 g to 50 to 60 ml. Care must be taken to ensure that the mix is free of air bubbles, since these may appear on the surface of the impression leading to inaccuracy.

25.1.3 Properties

(a) Accuracy
- (i) Plaster is excellent at recording fine detail since the mixed material is very fluid when inserted into the mouth.
- (ii) The dimensional changes on setting are small, due to anti-expansion additives.
- (iii) If there are undercuts present, the plaster impression will fracture on removal from the mouth.
- (iv) On storage of a plaster impression, the dimensional changes are small, though a small degree of drying shrinkage may occur.
- (v) Before casting a model in plaster or dental stone (Section 40.2), the plaster impression must be treated with a separating agent. An alginate mould seal (Section 33.3.3), a varnish or waterglass or soap solution may be used.

(b) Other properties
- (i) Impression plasters are non-toxic. However, they may be unpleasant for the patient, because they produce a dry sensation in the mouth.
- (ii) The setting time can be precisely controlled by use of the appropriate quantities of additives.
- (iii) Plaster is stable on storage over a long time, provided it is kept in a sealed container.

25.2 IMPRESSION COMPOSITION (COMPOUND)

25.2.1 Constituents and applications

These materials are generally composed of a mixture of natural resins (e.g. colophony and shellac and/or waxes), fillers (soapstone or talc) and lubricants (stearic acid or stearin). They are *thermoplastic*—that is, they soften when heated and harden when cooled, without the occurrence of a chemical reaction. The available materials may be classified into two types:

(a) Type I—lower fusing materials:

- (i) For recording prosthetic impressions, such as preliminary impressions of edentulous patients, supplied in sheets about 4 to 5 mm thick.
- (ii) Peripheral seal materials—see Section 25.5.1
- (iii) Supplied in stick form for copper band impressions for inlays and crowns and marginal additions to special trays, etc.

(b) Type II—higher fusing materials, used as tray materials, which are sufficiently rigid to support other impression materials.

25.2.2 Manipulation

(a) For prosthetic impressions the composition is heated in a water bath at 55 to 60°C. Since the material has a low thermal conductivity it must be immersed in the water bath for sufficient time to ensure complete softening. However, if it is left too long, some of the constituents may be leached out into the water bath, so altering the properties of the material. If the composition is kneaded in the water bath, water will become incorporated in the material, and act as a plasticiser. If the composition is too cool, it will not flow properly in the mouth; if it is too hot, the material becomes sticky. In all cases the water bath should be lined with a napkin, otherwise the material will adhere to the bath.

(b) For copper band impressions, e.g. for inlays and crowns, the stick of composition is heated in a flame. If overheating occurs, some of the constituents may be volatilised, with a consequent alteration of properties of the material.

25.2.3 Properties

(a) Accuracy

- (i) In general, this material, though plastic on insertion into the mouth, is not sufficiently fluid to record all the fine detail of the mouth.
- (ii) Impression composition has a high coefficient of thermal expansion; thus, on cooling during setting, there is considerable shrinkage. This can be minimised to some extent in prosthetic impressions by heating the surface of the set material in a flame and re-taking the impression. Since only

a small quantity of composition is contracting, the actual magnitude of the contraction is small. Shrinkage also occurs on cooling from mouth temperature to room temperature (about 1.5% by volume).

(iii) Impression composition will distort on removal over undercut areas.

(iv) Dimensional changes can occur on storing the impression in the laboratory. Stresses can be set up within the material, particularly if it is manipulated or deformed when it is not fully softened. Subsequently distortion can occur due to relief of these stresses, particularly if the impression is left for some time, in a warm atmosphere, before casting up the model.

(v) These materials are compatible with model and die materials.

(b) Other properties

Impression composition materials:

(i) are non-toxic and non-irritant,

(ii) harden in a reasonably acceptable time in the mouth, and,

(iii) their shelf-life is very adequate, but changes in shellac may cause deterioration over a long period.

25.3 ZINC OXIDE–EUGENOL AND SIMILAR PASTES

25.3.1 Chemistry

The reaction between zinc oxide and eugenol has already been discussed (Section 12.7.2). In these materials:

(a) The zinc oxide is supplied in paste form. This is achieved by the addition of an oil (e.g. olive oil, light mineral oil or linseed oil). The oil also acts as a plasticiser for the material. Hydrogenated rosin can also be incorporated; it quickens the setting and makes the impression paste more cohesive.

(b) The eugenol contains talc or kaolin as a filler, to form a paste.

(c) Either or both pastes may contain accelerators, such as zinc acetate.

(d) At least one proprietary paste contains a substitute for eugenol. This is a carboxylic acid, which can react with zinc hydroxide (possibly formed by the hydrolysis of zinc oxide) to form a salt as follows:

$$Zn(OH)_2 + 2RCOOH \rightarrow (RCOO)_2Zn + 2H_2O$$

25.3.2 Manipulation

The two pastes are provided in contrasting colours. The correct proportions (usually equal lengths of the two) are mixed together on a slab or mixing pad with a flexible spatula until a homogeneous colour is obtained.

25.3.3 Properties

(a) Accuracy
- (i) These impression materials are sufficiently fluid to record the fine detail in the mouth.
- (ii) There is probably little or no dimensional change associated with the setting process.
- (iii) The set material is not elastic, so will not record undercuts.
- (iv) The set material appears to be stable on storage in the laboratory.
- (v) Impression pastes are compatible with dental stone model materials. The paste can be removed from the stone by softening it in water at 60°C.

(b) Other properties
- (i) These materials are non-toxic, but those containing eugenol can be irritant, giving a tingling or burning sensation to the patient and leaving a persistent taste, which some people may regard as unpleasant. The paste can adhere to tissues, so the lips of the patient are usually coated with petroleum jelly.
- (ii) The setting time is usually satisfactory if the manufacturer's instructions are followed and the correct ratio of pastes used. The presence of water, and an increase in temperature, both reduce the setting time.
- (iii) The shelf-life of these materials is satisfactory.

25.3.4 Applications

This material is generally used in thin sections (2 to 3 mm) as a wash impression. A zinc oxide–eugenol impression can be taken using a close-fitting special tray, or in an existing denture, particularly one that is to be relined.

25.4 IMPRESSION WAXES

Waxes, sometimes in combination with resins of low melting point, can be used as impression materials. These materials differ from impression composition, in that they sometimes flow at mouth temperature. In contrast to the zinc oxide–eugenol pastes, they do not set by chemical reaction. Different combinations of waxes and resins can be blended to give a range of materials for different techniques.

A model should be cast up immediately from such an impression to avoid distortion (Section 41.3.4).

25.5 OTHER MATERIALS

25.5.1 Peripheral seal materials

In addition to impression composition (Section 25.2.1), alternative materials are available for outlining the denture-bearing area. These are monomer–polymer formulations, the monomer being n-butyl methacrylate containing a tertiary amine activator, and the polymer poly(ethyl methacrylate), with a peroxide initiator (Section 8.3.1). On mixing together, polymerisation occurs. The merits of this material are that it is simple and rapid to use. A conventional auto-polymerising acrylic is unsuitable for this application due to (a) the toxic effect of methyl methacrylate (b) the heat evolved during the exothermic polymerisation and (c) the speed of the reaction.

25.5.2 Gutta percha

Gutta percha softens at 60 to 65°C. At mouth temperature the material will flow if pressure is applied to it. It can be used for example, for impression taking for cleft palate patients, being moulded for a number of days by contact with the moving soft tissues.

26. Hydrocolloid impression materials

26.1 GENERAL PROPERTIES

A *colloid* must be distinguished from a *solution* and a *suspension*. A solution is a homogeneous mixture. For example, in an aqueous solution the solute exists as small molecules or ions in the solvent. In contrast to this, a *suspension* is heterogeneous, consisting of particles of at least sufficient size to be seen microscopically, dispersed in a medium. Thus a suspension is a two phase system.

Colloids fall between these two extremes. They are heterogeneous, (2-phase systems), like suspensions, but the particle size of the dispersed phase is smaller, usually in the range 1 to 200 nm. However, it is not always possible to distinguish between a colloid and a solution on the one hand and a colloid and a suspension on the other.

When the dispersion medium of a colloid is water, it is termed a *hydrocolloid*.

Colloids may exist in the *sol* and *gel* state. In the *sol* state, the material is a viscous liquid. A sol can be converted into a *gel*—a material of jelly-like consistency, due to agglomeration of the molecules of the dispersed phase, to form *fibrils*, or chains of molecules, in a network pattern. These fibrils enclose the dispersion medium, for example water.

A sol may be converted into a gel in one of two ways:

(a) By a reduction in temperature; such processes are reversible, since on heating, a sol is formed again; for example, agar (Section 26.2). In such a gel the fibrils are held together by Van der Waals forces.

(b) Other materials can form a gel by a chemical reaction, which is irreversible (for example, alginates, Section 26.3).

The strength or toughness of a gel depends on:

(a) The concentration of fibrils—the greater the concentration, the stronger the material.
(b) The concentration of fillers—inert powders can be added to a gel to render it less flexible.

A gel can lose or take up water or other fluids. Loss of water can occur by evaporation. *Syneresis* can also occur; this happens when the gel molecules are drawn closer together, for example by continuation of the setting reaction. As a result a fluid exudate appears on the surface of the gel. Uptake of water is called *imbibition*.

In the use of hydrocolloids for dental impressions, the material is inserted in the mouth in the sol state, when it is sufficiently fluid to record detail. No gelation should have occurred at this stage. It is removed from the tissues after the gel is formed, when it exhibits elastic properties.

Clearly syneresis and imbibition of the gel should be avoided, as the former is associated with shrinkage, and the latter results in expansion.

26.2 AGAR

26.2.1 Composition

This is recorded in Table 26.1

Table 26.1 Composition of agar impression materials

Constituent	Approximate percentage	Function
Agar	14	Colloid
Borax	0.2	Strengthens the gel, but retards the setting of dental stone model materials (Section 40.2.6)
Potassium sulphate	2	To accelerate the setting of stone (Section 40.2.6)
Water	83.8	Dispersion medium

26.2.2 Manipulation

(a) The material is supplied in sealed containers to prevent evaporation of water. It is brought to a fluid state by heating the tube in boiling water for about 10 minutes.
(b) It is mixed thoroughly by manipulation of the tube, allowed to cool to 45°C and then exuded from the tube into the impression tray.
(c) It is allowed to gel in the mouth after insertion and seating of the tray.

(d) The gel formation is rather slow, and may be speeded up by either:

- (i) spraying cold water on the tray, or
- (ii) having trays which contain channels in which cold water is circulated.

A higher temperature is required for the conversion of gel to sol than for the reverse reaction.

26.2.3 Properties

(a) Accuracy

- (i) Rheological properties: the material can be sufficiently fluid to record fine detail if it has been correctly manipulated.
- (ii) The first material to set is that which is in contact with the tray (contrast with alginates, Section 26.3.3) since this is cooler than the tissues. Thus the material in contact with the tissues stays liquid for the longest time, and can flow to compensate for any inaccuracy due to dimensional changes, or to inadvertent movement of the tray.
- (iii) The set material can be withdrawn over undercuts. The adhesion of agar to metal is poor, so perforated trays are used.
- (iv) Models should be cast up immediately from agar impressions, to avoid the possibility of syneresis or imbibition.
- (v) The compatibility with model materials depends on the chemicals in the impression material. Without an accelerator for the setting of stone (e.g. K_2SO_4) a soft surface may be obtained.

(b) Other properties

- (i) These materials are non-toxic and non-irritant.
- (ii) Their setting time is rather slow, unless efficient cooling is achieved.
- (iii) Their shelf-life is adequate. The material can be reused and can be sterilised. Loss of water, with an increase in viscosity of the sol, may occur. Water can be added if required.

26.2.4 Applications

These materials may be used to some extent for prosthetic impressions, and in crown and bridge work. They have been largely superseded by alginates (Section 26.3) and elastomers (Chapter 27) for clinical use. Agars can be employed in the laboratory, for model duplication, since they can be re-used many times, due to the reversible nature of the reaction. Recently, techniques have been reported on the use of agar in conjunction with alginates—See Section 26.3.5(c).

26.3 ALGINATES

26.3.1 Composition and setting

The composition of these materials is given in Table 26.2.

Table 26.2 Composition of alginate impression materials

Constituent	Approx. %	Function
Soluble salt of alginic acid (a polysaccharide, (Appendix III) e.g. sodium, potassium or ammonium alginate*	12	Reacts with Ca^{2+} to give calcium alginate gel (equation (1)
Slowly soluble calcium salt (e.g. $CaSO_4, 2H_2O$)	12	Releases Ca^{2+} to react with alginate
Trisodium phosphate	2	Reacts with Ca^{2+} to give $Ca_3(PO_4)_2$ (equation (2), to delay gel formation
Filler (e.g. diatomaceous earth)	70	Increases cohesion of mix and strengthens gel
Silico fluorides, or fluorides	Small quantity	Improves surface of stone model
Flavouring agents	Small quantity	Makes material more acceptable to patient
Chemical indicator present in some materials	Small quantity	Changes colour with pH change, to indicate different stages in manipulation, e.g. violet colour during spatulation, pink when ready to load the tray, white when ready for insertion into the mouth.

* Alternative materials have been suggested—e.g. the triethanol amine salt of alginic acid

On mixing the powder with water a sol is formed, and the alginate, the calcium salt and the phosphate begin to dissolve. The following reaction occurs to form an elastic gel of calcium alginate:

$$Na_nAlg + \frac{n}{2} CaSO_4 \longrightarrow \frac{n}{2} Na_2SO_4 + Ca_{n/2}Alg \quad \ldots (1)$$

Only the outer layer of each particle of sodium alginate dissolves and reacts.

However, the above reaction is liable to occur during the mixing and tray-loading procedures. This is obviously undesirable, since the material should deform plastically, not elastically, on insertion into the mouth. Gel formation is delayed by trisodium phosphate, which reacts with the calcium sulphate to give a precipitate of calcium phosphate, as follows:

$$2Na_3PO_4 + 3CaSO_4 \longrightarrow Ca_3(PO_4)_2 + 3Na_2SO_4 \quad \ldots . (2)$$

This latter reaction does not contribute any elastic properties to the material.

Reaction (2) occurs in preference to (1); no substantial quantity of calcium alginate gel is formed until the trisodium phosphate is used up. The manufacturer can therefore control the setting time of his product by adjusting the quantity of this constituent.

The fibrils of the set gel are linked together by the calcium ions; each divalent Ca^{2+} ion is linked to two carboxyl ($—COO^-$) groups, each from a different polysaccharide molecule.

26.3.2 Manipulation

The following points should be observed in order to obtain the best results:

(a) The container of powder should be shaken before use to get an even distribution of constituents.

(b) The powder and water should be measured, as directed by the manufacturer. One brand of powder has been supplied in water soluble sachets, which helps to ensure a uniform consistency of mix.

(c) Room-temperature water is usually used; slower or faster setting times can be achieved, if required, by using cooler or warmer water respectively.

(d) Retention to the tray is achieved by one or both of two means:

(i) perforated trays,

(ii) an adhesive such as molten sticky wax or methyl cellulose.

(e) There should be vigorous mixing—by spreading the material against the side of the bowl—for the stipulated time, usually one minute.

(f) An alginate impression should be displaced sharply from the tissues—this sudden displacement ensures the best elastic behaviour. The impression is removed about two minutes after it first appears to be elastic.

(g) On removal from the mouth, the impression should be:
  (i) washed with cold water to remove saliva,
  (ii) covered with a damp napkin to prevent syneresis, and,
  (iii) cast up as soon as possible, preferably not more than 15 minutes after taking the impression.

26.3.3 Properties

(a) Accuracy
  (i) Rheological properties: alginates are sufficiently fluid to record fine detail in the mouth. The viscosity-time curve shows a well defined working time, during which there is no viscosity change (Fig. 26.1).
  (ii) During setting of the material it is important that the impression should not be moved. The reaction is faster at higher temperatures (Fig. 26.1) and so the material in contact with the tissues sets first (contrast with agar materials, Section 26.2.3). Any pressure on the gel due to movement of the tray will set up stresses within the material, which will distort the alginate after its removal from the mouth.

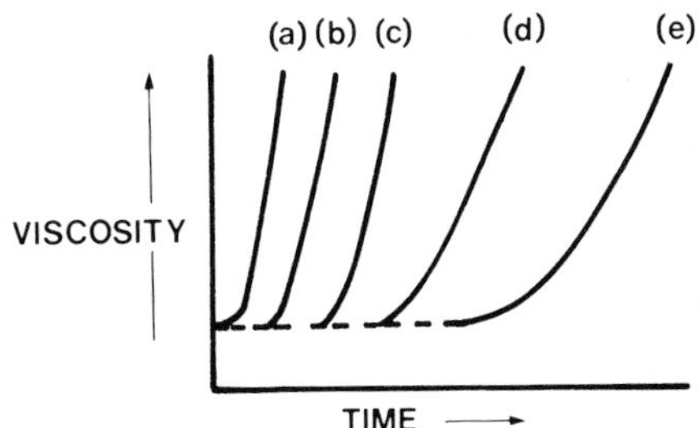

Fig. 26.1 Viscosity-time curves for an alginate impression material at various temperatures (a) 37°C (b) 20°C (c) 15.5°C (d) 11.5°C (e) 7°C. (After Fish and Braden. 1964 J. Dent. Res., 43: 107)

  (iii) The material is sufficiently elastic to be withdrawn over undercuts; occasionally tearing of the impression material may occur with servere undercuts. Adhesion to the tray has already been considered (Section 26.3.2); the cellulose adhesives, though often effective, can be difficult to clean from the tray.
  (iv) Alginates are not dimensionally stable on storage, due to syneresis.

(v) Compatibility with plaster and stone can be good; some alginates give a powdery surface on models from some dental stones.

(b) Other properties

(i) The materials are non-toxic and non-irritant; their taste and odour is usually acceptable.

(ii) The setting time depends on the composition (e.g. the trisodium phosphate content), and on the temperature of mixing.

(iii) The alginate powder is not stable on storage in the presence of moisture or in conditions warmer than room temperature.

26.3.4 Applications

These materials are not generally used for impressions for inlay, crown and bridge work, but are applied with great success for prosthetic and orthodontic purposes. Alginates are dimensionally less stable than the elastomers (Chapter 27).

26.3.5 Recent developments

(a) Dustless alginates. Some recent materials have been developed which give off little or no dust particles, so avoiding dust inhalation. This can be achieved by coating the material with a glycol.
(b) Siliconised alginates. Two paste alginates have been developed, which incorporate a silicone polymer component. These materials have superior resistance to tearing compared to unmodified alginates.
(c) A combination reversible hydrocolloid/alginate impression technique has been developed, for example, for inlay impressions. The agar material is injected on to the preparation, and an alginate on an impression tray positioned over it. The alginate assists the cooling of the agar. Good bonding between the hydrocolloids is essential. It is claimed that this technique eliminates the need for water cooled trays (Section 26.2.2).

READING REFERENCE

Braden M 1975 Impression materials. Inivon Fraunhafer J A (ed) Scientific aspects of dental materials Butterworth London, ch 13

The opening section of this chapter deals with the composition of, and recent developments in, alginate impression materials.

Miller M 1975 Syneresis in alginate impression materials. British Dental Journal 139: 425

This paper discusses the causes of syneresis, and gives data on the magnitude of this effect for currently available materials.

27. Elastomeric materials

27.1 CHEMISTRY OF THE POLYSULPHIDES

(Alternative names: rubber-base, mercaptan, thiokol.)

27.1.1 Composition

These materials are supplied as two pastes.

(a) The base paste contains:

(i) A polysulphide, such as:

$$HS\!-\!(CH_2\!-\!CH_2\!-\!O\!-\!CH_2\!-\!CH_2\!-\!S\!-\!S)_n\!-\!\underset{\displaystyle SH}{\overset{\displaystyle C_2H_5}{\underset{|}{\overset{|}{C}}}}\!-\!(S\!-\!S\!-\!CH_2\!-\!CH_2\!-\!O\!-\!CH_2\!-\!CH_2)_m\!-\!SH$$

This may be called a mercaptan, since it contains -SH groups. Two of these groups are *terminal*, one is *pendant*.

(ii) A filler, between 11 to 54%, for different materials, are not zinc oxide and calcium sulphate, as reported in the earlier dental literature; titanium dioxide is one example of a filler. The base paste is usually coloured white, due to the colour of the filler.

(b) The reactor paste (sometimes called 'accelerator' or 'catalyst' paste). This contains:

(i) Lead dioxide (PbO_2)—this causes polymerisation and

cross-linking, by oxidation of -SH groups (see below). Copper salts are present in one product.
(ii) Sulphur, which facilitates the reaction.
(iii) An oil, (an ester or chlorinated paraffin) to make a paste, but not castor oil as once believed.

This paste is brown coloured due to the lead dioxide.

27.1.2 Setting

The -SH groups can be oxidised by PbO_2, giving S—S linkages, as follows:

$$SH \; HS \longrightarrow -S-S- \; + \; H_2O$$

This means that the polysulphide paste will:

(i) Polymerise further, due to oxidation of the terminal-SH groups.
(ii) Cross-link, due to oxidation of pendant -SH groups; it has already been shown that some cross-linking is necessary for an elastomer (Section 8.5 and 8.6.2). The percentage of cross-links will depend on the values of m and n in the formula of the polysulphide above, that is, on the initial chain length of the polysulphide.

27.1.3 Modifications

(a) One material avoids the use of PbO_2, and replaces it by an organic reactor, such as cumene hydroperoxide or t-butyl hydroperoxide. However, this constituent is volatile, and its loss by evaporation leads to shrinkage of the set mass.
(b) A recently developed polysulphide replaces the lead dioxide by a zinc carbonate/organic accelerator system. It is claimed that this is much cleaner to handle than a conventional polysulphide.

27.2 CHEMISTRY OF THE SILICONES

27.2.1 Composition

(a) The base paste contains:

(i) a silicone polymer with terminal hydroxy groups, for example:

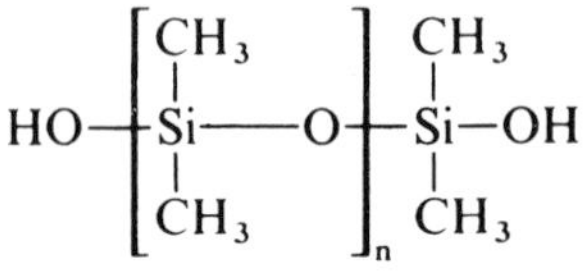

$$HO-\left[\begin{array}{c} CH_3 \\ | \\ Si \\ | \\ CH_3 \end{array}-O\right]_n-\begin{array}{c} CH_3 \\ | \\ Si \\ | \\ CH_3 \end{array}-OH$$

(ii) a filler.

(b) The reactor paste (or liquid) contains:

(i) A cross-linking agent; either an alkoxy ortho-silicate (or a polymer of it), or an organohydrogen siloxane, for example:

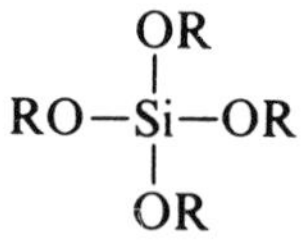

$$RO-\begin{array}{c} OR \\ | \\ Si \\ | \\ OR \end{array}-OR$$

(alkoxy ortho-silicate)

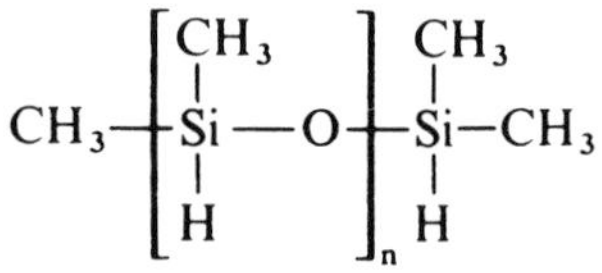

$$CH_3-\left[\begin{array}{c} CH_3 \\ | \\ Si \\ | \\ H \end{array}-O\right]_n-\begin{array}{c} CH_3 \\ | \\ Si \\ | \\ H \end{array}-CH_3$$

(organohydrogen siloxane)

This latter compound may be written in a simplified form:

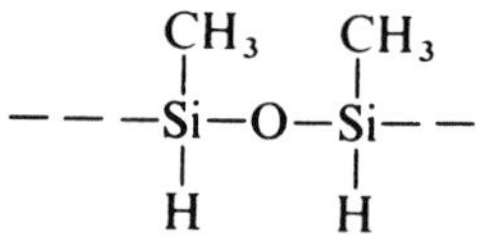

$$---\begin{array}{c} CH_3 \\ | \\ Si \\ | \\ H \end{array}-O-\begin{array}{c} CH_3 \\ | \\ Si \\ | \\ H \end{array}--$$

(ii) An activator usually an organo-tin compound, such as dibutyl-tin dilaurate.

27.2.2 Setting reactions

Cross-linking occurs on mixing the two materials together, e.g. either

~~~~OH + OR OR Si OR OR + HO~~~~
~~~~OH

(2 chains of silicone polymer) + (cross linking agent) + (one chain of silicone polymer)

⟶ ~~~~O O~~~~ Si ~~~~O OR + 3ROH

(3 chains linked together) + (alcohol)

or:

~~~~OH H—Si—CH$_3$ ⟶ ~~~~O—Si—CH$_3$ + H_2

+ O ⟶ O

~~~~OH H—Si—CH$_3$ ⟶ ~~~~O—Si—CH$_3$ + H_2

(2 chains of silicone polymer) + (organohydrogen siloxane)

27.2.3 New products

The above two cross-linking reactions occur with elimination of by-products. In the first reaction, alcohol is formed; volatilisation of this can contribute to lack of dimensional stability (Section 27.5). In the other reaction, hydrogen is produced, which can cause pitting of a dental stone surface (Section 27.5).

New products are available which polymerise by an addition reaction, so no by-products are formed. The reaction is between an organo-hydrogen siloxane and a compound with a vinyl silane group, in the presence of a precious metal catalyst (H_2PtCl_6):

$$\sim\!\sim O-\underset{CH_3}{\overset{CH_3}{|}}{Si}-H \quad + \quad CH_2=CH-\underset{CH_3}{\overset{CH_3}{|}}{Si}-O\sim\!\sim$$

(organohydrogen siloxane) (vinyl silane compound)

$$\longrightarrow \sim\!\sim O-\underset{CH_3}{\overset{CH_3}{|}}{Si}-CH_2-CH_2-\underset{CH_3}{\overset{CH_3}{|}}{Si}-O\sim\!\sim$$

Such reactions can lead to the formation of a cross-linked silicone rubber:

$$\begin{array}{l}\sim\!\sim O-\underset{R}{\overset{R}{Si}}-CH=CH_2 \;+\; H-\overset{\wr}{Si}-R \\ \qquad\qquad\qquad\qquad\qquad\quad | \\ \qquad\qquad\qquad\qquad\qquad\quad O \\ \qquad\qquad\qquad\qquad\qquad\quad | \\ \qquad\qquad\qquad\qquad\quad R-Si-H \;+\; CH_2=CH-\underset{R}{\overset{R}{Si}}-O\sim\!\sim \\ \qquad\qquad\qquad\qquad\qquad\quad | \\ \qquad\qquad\qquad\qquad\qquad\quad O \\ \qquad\qquad\qquad\qquad\qquad\quad | \\ \sim\!\sim O-\underset{R}{\overset{R}{Si}}-CH=CH_2 \;+\; H-\underset{\wr}{Si}-R\end{array}$$

$$\xrightarrow[\text{salt}]{\text{Pt}} \begin{array}{l}\sim\!\sim O-\underset{R}{\overset{R}{Si}}-CH_2-CH_2-\overset{\wr}{Si}-R \\ \qquad\qquad\qquad\qquad\qquad\qquad\quad | \\ \qquad\qquad\qquad\qquad\qquad\qquad\quad O \\ \qquad\qquad\qquad\qquad\qquad\qquad\quad | \\ \qquad\qquad\qquad\qquad\qquad\qquad\quad Si-CH_2-CH_2-\underset{R}{\overset{R}{Si}}-O\sim\!\sim \\ \qquad\qquad\qquad\qquad\qquad\qquad\quad | \\ \qquad\qquad\qquad\qquad\qquad\qquad\quad O \\ \qquad\qquad\qquad\qquad\qquad\qquad\quad | \\ \sim\!\sim O-\underset{R}{\overset{R}{Si}}-CH_2-CH_2-\underset{\wr}{Si}-R\end{array}$$

27.3 POLYETHERS

These elastomers have a *base paste* containing an unsaturated polyether with imine end groups (Appendix III, no. 14), a plasticiser and a filler. The *reactor paste* has an aromatic sulphonate as its chief constituent, together with a plasticiser and an inorganic filler. Setting occurs by a cross-linking reaction of the imine groups; this is a cationic polymerisation reaction (Section 8.4.2).

27.4 MANIPULATION

(a) Uniform mixing (as with zinc oxide–eugenol pastes, Section 25.3), is required.
(b) Retention of the material on the tray is achieved by use of an adhesive, such as a rubber solution.
(c) Ideally there should be a uniform thickness (2 to 3 mm) of impression material.
(d) Elastomers should be displaced sharply from the tissues to ensure elastic behaviour.

27.5 PROPERTIES

The general properties of elastomers are discussed in Section 8.6.2.
(a) Accuracy
 (i) The fluidity of these materials depends largely on their composition. Some polysulphides are supplied in a range of viscosities, for example, light bodied for injection by a syringe, and medium and heavy bodied for use on a tray. Some materials are supplied with a diluent to enable the operator to alter the viscosity of the mixed material as required. Silicones are also supplied with a range of consistencies including putty type and lower viscosity materials. (Table 27.1) In general, elastomers can record fine detail.

Table 27.1 Apparent viscosities of unmixed impression pastes at a shear rate of 65 s^{-1} and 25°C

Grade of material	Typical range of apparent viscosity values (Nsm^{-2})
Putty	400–700
Heavy bodied	200–300
Regular	40–150
Light bodied and wash materials	10– 70

* from Combe and Moser, J. Dent. Res., 57, 233, 1978.

Unmixed elastomer pastes are usually pseudoplastic in nature.

(ii) There is a small contraction on setting of these materials, due to polymerisation shrinkage. Contraction also occurs on cooling the impression from mouth to room temperature. The coefficient of thermal expansion of these materials is in the order:

$$\text{polyether} > \text{silicone} > \text{polysulphide}$$

The magnitude of the thermal shrinkage is reduced by the adhesion of the material to the tray.

(iii) These materials are sufficiently elastic to be withdrawn over undercuts, and are usually tougher and less likely to tear than the alginates. Polyether materials are stiffer than the other elastomers, therefore are more difficult to withdraw. Adhesives are supplied with most materials.

(iv) On storage, contraction can result from further polymerisation of the material. Evaporation of volatile by-products (e.g. alcohol, Section 27.2.2) is another source of shrinkage. The dimensional stability of polyethers is poor in the presence of moisture.

(v) These materials are in general compatible with model and die materials, though they can cause a small degree of softening of a dental stone surface (Section 40.2.10). In early silicones evolution of hydrogen from materials containing an organo-hydrogen siloxane caused pitting of stone surfaces. Present day silicones either do not use this system, or contain a compound to react with hydrogen as soon as it is generated. These impression materials can be electroplated, to give metal coated dies (Section 40.3.5).

(b) Other properties

(i) In general these materials are non-toxic and non-irritant. The odour and taste of some pastes containing lead dioxide is not pleasant.

(ii) The setting time depends on the composition of the material (for example, the quantity of reactors, etc.). Also, the presence of water, and high temperatures accelerate the setting of polysulphides.

(iii) Stability on storage of the unmixed materials is not always ideal; some of the reactors are unstable over a two-year period, but keep better if stored in a refrigerator.

27.6 APPLICATIONS

The chief use of elastomers is in impressions for inlays, crowns and bridges, or for partial dentures when the under-cuts are so severe that alginates would tear on removal from the tissues. Because of their expense, these materials are not frequently used in impressions requiring large quantities of material.

27.7 SUGGESTED NEW MATERIALS

It has been suggested that polyolefine rubbers could be used for dental applications. Research is being conducted to obtain a very elastic material which can be cross-linked with small dimensional changes and without the formation of volatile by-products.

READING REFERENCES

Braden M, Causton B, Clarke R L 1972 A polyether impression rubber. Journal of dental research 51: 889

The composition and properties of polyethers are discussed.

Braden M 1975 Impression materials. In: von Fraunhofer J A (ed) Scientific aspects of dental materials. Butterworth, London, Ch 13

A section of this chapter gives extensive information on the chemistry, formulation, setting and properties of impression rubbers.

Braden M 1976 The quest for a new impression rubber. Journal of dentistry 4: 1

This paper deals with the chemical development of elastomers, including polyethers, developments in polysulphides and new silicones. Materials not yet used in dentistry, but which have promising properties, are considered.

Brown D 1973 Factors influencing the dimensional stability of elastic impression materials. Journal of dentistry 1: 265

As analysis of all the factors that can affect dimensional accuracy and stability of elastic impression materials.

SECTION V

Inlay, crown and bridge materials

28. Dental porcelain

28.1 APPLICATIONS OF PORCELAIN

Porcelain is used:

(a) For the construction of jacket crowns
(b) As a veneer over metallic restorations (Ch. 30)
(c) As a tooth material for dentures (Ch. 37)

28.2 CLASSIFICATION AND COMPOSITION

28.2.1 Introduction

Traditionally household porcelain is made from about 50% by mass, kaolin, 25% feldspar and 25% quartz. The functions of these ceramic raw materials are discussed in Section 12.2.

Dental products differ from the above in that little or no kaolin is present. They may thus be more accurately described as glasses than porcelains. The dental laboratory is supplied with a powdered material. This is a *frit*, which has been prepared by the manufacturer by (i) blending the raw materials (ii) melting them together in a refractory crucible, during which procedure the fluxes partially combine with the silica—these high temperature reactions are termed *pyrochemical reactions*; and (iii) quenching the red-hot glass to break it up.

28.2.2 Methods of classificaton

The porcelain powder is mixed with water to form a slurry which is adapted as a plastic mass to the requisite shape prior to firing in an oven (Sections 12.3.1 and 28.3).

According to a standard specification, the available materials may be classified according to their temperatures of fusion in the dental laboratory:

(a) high-fusing 1200–1400°C
(b) medium-fusing 1050–1200°C
(c) low-fusing 800–1050°C

However, it is now rare to find a porcelain with a firing temperature in excess of 1200°C.

Classification can also be made according to applicaton:

(a) Core porcelain—the basis of a porcelain jacket crown; must have good mechanical properties.
(b) Dentine or body porcelain—more translucent than the above; this largely governs the shape and colour of the restoration.
(c) Enamel porcelain forms the outer part of the crown, and is quite translucent.

Another difference between materials is in the method of firing:

(a) at atmospheric pressure
(b) at reduced pressure—vacuum firing.

28.2.3 Composition

A typical modern porcelain, medium-fusing, for vacuum firing will contain the following oxide composition (figures are % by mass): SiO_2 65; Al_2O_3 19; fluxes (B_2O_3, K_2O, Na_2O, MgO, Li_2O, P_2O_5) 16.

The above material is *non-aluminous*. Although Al_2O_3 is present, there is no free alumina, since it is part of the glass network. In the 1960's, *aluminous porcelain* was developed. This is a material, similar to the above, but strengthened by the incorporation of 40 to 50% by mass by crystalline alumina (Section 12.2). Alumina has a higher compressive, tensile and flexural strength than conventional porcelain. Its incorporation hinders crack propagation within the material, so acting as a strengthening agent.

28.2.4 Other components

(a) Pigments are present to give the required colour; these are fused in the glassy material. Examples: the oxides of chromium, cobalt, nickel, titanium and iron (II) oxide.
(b) Oxides such as that of titanium can be used to opacify the material.
(c) Glazes and stains may also be used to achieve required aesthetic effects (Section 12.3.2).
(d) Sugar or starch may be included to act as a binder.

28.3 MANIPULATION

28.3.1 Compacting (or condensation)

In the construction of a porcelain jacket crown, the plastic mass of powder and water is applied to the die which has been coated with platinum foil. Compacting is carried out for the following reasons:
(a) To adapt the material to the requisite shape.
(b) To remove as much water from the material as possible. On firing there is a volumetric shrinkage of 30 to 40%; the more water removed, the less is this contraction.

The following methods of compacting have been suggested for use:
(a) Dry powder can be sprinkled on to the surface of the wet material. This helps to remove water by capillary action.
(b) Excess water can be blotted off the material after compressing it, or whipping it with a brush.
(c) Vibration may be used to help the powder particles settle; this method is also used in the construction of artificial teeth (Section 37.2).

The success of compacting depends not only on the skill of the operator, but also on the range of sizes of the powder particles. It has been shown theoretically that if all the particles are of approximately the same size, 45% of a given volume will consist of voids (Fig. 28.1). If a number of smaller particles are blended with larger ones, the void space is considerably reduced (Fig. 28.2). Three or more particle sizes achieve an even greater degree of compaction (Fig. 28.3).

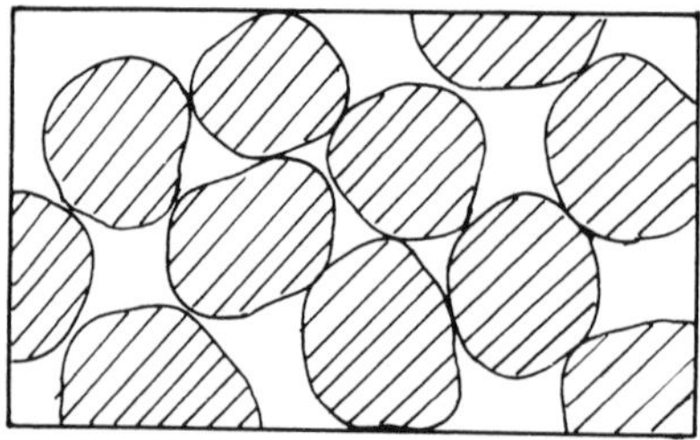

Fig. 28.1 Packing of particles of approximately the same size; the voids occupy approximately 45%.

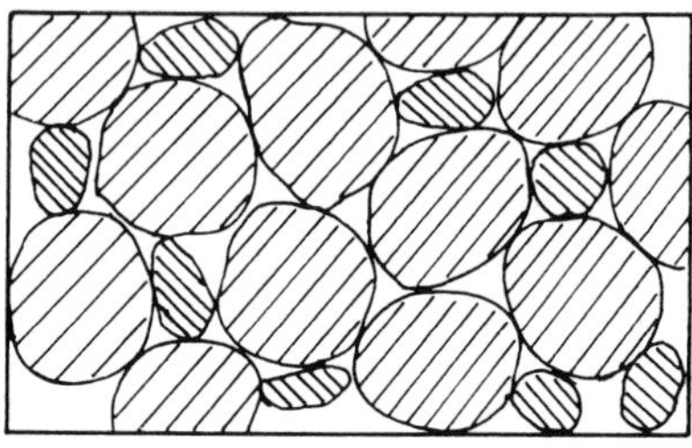

Fig. 28.2 Packing of particles of two different sizes—volume of voids considerably less.

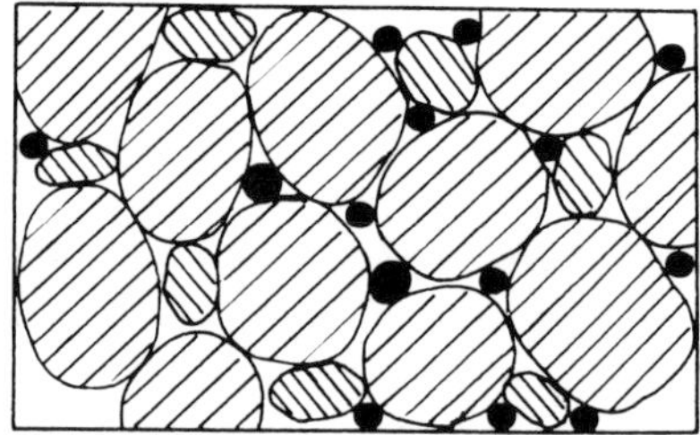

Fig. 28.3 Packing of particles of three different sizes—much greater degree of compaction.

28.3.2 Firing

This is carried out in an electrically heated muffle furnace. The heating element may be made of:

(a) Nickle-chromium alloys, suitable for the lower fusing porcelains.

(b) Platinum or platinum alloys, where higher temperatures are required,

The following practical points are important:

(a) The compacted porcelain should be placed on a fire-clay tray, and not be permitted to come into contact with the floor or walls of

the furnace. The heating element will become brittle if porcelain fuses on to it.
(b) The initial rates of heating should be slow, otherwise the water will be converted to steam so rapidly that the unfired restoration will crumble.
(c) Uniform heating is desirable. Since the thermal conductivity of porcelain is low, slow heating is desirable to give sufficient time for the interior of the porcelain to heat up.
(d) Initially the furnace door should be left open to allow steam and the combustion products of any binders to escape.

The following stages can be recognised in firing porcelain:
(a) *Low bisque* or *low biscuit* stage, when the material develops some rigidity and the fluxes have started to flow.
(b) *Medium bisque* or *medium biscuit* stage, when some shrinkage has occurred and there is greater cohesion between the particles.
(c) *High bisque* or *high biscuit* stage—at this stage no further shrinkage will occur.

28.3.3 Cooling

Cooling must be carried out slowly and uniformly, otherwise different portions will shrink to different extents, leading to stresses which can cause cracking and a loss in strength.

28.3.4 Glazes and stains

The firing shrinkage is compensated for by adding more porcelain to the fired restoration and re-firing. When the final desired size is achieved, a smooth surface is desirable to prevent food clinging to the restoration. Polishing may not achieve a satisfactory surface due to the presence of porosity (Section 28.4.2).

The desired surface finish can be achieved by either:
(a) Heating under controlled conditions (rapid heat up to the fusion temperature, this temperature maintained for about five minutes) which causes the surface to flow and become smooth. Prolonged heating can result in *pyroplastic flow*—flow of the material at high temperatures, which causes rounding of sharp angles and edges of the restoration.

or: Gross overheating may result in complete loss of form;
(b) Applying a *glaze*, an almost transparent ceramic, to the surface, and re-firing. A glaze is composed of low fusing fluxes and silica. Before glazing, a *stain* may be painted on to the porcelain surface, to

imitate stains or developmental faults and features of the natural teeth. The stain is suspended in a liquid which will evaporate during firing.

28.4 PROPERTIES

28.4.1 Shrinkage on firing

During firing any residual water is lost from the material (as already discussed, Section 28.3.1), accompanied by loss of any binders which may be present. Volume shrinkage is of the order of 30 to 40%, principally due to elimination of voids during sintering. Porcelain is not popular for inlay constuction because of the great difficulty of achieving the required degree of accuracy.

28.4.2 Porosity

Inevitably in a fired porcelain there are present numerous air bubbles. This can weaken the material, and reduce its translucency. Research workers have suggested the following methods of reducing porosity, the first of which is frequently used in the dental laboratory:

(a) Firing in a vacuum to remove air.
(b) Firing in the presence of a gas which will be able to diffuse out of the porcelain.
(c) Cooling under pressure to reduce the magnitude of the pores.

28.4.3 Chemical properties

One of the chief attractions of porcelain as a dental material is that it is chemically indestructible in most environments (Section 12.9.1).

28.4.4 Mechanical properties

As outlined in Section 12.9.2, porcelain is essentially a brittle material; developments in ceramics over the last few years have been directed to the attainment of improved mechanical properties as in the aluminous materials (Section 28.2.3).

28.4.5 Thermal properties

The low thermal conductivity of porcelain has been referred to earlier (Section 12.9.3 and 28.3.2). The coefficient of thermal expansion is close to that of enamel and dentine (Section 12.9.3 and Appendix II).

28.4.6 Aesthetics

The aesthetics of porcelain itself are excellent (Section 12.9.4). Nevertheless, if the cement dissolves, the crevice formed at the margin of the restoration will be discoloured by debris.

28.5 RECENT DEVELOPMENTS

28.5.1 Castable glass-ceramics

Castable glass-ceramics (section 12.5) are being used for full veneer crown work.

28.5.2 Non-shrink alumina ceramics

These products contain aluminium oxide, magnesium oxide and a barium glass.

On firing, a magnesium aluminate spinel is formed, and the expansion associated with this compositional change can compensate for firing shrinkage (Section 28.4.1). (*Spinel* is the name given to the mineral $MgAl_2O_4$.)

28.5.3 Critique

Both the above materials have the merit of producing very accurate restorations. At the time of writing, two limitations should be noted:
(a) Neither material appears to be strong enough for use in the molar area or for bridgework.
(b) Aesthetic problems may arise; it is difficult to obtain colour control for glass-ceramics, whilst the alumina ceramics are quite opaque.

READING REFERENCE

British Standards Institution 1982 Guide to the use of dental materials. BSI PD 6502: 1982

Secton 24 of this guide gives valuable information on the composition, manipulation and properties of dental porcelain.

Southan D E 1970 The development and characteristics of dental porcelain. Australian Dental Journal 15: 103

A historical background to the development of dental porcelain.

McLean J W 1979 The science and art of dental ceramics, Vol. 1, The nature of ceramics and their clinical use. Quintessence, Chicago

This book contains four monographs:
I The nature of dental ceramics
II Strengthening of dental porcelain
III Aesthetics of dental porcelain
IV Porcelain as a restorative material.

29. Alloys for inlays, crowns and bridges

29.1 REQUIREMENTS

In this chapter, alloys for casting inlays, crowns and bridges are considered. In chapters 30 and 35, other casting alloys are discussed. Before reading this chapter, the principles of metallurgy should be thoroughly studied (Chs. 9–11); in particular, the sections on the effects of alloying elements on gold (Sections 10.4 and 10.5). The reader should also be familiar with the principles of metal casting, and faults which can occur in this procedure (Ch. 43).

Casting alloys should have the following desirable properties:

(a) Biocompatibility; specifically, they should be non-allergenic, and should not contain toxic components which can be dangerous in the dental laboratory during grinding and polishing procedures.

(b) Good corrosion and tarnish resistance.

(c) Suitable mechanical properties, for example:

- (i) High yield stress if the cast restoration is to be subjected to large forces *in situ*.
- (ii) If the alloy is insufficiently ductile, it may fracture during burnishing procedures (Section 45.4).
- (iii) Hardness of the alloys is an indication of the difficulty of grinding and finishing of the alloy.

(d) Ease of casting—alloys of high density and good fluidity when molten are easier to cast.

(e) Cost—ideally, alloys should be inexpensive, both in terms of material and labour costs.

29.2 GOLD ALLOYS WITH AT LEAST 75% NOBLE METALS

29.2.1 Introduction

The proportion of gold in alloy may be designated in one of two ways:

(a) The *carat* rating expresses the number of 24th parts of gold in the alloy: for example, 24 carat gold is pure gold, 18 carat gold contains 18/24th or 75% gold.

(b) The *fineness* rating is the parts per thousand of gold; for example, 24 carat gold is 1000 fine, and 18 carat gold is 750 fine.

29.2.2 Classification and composition

Table 29.1 shows the approximate compositions of the various types of dental gold alloys.

29.2.3 Dental uses

(a) Type I alloys are used in situations where they are not subjected to great stress, as in Class III and Class V cavities.

(b) Type II alloys are widely used for most types of inlay.

(c) Type III alloys are used for crowns and bridges, and in situations where there may be great stresses involved.

(d) Type IV alloys are used for cast partial dentures and clasps; these are discussed further in Section 35.2.

29.2.4 Heat treatment

The properties of an alloy depend on:

(a) its composition, as in Table 29.1,

(b) its mechanical history, for example, the extent to which it has been work hardened (Section 9.6), and,

(c) its thermal history, for example, the temperature to which it has been heated, and its rate of cooling.

Heat treatments can be carried out on some gold alloys to improve their mechanical properties. This is carried out for class IV alloys, and is discussed in detail in Section 35.2.3. Type I and II alloys, in the as-cast condition, have usually adequate mechanical properties for their various applications. The properties of type III alloys can be improved by heat treatment.

Table 29.1* Dental gold alloys

Type	Description	Minimum total amount of noble metals (%)	Au(%)	Ag(%)	Cu(%)	Pt(%)	Pd(%)	Zn(%)
I (or A)	Soft	83	80–90	3–12	2–5	Little or none	Little or none	Little or none
II (or B)	Medium	78	75–78	12–15	7–10	0–1	1–4	0–1
III (or C)	Hard	78	62–78	8–26	8–11	0–3	2–4	1
IV (or D)	Extra hard	75	60–70	4–20	11–16	0–4	0–5	1–2

* Data adapted from Crowell W S 1961 Gold alloys in dentistry. Metals Handbook. 8th edn., vol. I. Properties and selection of metals. American Society for Metals, Metals Park, Ohio, p 1188-1189

29.2.5 Mechanical properties

Table 29.2 gives the mechanical properties of types I and III alloys. For comparison, data is given for heat hardened alloys of type III. Similar data for type IV alloys is in Table 35.1.

Table 29.2* Mechanical properties of gold alloys

Type	Proportional limit (MN/m^2)	Ultimate tensile strength (MN/m^2)	Elongation (%)	Hardness (BHN)
I (as cast)	85	200	25	40–75
II (as cast)	160	345	24	70–100
III (softened)	195	365	20	90–140
III (hardened)	290	445	10	120–170

* See Crowell, W. S. (1961) Gold alloys in dentistry. Metal Handbook, 8th edn., vol. I. Properties and Selection of Metals, pp. 1188–1189. Metals Park, Ohio: American Society for Metals.

29.2.6 Some practical precautions

To obtain a successful cast restoration, attention must be given to manipulative variables associated with the impression and die materials (as in the indirect technique), inlay wax (in both the direct and indirect technique) and investment materials. The following points in relation to the manipulation of gold alloys are important:

(a) Melting can be carried out by an air/gas torch. It is important that:
   (i) the alloy is sufficiently heated to render it completely molten, otherwise an incomplete casting may result,
   (ii) overheating is avoided to reduce the likelihood of contamination of castings as a result of oxidation,
   (iii) the reducing zone of the flame is used, and,
   (iv) flux should be applied to prevent oxidation.

(b) Re-use of surplus alloy. Inevitably there is surplus alloy removed from a casting. This alloy can be re-used, provided that:
   (i) surplus alloys of different types are not mixed, and,
   (ii) the alloy is not melted more than two or three times, otherwise zinc (a scavenger for oxygen) may be lost by volatilisation.

A mixture of new and used alloy is commonly used.

29.2.7 Critique

In most respects, gold alloys are ideal for oral use. However, in recent years, economic considerations have led to the quest for less expensive materials as detailed in the Sections below.

29.3 OTHER ALLOYS

29.3.1 Medium and low gold alloys

Medium gold alloys contain around 50% gold, with palladium, silver, copper and zinc. Other alloys contain lesser amounts of gold—see Section 29.3.2. There is an approximate linear relationship between gold content and density—see reference at the end of the chapter. The alloys with less gold content are more prone to show tarnish, although few comparative data are available.

29.3.2 Silver palladium alloys

These alloys contain silver, palladium (at least 25%), and gold, copper, indium and zinc. They are more difficult to cast than gold alloys, owing to their density, and to the dissolution of oxygen by molten alloys, resulting in porosity in casting.

29.3.3 Nickel–chromium alloys

These alloys contain about 75% nickel and 20% chromium. They are used in resin bonded techniques (Section 31.3), and can also be applied for porcelain bonding; a critique of them is given in Section 30.2.6.

29.3.4 Miscellaneous materials

Other alloys which are being used, or which have been suggested include:

(a) Copper–zinc (brass) with indium and nickel
(b) Silver–indium with palladium
(c) Aluminium bronze.

READING REFERENCE

Cruickshanks–Boyd O W 1981 Alternatives to gold 1. Non-porcelain alloys Dental Update 8: 17

This is a comprehensive review of the desirable properties of alloys, with much detailed information on the composition and properties of individual alloys, and a critique of the available materials.

30. Porcelain bonded to alloys

30.1 INTRODUCTION

In general, alloys have good mechanical properties, and porcelain can have excellent aesthetics. Techniques are available in which porcelain is fired on to a surface of a cast restoration, in attempts to obtain a strong and aesthetic restoration.

30.2 TYPES OF ALLOY

30.2.1 Requirements

(a) Good corrosion resistance.
(b) High melting range, so that no melting or permanent deformation will occur during fusion of the porcelain.
(c) Close matching of thermal properties of alloy and porcelain (see below).
(d) High modulus of elasticity (minimum elastic deformation) and high yield stress (no plastic deformation), to avoid excess stress on the porcelain, which is brittle (Section 28.4.4).
(e) Discolouration could occur due to the presence of copper in certain alloys. However, greening of porcelain is a common problem encountered with alloys containing silver. It should also be noted that the composition of the porcelain plays a part, some porcelains being less susceptible to silver greening than others.

30.2.2 High gold alloys

(a) Composition: 80 to 90% gold, with platinium and/or palladium to harden it (Section 10.5.2); they may contain small amounts of silver, iron, tin and indium. Iron can produce a precipitate of $FePt_3$, which has a strengthening effect. Tin and indium migrate to the surface on heating and produce oxides which aid chemical bonding of porcelain to alloy (Section 30.4.1).

(b) Merits:
  (i) good corrosion resistance
  (ii) good bonding to porcelain

(c) Limitations:
  (i) creep of alloy may occur during firing of porcelain, since alloys have a comparatively low melting range
  (ii) low modulus, thus minimum alloy thickness of 0.5 mm required.

30.2.3 Gold-palladium

(a) Composition: 50% (approx.) gold, 30% palladium, 10% tin and indium; remainder, silver.

(b) Properties:
  (i) better resistance to creep than high gold alloys,
  (ii) more economical than high gold alloys.

30.2.4 Palladium-silver

(a) Composition: 60% palladium, 30% silver and 10% indium and tin.

(b) Properties:
  (i) mechanical properties similar to high gold alloys,
  (ii) difficult to cast: may occlude gases; low density; high shrinkage,
  (iii) problems with 'greening' can occur when used with certain porcelain.

30.2.5 High palladium alloys

(a) Composition: at least 80% palladium with 10 to 12% tin. The alloys also contain gallium, but do not contain gold or silver.

(b) Properties:
  (i) considerably cheaper than high gold alloys; the absence of gold from the composition gives a stable price,
  (ii) silver-free, so no greening problems with porcelain,
  (iii) low density,

(iv) somewhat technique sensitive in obtaining a good bond with porcelain.

30.2.6 Nickel chromium

(a) Composition: nickel 70 to 80% (may be partially replaced by cobalt), chromium 10 to 25%; may also contain molybdenum, tungsten, manganese and beryllium and other minor components.
(b) Merits:
- (i) corrosion resistance good, owing to the passivating effect of chromium (Section 11.2.7);
- (ii) low creep during porcelain firing;
- (iii) high modulus of elasticity, so can be used in thin sections (e.g. 0.3 mm);
- (iv) high yield strength.

(c) Limitations:
- (i) nickel is allergenic;
- (ii) beryllium is toxic, so hazards arise in the laboratory when casting the alloys, and also when grinding the cast alloys;
- (iii) may be difficult to cast because of their low density and high shrinkage on cooling;
- (iv) difficult to finish because of their hardness;
- (v) adhesive failure of porcelain bond may occur (Section 30.4.2).

Note: These alloys are used in resin-bonded bridge techniques (Ch. 31).

30.3 CHOICE OF CERAMIC MATERIAL

When a porcelain (or more correctly, a glass) is used to veneer a restoration, it is important that:
(a) The porcelain should fuse at a temperature lower than the melting point of the alloy.
(b) Because it is not possible to obtain an exact match of coefficients of thermal expansion between porcelain and alloy, the latter should contract slightly more than the former, giving a degree of compressive bonding.

30.4 NATURE OF THE CERAMO-METALLIC BOND

30.4.1 Gold-porcelain bond

The observed bond between gold alloys and porcelain is believed to

result from a combination of three factors:
(a) Mechanical bonding. If the fused porcelain is able to wet the metal surface efficiently, it will flow into small irregularities on the surface, resulting in mechanical interlocking.
(b) Chemical bonding. Evidence suggests that if tin or indium is present in the alloy, it will form a surface film of oxide which can react with porcelain to give a chemical bond. In contrast to this, poorer bonding results from treating the alloy surface by acids which remove elements capable of being oxidised.
(c) Compressive bonding. If the porcelain contracts less than the alloy on cooling, in the resultant restoration the ceramic material will have a residual compressive stress. Consequently a higher applied stress is necessary to cause tensile failure of the bond.

In practice, with careful attention to detail (Section 30.5), strong bonds can be formed between gold alloys and porcelain. In testing such bonds, cohesive failure of the ceramic is usual, indicating the presence of good adhesion between the two materials.

30.4.2 Base metal alloy-porcelain bond

Strong bonds can also be formed between nickel-chromium alloys and porcelain. In contrast to the above, however, failure of such bonds occurs at the interface between metal and ceramic (that is, adhesive failure). Sudden failure of such restorations may occur because of the high degree of residual stress at the bond, or due to excessive oxidation of the alloy at the interface with the porcelain.

30.5 PRACTICAL POINTS

To obtain good bonding between gold and porcelain, it is essential:
(a) that the metal surface is degassed and free if grease and other contaminants,
(b) that strong acids are not used to clean the casting (Section 30.4.1), and,
(c) that the surface is sandblasted to aid mechanical bonding.

30.6 PORCELAIN BONDED TO PLATINUM FOIL

As an alternative to the techniques described above, porcelain can be bonded to platinum foil. The die is covered with a layer of platinum foil, as mentioned in Section 28.3.1. Then a second layer of foil is placed over all the die surfaces except the shoulder. This second layer, is bonded to the porcelain, the following procedures being carried out to both outer and inner surfaces of the foil:

(i) light abrasion to increase surface area
(ii) degreasing using sodium hydroxide solution
(iii) neutralisation of the caustic solution and thorough washing
(iv) tin plating, using a stannous sulphate solution
(v) heating *in vacuo* up to 1000°C so that the tin will alloy with the platinum
(vi) oxidation of the tin when air is permitted to enter the furnace

A porcelain crown is constructed over the double foil matrix, using a special core material developed for this procedure. The dark colour of the platinum is effectively masked by this opaque core porcelain.

The oxidised tin coating has two functions:

(i) on the outer surface, it enhances bonding to the porcelain
(ii) on the inner surface, it enables adhesion to occur between the restoration and a cement containing poly (acrylic acid) — e.g. polycarboxylate and glass-ionomer cements (Sections 17.3 and 18.3).

The technique of bonding porcelain to platinum can lead to the production of single unit crowns of good mechanical properties. The platinum can contribute to the strength of the restoration by hindering crack propagation.

READING REFERENCES

Cruikshanks-Boyd D W 1981 Alternatives to gold. 2. Porcelain bonding alloys. Dental Update 8: 111

The reader is referred to this article for detailed information on composition and properties of bonding alloys, and for an excellent critique of the available materials.

McLean J W 1975 The ceramo-metallic bond. In: von Fraunhofer J A (ed) Scientific aspects of dental materials. Butterworth, London, Ch 10

This chapter discusses the nature of the bond between gold and porcelain, in terms of mechanical, chemical and compression bonding. Such bonds are contrasted with those between base metals and porcelain. Some important technical considerations are also given.

McLean J W 1979 The science and art of dental ceramics, vol 1 the nature of ceramics and their clinical use. Quintessence, Chicago

Monograph II in this book deals specifically with strengthening of dental porcelain, including metal-ceramic systems.

31. Resin-bonded bridges

31.1 INTRODUCTION

Bridges can be bonded by composite resins to etched enamel. Three factors need to be considered in relation to the strength of the bond:
(a) The bond of composite to acid etched enamel.
(b) The strength of the composite.
(c) The strength of the bond of resin to metal.

Bonding is achieved in one of two ways:
(i) perforated castings—the so-called 'Rochette' technique. (Section 31.2)
(ii) acid etched castings—the 'Maryland' technique (Section 31.3)

31.2 PERFORATED CASTINGS (Rochette technique)

To provide mechanical locking of composite to the casting (typically of nickel–chromium alloy—Section 30.2.6), the flanges are perforated using a small rose-head tungsten carbide bur, prior to firing of porcelain on to the pontic framework.

31.3 ETCHED CASTINGS (Maryland technique)

Mechanical retention between nickel–chromium alloy and resin is achieved by electrolytic etching of the alloy (Fig. 31.1). After cleaning the alloy in ethanol, it is immersed in 0.5 nitric acid and is the anode in an electrolytic cell, the current density being 250 mA/cm^2. A stainless steel cathode is used, and an etching time of 5 minutes is required. Good bonding between metal and resin is claimed (Table 31.1).

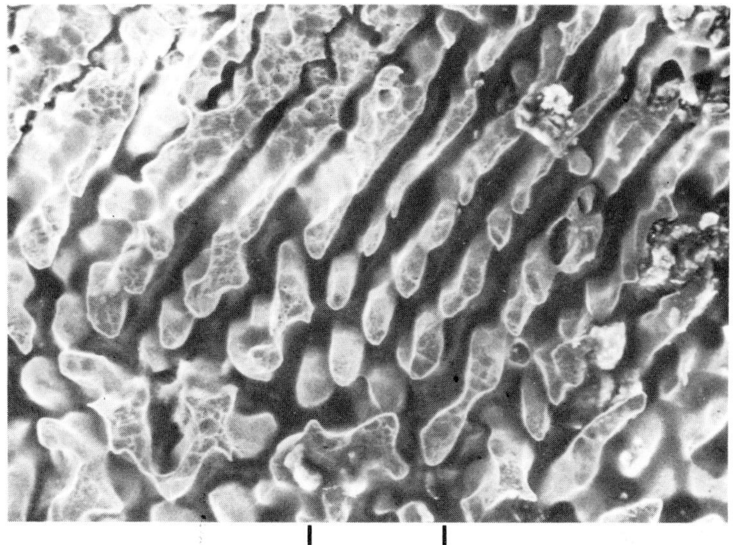

Fig. 31.1 SEM photograph of etched nickel–chromium alloy for Maryland technique.

Table 31.1 Factors involved in the strength of bond of resin to etched nickel–chromium alloy

	Tensile strength MN/m^2
Resin–enamel bond	8.5–9.9*
Composite resin	33–60**
Resin-etched metal bond	c. 27*

* Data from Livaditis G J, Thompson V P 1982 Journal of Prosthetic Dentistry 47: 52

** Data from Combe and Hannah 1976 British Dental Journal 140: 167

31.4 CEMENTATION

The composite resin cements for these applications require the following characteristics:

(a) Low film thickness.
(b) Good mechanical properties.
(c) Opacity to mask metal flanges.

31.5 APPLICATIONS

(a) To replace missing teeth.
(b) Periodontal splinting.
(c) Orthodontic retention.

31.6 CRITIQUE

(a) Minimal tooth preparation with no dentinal or pulpal involvement.
(b) Good aesthetics can be achieved.
(c) Simple fabrication technique.

REFERENCES

Livaditis G J, Thompson V P 1982 Etched castings: an improved retentive mechanism for resin-bonded retainers. Journal of Prosthetic Dentistry, 47: 52

Detailed information on the Maryland technique (Section 31.3).

Tay W M, Shaw M J 1979 The 'Rochette' adhesive bridge. Dental Update 6: 153

Detailed information on the Rochette technique (Section 31.2).

32. Polymeric crown and bridge materials

32.1 INTRODUCTION

Temporary crown and bridge materials are required during the interval between tooth preparation and cementation of the final restoration. The presence of such a material is advantageous in terms of:

(i) protection of the prepared tooth or teeth from thermal stimuli and irritant effects of chemicals
(ii) aesthetics
(iii) masticatory function
(iv) maintenance of the relationship between the prepared teeth and other teeth.

The available materials may be either:

(i) preformed, e.g. polycarbonates (Section 32.3)
(ii) fabricated from room temperature polymerising materials (Section 32.4)

32.2 REQUIREMENTS

(a) Biological considerations: non-irritant to soft tissue and the pulp.
(b) Mechanical properties: sufficiently strong to withstand the forces of mastication for a short period of time.
(c) Thermal properties: low thermal diffusivity.
(d) Manipulative characteristics: easy to manipulate in a crown former.
(e) The dimensional change on setting should be low, and the reaction should not be highly exothermic.

32.3 POLYCARBONATES

Pre-formed crowns are supplied which are made of polycarbonate (formula in Appendix III no. 30). This is a polymer with high impact resistance. These temporary crowns can be cemented in place with a self-cured acrylic polymer.

32.4 OTHER CROWN AND BRIDGE MATERIALS

32.4.1 Polymer systems

There are four types of material currently available:
(a) Poly(methyl methacrylate)—similar to the self cured acrylic filling materials (Section 19.1).
(b) Epimine resin, supplied as two components:
- (i) A base paste consisting of an ethylene imine derivative of bisphenol-A (Appendix III no. 14) with 25% powdered nylon filler.
- (ii) A 'catalyst' liquid which is an aromatic sulphonate ester.

On mixing the two together, cationic polymerisation (Section 8.4.2) occurs giving a cross-linked polymer.
(c) Two systems based on higher methacrylates—poly(ethyl methacrylate) powder plus butyl methacrylate liquid. One such system uses n-butyl methacrylate and the other has the iso-butyl compound.

32.4.2 Comparative properties

These are detailed in Table 32.1
(a) Poly(methyl methacrylate)
- (i) Disadvantages: irritant monomer; large polymerisation shrinkage; high exotherm.
- (ii) Advantage: acceptable mechanical properties.

(b) Epimine
- (i) Disadvantages: possible hypersensitivity in soft tissue; poor impact properties.
- (ii) Advantages: low polymerisation shrinkage; low exotherm.

(c) Higher methacrylate systems
- (i) Disadvantages: high polymerisation shrinkage; lower tensile strength.
- (ii) Advantages: low exotherm; more flexible and tougher than other materials.

Table 32.1 Comparative properties of temporary crown and bridge materials*

	PMMA/MMA**	Epimine	Higher methacrylate systems PEMA/n-BMA*	PEMA/iso-BMA**
Biological properties	Monomer is irritant to soft tissue and pulp.	Hypersensitivity in soft tissue has been reported.	Less pulpal response than materials with MMA	Less pulpal response than materials with MMA
Linear polymerisation shrinkage (%)	1.9	0.4	1.95	2.0
Flexural strength (MN/m^2)				
at 24 hours	60	76	104	58
at one month	43	65	107	49
Tensile strength (MN/m^2)				
at 24 hours	47	33	25	23
at one month	36	33	20	18
Impact energy (MJ/m^3)				
at 24 hours	0.46	0.28	0.58	—
Young's modulus (GN/m^2)				
at 24 hours	2.3	1.9	1.1	1.2
at one month	2.0	1.5	0.9	0.9
Approximate temperature rise on setting (°C)	46	20	20	20

* Data from Braden et al 1976 Brit Dent J., 141: 269

** MMA = methyl methacrylate; n-BMA = n-butyl methacrylate; iso-BMA = iso-butyl methacrylate; PMMA = poly(methyl methacrylate); PEMA = poly(ethyl methacrylate).

READING REFERENCE

Braden M, Clarke R L, Pearson G J, Keys W C 1976 A new temporary crown and bridge resin. British Dental Journal 141: 269

This paper describes the poly(ethyl methacrylate)—n-butyl methacrylate system and compares it with other polymers for temporary crown and bridge construction.

SECTION VI

Materials for dental protheses

33. Polymeric denture base materials

33.1 REQUIREMENTS OF POLYMERIC DENTURE BASE MATERIALS

Ideally a denture base material should possess the following properties:

(a) It should be non-toxic and non-irritant.

(b) It should be unaffected by oral fluids, that is, it should be insoluble, non-absorbent and inert.

(c) It should have adequate mechanical properties, for example:
- (i) a high modulus of elasticity, so that greater rigidity can be achieved, even in comparatively thin sections of material,
- (ii) a high proportional limit, so that the denture will not easily undergo permanent deformation when stressed,
- (iii) great strength—this is frequently measured as the transverse strength (Section 4.2),
- (iv) sufficient resilience,
- (v) high impact strength, so that the denture will not fracture if accidentally dropped, or fracture if the wearer is involved in an accident,
- (vi) high fatigue strength, and
- (vii) hard and with good abrasion resistance, so that the material will not wear appreciably, but will take and retain a high polish.

(d) The other physical properties such materials should have are:

(i) the thermal expansion of the denture base should match that of the tooth material,

(ii) the thermal conductivity should be high,

(iii) the density should be low, to assist in the retention of an upper denture, and,

(iv) the softening temperature should be higher than the temperature of liquids and foods in the mouth.

(e) It should be aesthetically satisfactory—a matter of prime importance. The material should be transparent or translucent, and easily pigmented. The colour should be permanent.

(f) Other considerations for denture base materials are:

(i) radio-opacity—if a denture or a fragment of a broken denture is accidentally inhaled or ingested, it should be capable of detection by X-rays.

(ii) a denture base material should be easy to process with the minimum of expense and equipment,

(iii) it should be easy to repair if accidentally fractured,

(iv) there should be no dimensional changes (expansion, contraction or warpage) either on processing the denture, or while it is in service, and

(v) the material should be easy to clean; the topic of denture cleansers is dealt with in Chapter 51.

No known denture material adequately fulfills all these requirements.

33.2 FORMERLY USED MATERIALS

33.2.1 Vulcanite (vulcanised rubber)

Molecules of pure rubber are long coiled chains of polyisoprene (Appendix III no. 32). The properties of rubber are altered by the addition of sulphur, which can react at a temperature of around 160°C with the double bonds of polyisoprene and also cause cross-linking, with alteration in properties. For example, with 32% sulphur, *vulcanite* is obtained; this material is sufficiently hard to be polished.

Vulcanite for dental use contains rubber with 32% sulphur, and metallic oxides to pigment the material. Vulcanisation is carried out under steam pressure of about 620 kN/m^2 (168°C).

Although vulcanite is non-toxic and non-irritant, and has in many ways excellent mechanical properties, it has the following limitations:

(a) It absorbs saliva and becomes unhygienic due to bacterial proliferation.
(b) The aesthetics are poor, due to the opacity of rubber. No matter what colouring agent is used, the denture has never a natural appearance.
(c) Dimensional changes occur:
  (i) thermal expansion during heating in the vulcaniser, and,
  (ii) contraction of 2 to 4% by volume during addition of the sulphur to the rubber.

33.2.2 Other polymers

(a) Bakelite—a condensation polymer formed by the reaction between phenol and formaldehyde (Section 8.2 and Appendix III no. 4). This material was never widely used because:
  (i) the polymer is hard, but too brittle due to extensive cross-linking, and,
  (ii) it is difficult to mould, because water (the by-product of the condensation reaction, Appendix III no. 4) has to be eliminated from the material during the reaction.
(b) Cellulose nitrate (celluloid) was tried, but was unsuccessful because of:
  (i) excessive warpage,
  (ii) high water absorption,
  (iii) poor colour stability, and,
  (iv) camphor was used as a plasticiser—it has an unpleasant taste.
(c) Nylon (Section 8.2) has also been used, but water absorption is high, resulting in swelling and softening of the denture.
(d) Epoxy resins (Section 8.2) have also been used for denture construction, but some of the curing agents (polyamines) for these are believed to be toxic.
(e) Vinyl polymers, for example, poly(vinyl chloride), poly(vinyl acetate) and styrene were tried as denture base materials, but were unsuccessful due to difficulty in processing, and to the tendency for warpage to occur in service.
(f) Polycarbonates (formula in Appendix III No. 30) containing up to 10% glass fibres of 150 μm length and 10 μm diameter have been used for denture construction. These polymers have remarkably good impact properties—up to nine times better than poly(methyl methacrylate). These materials are more difficult to mould dentally than acrylics, since injection moulding is required.

33.3 HEAT-CURED ACRYLIC MATERIALS

33.3.1 Introduction

These are the most widely used polymeric denture materials today. The chemistry of their polymerisation is discussed in Section 8.3.

33.3.2 Composition

(a) Powder
- (i) Polymer—poly(methyl methacrylate)—either beads produced by polymerising methyl methacrylate in water, or irregular particles ground from a block of polymer.
- (ii) Peroxide initiator—0.2 to 0.5% benzoyl peroxide.
- (iii) Pigment, about 1%, ground into the polymer particles.

(b) Liquid
- (i) Monomer—methyl methacrylate.
- (ii) A stabiliser—about 0.006% hydroquinone to prevent polymerisation on storage.
- (iii) A cross-linking agent may sometimes be present, such as ethylene glycol dimethacrylate (Section 8.5).

33.3.3 Manipulation

(a) Polymer/monomer ratio. This is usually 3 to 3.5/1 by volume, or 2.5/1 by weight. Use of the correct ratio is important:
- (i) If it is too high, not all the polymer will be wetted by monomer, and the cured acrylic will be granular.
- (ii) It should not be too low. There is a shrinkage on polymerisation of about 21% by volume for pure monomer. In a correctly proportioned acrylic dough this is about 7%. If there is too much monomer there will be greater shrinkage.

(b) Mixing. The correct proportions are mixed and allowed to stand in a closed container until the dough stage is reached.

(c) Observations after mixing monomer and polymer. The material goes through the following pages:
- (i) Initially a wet sand-like mixture is formed.
- (ii) The material becomes tacky as the polymer begins to dissolve in the monomer.
- (iii) A smooth dough-like material then results, which does not stick to the mixing jar; this is the correct *dough stage* for packing the material.

(iv) If the mix is left too long it becomes too rubbery and stiff to be moulded properly.

(d) The dough time depends on:

(i) The particle size of the polymer; the smaller the particles, the more rapid is the dissolution and dough formation.

(ii) The molecular weight of the polymer; the lower this is, the faster is the dough formation.

(iii) A plasticiser is present in some materials—this reduces the dough time.

(iv) The temperature is important; for example, dough formation can be delayed by refrigeration of the mix.

(v) The polymer/monomer ratio—if this is high, there is shorter dough time.

(e) Mould lining. After the wax is completely removed from the mould by flushing with boiling water and detergent, the walls of the mould must be lined:

(i) To prevent monomer penetrating into the mould material and polymerising there, producing a rough surface with adherent mould material.

(ii) To prevent water from the mould entering into the acrylic resin (Section 33.3.4).

Formerly tin foil was widely used to line the moulds. This is a time consuming and difficult process. Tin foil substitutes are mainly used today. These are usually a solution of an alginate, such as potassium, sodium or ammonium alginate. They react with the calcium of the plaster or stone mould material to form a film of insoluble calcium alginate. These substitues are used with great success, though they are not entirely satisfactory in preventing water from the mould entering the acrylic. This may lead to crazing (Section 33.3.4).

(f) Packing. It is important to ensure:

(i) that the mould is full, and,

(ii) that there is sufficient pressure on the mould—this is achieved by packing excess dough into the mould causing it to deform. On polymerisation there is contraction which reduces the pressure in the mould. Under-packing can lead to shrinkage porosity (Section 33.3.4).

(g) Curing. The packed mould is heated in an oven or water-bath; both the temperature and time of heating must be controlled. The following principles are important:

(i) If the material is under-cured the denture may have a high residual monomer content. It is important that this is avoided (Section 33.3.4).

(ii) The rate of tempeature rise must not be too high. Monomer boils at 100.3°C. The resin must not reach this temperature while there is a substantial quantity of unreacted monomer left. The polymerisation reaction is exothermic. Thus if a large mass of uncured material is suddenly plunged into boiling water, the temperature of the resin may rise above 100.3°C, so vapourising the monomer. This causes gaseous porosity (Section 33.3.4).

Two alternative heating techniques are used:

(i) Heat at 72°C for at least 16 hours; or,

(ii) Heat at 72°C for 2 hours, by which time most of the monomer has reacted, although the residual monomer content is still above acceptable limits; the temperature is then raised to 100°C and heating continued for a further 2 hours. This latter technique obviously enables a denture to be produced in a shorter time, but there is more likelihood of warpage of the denture on deflasking (see below).

(h) Cooling. The flask should be cooled slowly on the bench, or in the oven or water bath. There should never be sudden cooling. On cooling, there is a difference of contraction between the mould material and acrylic, which causes stresses within the polymer. Slow cooling permits relief of these stresses by plastic deformation. Materials cured at higher temperatures will have greater residual stresses, to will be more likely to warp.

(i) Deflasking. This has to be done with care to avoid flexing and breaking the denture.

(j) Finishing and polishing. A suspension of finely ground pumice in water is commonly used. Final polishing is done with, for example, whiting, used as a suspension on a wet soft mop. Sometimes dry polishing techniques are used; care must be taken not to overheat the denture.

33.3.4 Properties

(a) Molecular weight

(i) Of polymer powder, as supplied, up to 500 000 to 1 000 000 (in the literature lower values, for example, 3 500 to 36 000 have been wrongly quoted).

(ii) Of monomer, 100.

(iii) Of the cured polymer, up to 1 200 000 (again lower values have sometimes been quoted, for example, between 10 000 and 40 000).

(b) Residual monomer. This has a pronounced effect on the average molecular weight. Even in a properly cured acrylic, 0.2 to 0.5% remains. Processing at too low a temperature or for too short a time, gives higher residual monomer values. This should be avoided because:

(i) Free monomer may be released from the denture and irritate the oral tissues.

(ii) Residual monomer will act as a plasticiser and make the resin weaker and more flexible.

(c) Porosity. This may have undesirable effects on the strength and optical properties of the acrylic.

(i) Shrinkage porosity appears as irregular voids throughout, and on the surface of the denture.

(ii) Gaseous porosity shows as fine uniform bubbles, particularly in thicker sections of the denture remote from the external heating source.

(d) Water absorption. Immediately after processing, a denture produced in a mould with tin foil substitutes, contains some water. In service, further water absorption can occur up to an equilibrium value of about 2%. It has been claimed that each 1% increase in weight of the resin due to water absorption causes a linear expansion of 0.23%. Similarly, drying out of the material is associated with shrinkage. For this reason dentures should at all times be kept wet when not in service.

(e) Crazing. Cracks may appear on the surface of the resin. This is believed to be due to tensile stresses causing separation of the polymer molecules. Such *crazing* may result from:

(i) Mechanical stresses on repeated drying and wetting of the denture, causing alternate contraction and expansion. The use of tin-foil substitutes for mould lining permits the cured denture to contain water. Subsequent loss of this water may lead to crazing.

(ii) Stresses due to differences in the coefficients of thermal expansion between porcelain teeth or other inserts, such as clasps, and the acrylic denture base; cracks may appear around the insert.

(iii) Solvent action—for example, when a denture is being repaired, some monomer comes in contact with the resin and may cause crazing.

Crazing has a weakening effect on a denture. Cross-linked resins are less likely to craze (see Section 37.1 on acrylic teeth).

(f) Dimensional accuracy. The following factors must be taken into account:

- (i) the mould expansion on packing (Section 33.3.3),
- (ii) thermal expansion of the acrylic dough,
- (iii) polymerisation shrinkage—approximately 7% by volume for the polymerisation of the dough, or about 2% linear contraction.
- (iv) thermal shrinkage on cooling—the coefficient of thermal expansion of acrylic is $81 \times 10^{-6}/°C$, it can be shown that there is 0.44% shrinkage on cooling from 75 to 20°C. This may be a cause of palatal discrepancies in upper dentures, and,
- (v) if excess heat is generated during polishing the denture, this may cause warpage due to release of stresses within the material.

(g) Dimensional stability. This is related to:

- (i) water absorption, as discussed above, and,
- (ii) relief of internal stresses may occur while the denture is in service. This effect is probably small and not of clinical significance.

(h) Fracture. Dentures may break:

- (i) on impact, for example, if dropped on a hard surface, or,
- (ii) due to fatigue, from repeated bending of the denture in service.

It is possible to determine the cause of fracture by observing the fracture surfaces with a magnifying glass. If there are parallel cracks within the material the breakage was probably due to fatigue.

The 'strength' of a denture depends on:

- (i) The design of the denture, as discussed in texts on dental mechanics and prosthetics; for example, stress concentration around a notch may occur (e.g. the fraenal notch) leading to midline fracture. Surface irregularities also lead to stress concentration.
- (ii) The strength of the acrylic, which depends on the molecular weight of the cured polymer, the residual monomer content, porosity and inclusions of foreign matter.

(i) Acrylic resin is radiolucent. Several experimental approaches have been tried to solve this problem, with as yet little success:

- (i) The incorporation of metal wire or mesh into acrylic; this weakens the material by causing stress concentration.

(ii) The addition of halogen compounds, particularly those containing bromine and iodine.

(iii) The use of heavy metal compounds, for example, bismuth glasses and poly(barium acrylate).

So called radio-opaque materials have been produced containing 8 to 10% barium sulphate in the powder. This quantity of additive probably does not render the denture sufficiently radio-opaque, yet any greater quantity of the barium salt causes a deterioration of the mechanical properties of the materials.

33.3.5 Critique of heat-cured acrylic denture base materials

How do these materials compare with the list of ideal properties given in Section 33.1?

(a) They are non-toxic, and, if properly manipulated, non-irritant.

(b) They are insoluble and inert in oral fluids, though they show a degree of water absorption.

(c) In terms of mechanical properties the impact and fatigue properties of acrylic are not ideal (Section 33.6). Also, although the material can take a good polish, its abrasion resistance is not good.

(d) The other physical properties of acrylic are:

(i) the coefficient of thermal expansion is $81 \times 10^{-6}/°C$, similar to that of acrylic teeth, but very much greater than that of porcelain teeth.

(ii) the thermal conductivity is low, in common with other polymers.

(iii) its density is 1.18 g/cm^3—this is comparatively low, and,

(iv) the softening temperature is about 75°C, higher than the temperature of hot foods and liquids.

(e) One of the chief merits of acrylic is that it can provide good aesthetics; the polymer is translucent and easily pigmented. Colour stability is good (in contrast to self-cured acrylics, Section 33.4).

(f) Other factors are:

(i) Acrylics are radiolucent as discussed above.

(ii) They are easily to process with simple equipment; no expensive injection moulding equipment is required.

(iii) Acrylic dentures are easy to repair if accidentally fractured (Section 33.5.1).

(iv) Dimensional changes can occur (Section 33.3.4).

33.4 SELF-CURED ACRYLIC MATERIALS

33.4.1 Introduction

The chemistry of these materials is given in Section 8.3. Their composition is similar to heat-cured materials (Section 33.3.2) except that the liquid contains an activator, such as dimethyl-p-toluidine. They are sometimes called *cold-curing*, *auto-polymerising* or *chemically activated* materials.

33.4.2 Comparison with heat-cured materials

(a) They differ in method of activation, as mentioned above.
(b) The porosity of self-cured materials is greater, though this is not easy to see in pigmented resins. This may be due to air dissolved in the monomer which is not soluble in the polymer at room temperature.
(c) In general, self-cured materials have lower average molecular weights, and higher residual monomer contents—of the order of 2 to 5%.
(d) Self-cured materials are not as strong; the transverse strength is about 80% of that of the heat-cured materials. They may be related to their lower molecular weight.
(e) In terms of rheological properties, self-cured materials are less desirable, since they show greater distortion in use. In measurements on creep of poly(methyl methacrylate), heat-cured polymers had less initial deformation, less creep and quicker recovery than self-cured materials (Fig. 33.1).
(f) The colour stability of self-cured materials is poorer; if a tertiary amine activator is used, yellowing over a period of time can occur.

33.4.3 'Pour-and-cure' resins

A technique is available whereby a fluid mix of a self-curing acrylic is poured into an agar mould to form a denture. Such dentures may be dimensionally less accurate, more porous and weaker and show greater creep (Fig. 33.1) than those prepared from conventional heat-cured materials.

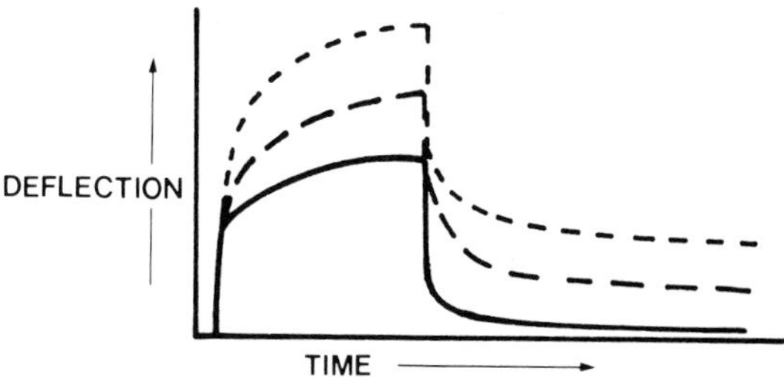

Fig. 33.1 Comparative creep of denture base polymers.
——————— heat cured acrylic
— — — — self cured acrylic
- - - - - 'pour and cure' resin
Each curve is in four parts: an immediate deformation on applying load, followed by a period of creep; on removal of load, an initial rapid partial recovery is followed by a period of slower recovery.
(after Glantz and Bates, 1973 Odont Revy 24: 283)

33.4.4 Other applications

Self-cured acrylics are used:
(a) Occasionally as restorative materials, as discussed in Chapter 19.
(b) With inert fillers, for the construction of special trays for impression taking (Section 24.4).
(c) For denture repair, relining and rebasing (Section 33.5).
(d) In removable orthodontic appliances.
(e) For adding a post-dam to an adjusted upper denture.

33.5 DENTURE REPAIR, REBASING AND RELINING

33.5.1 Denture repair

(a) Self-cured repairs. The following practical points are important to ensure a successful repair:

(i) The parts of the broken denture are held together with sticky wax and wires, and a model cast up in plaster.

(ii) When the denture parts are removed from the model, the fracture surfaces are finished with a smooth rounded contour with 3 to 5 mm separation. V-shaped edges should be avoided, as they will give stress concentration.

(iii) The alginate separating medium (tin foil substitute—Section 33.3.3) or tin foil is applied to the model, and the denture parts replaced on it.

(iv) The self-curing acrylic repair material is mixed to a fluid consistency and applied to the repair area.

(v) The porosity of the self-curing acrylic will be less if it is polymerised under a hydraulic pressure of up to 250 kN/m^2, and at a temperature of 40 to 45°C.

(b) Heat-cured repairs are often advocated for all but minor repairs. A problem is that warpage of the denture base is liable to occur. This can be overcome by replacing the palate of the denture with new heat-cured material.

33.5.2 Rebasing and relining

Dentures sometimes require adjustment of their fitting surfaces to accommodate changes in the soft tissues. This may be carried out by constructing a new denture (*rebasing*), or a new fitting surface for the denture (*relining*). The use of soft or resilient lining materials is discussed separately in Chapter 34.

33.6 MODIFIED ACRYLICS

There is a need for materials with greater impact and fatigue strength. These materials include vinyl co-polymers and rubber-acrylic graft co-polymers. Several such products are available, some of them requiring injection moulding. The graft co-polymers have better impact resistance properties than conventional acrylic materials.

One group of such materials is essentially emulsion polymerised beads of poly(methyl methacrylate) to which are grafted a rubbery butadiene-styrene layer that are then coated with poly(methyl methacrylate). These beads are then mixed with monomer which is composed of methyl methacrylate, a cross linking agent and an inhibitor. These materials show a greater resistance to crack formation, causing deceleration of the crack when it reaches the rubber phase. Rubber modified resins have better impact and fatigue properties.

One experimental approach to the developement of stronger denture base materials is to incorporate whiskers of, for example, alumina (Section 13.3.1) into acrylic. Carbon fibres suitably treated have also been used experimentally as an additive, and although this improves the strength properties, the black colour of the fibres may render the resultant resin unaesthetic.

Another product is a co-polymer of methyl methacrylate and

hydroxyethyl methacrylate (formula in Appendix III no. 19). It is claimed that this material is easily wetted, so that enhanced denture retention is obtained. However, when the material is saturated with water, it has poorer mechanical properties than poly(methyl methacrylate).

33.7 LIGHT-CURED DENTURE BASE MATERIALS

Free radical addition polymerisation can be initiated by visible light (Section 8.3.1). This technique has becomes widely used for composite restorative materials (Section 19.6.3) and has recently been suggested for denture base applications. One such system is currently being evaluated. It comprises:

(a) A denture base material with acrylic copolymers, microfine silica and high molecular weight acrylic monomers; no methyl methacrylate is present.

(b) A coating for the denture base material that helps to eliminate surface inhibition of polymerisation by oxygen.

(c) Arch form teeth, in four arch sizes.

(d) A bonding agent, which is cured by visible light, to aid bonding between base and teeth. This agent contains a mixture of acrylic monomers, including methyl methacrylate.

(e) A curing unit, with four tungsten halogen lamps, giving light of wavelength 400–500 nm.

READING REFERENCES

Paffenbarger G C, Woelfel J B, Sweeney A B 1965 Resins and technics used in the construction of dentures. Dental Clinics of North America, March, p 251

Woelfel J B, Paffenbarger G C, Sweeney A B 1965 Clinical evaluation of complete dentures made of 11 different types of denture base materials. Journal of the American Dental Association 70: 1170

These two papers review and compare the properties of a number of different polymer types for denture construction, including various co-polymer systems.

Stafford G D, Huggett R 1978 Creep and hardness testing of some denture base polymers. Journal of Prosthetic Dentistry 39: 682

This paper emphasises the importance of measuring creep behaviour of denture base resins as part of the assessment of their viscoelastic behaviour.

Bates J F, Stafford G D, Huggett R, Handley R W 1977 Current status of pour type denture base resins. Journal of Dentistry 5: 177

A review of the properties of eight pour type denture base resins in which their properties are contrasted with a standard heat cured resin.

34. Tissue conditioners: functional impression materials; resilient linings for dentures

34.1 INTRODUCTION

34.1.1 Indications and applications

An acrylic denture may have a soft lining, either as a temporary measure, or intended for permanent use.

(a) A temporary lining may be used for one of two purposes:

- (i) As a *tissue conditioner*; this may be defined as a soft material which is applied temporarily to the fitting surface of a denture in order to allow a more equal distribution of load, to permit the mucosal tissues to assume a more normal position.
- (ii) As a *functional impression material*—one which is applied to the fitting surface of a denture in order to secure an impression under functional stresses.

(b) A permanent resilient lining may be used in the following cases:

- (i) Where the tissues of the denture bearing area show evidence of atrophy, a soft lining may be used to avoid pain through pressure from, or movement of, the denture under masticatory load.
- (ii) A resilient material can utilise undercut areas to achieve maximum retention of the denture.

These resilient lining materials can also be used for:

(i) obturators, and
(ii) other prostheses, for example, facial prostheses.

34.1.2 General principles

The above applications require polymers that are soft at mouth temperature—in other words, their glass transition temperature (T_g) must be below 37°C (Section 8.6.2). The following type of materials are used:
(a) Acrylic polymers with a solvent, as in Section 34.2.2.
(b) Acrylic polymers or co-polymers with an inert ester as plasticiser (Section 34.3.2). Poly(ethyl methacrylate) is frequently used, as it has a lower glass transition temperature than poly(methyl methacrylate), so requires less plasticiser.
(c) Silicones, as in Section 34.3.2, similar to the impression materials described in Section 27.2.

34.2 TISSUE CONDITIONERS AND FUNCTIONAL IMPRESSION MATERIALS

34.2.1 Requirements

(a) General properties—obviously these materials should have no irritant or toxic effect.
(b) The set material—each of the two applications being considered has different requirements:
- (i) A tissue conditioner must be soft, and it must not undergo substantial permanent deformation—that is, it must be *elastic*. The softness and elasticity must be maintained for a sufficient length of time.
- (ii) A functional impression material should also be soft, but must deform plastically to record the impression.

N.B. Many of the materials used for these applications are *visco-elastic*—that is, they flow under a steady pressure, but are resilient under dynamic forces such as chewing.

34.2.2 Composition and properties

(a) Power/liquid materials contain:
- (i) Powder—acrylic polymers, for example, poly(ethyl methacrylate) or co-polymers.
- (ii) Liquid—usually a mixture of ethyl alcohol and an aromatic ester (for example, butyl phthalyl butyl glycolate).

On mixing the two together, a slurry is formed. The liquid then penetrates between the molecules of the powder, a process accelerated by the ethyl alcohol present, and the whole material becomes

stiffer, until a gel is formed. The setting, therefore, is a physical process, there being no chemical reaction involved. Note that these materials do not contain any monomeric substances.
(b) Preformed sheets of acrylic gel are also available, which can be adapted to the surfaces of the denture.
(c) The available commercial materials vary considerably in their precise composition and properties. Some of them are more suitable for tissue conditioning, others for functional impressions.

34.3 RESILIENT LININGS

34.3.1 Requirements

The following is a list of desirable properties of resilient linings:
(a) Non-toxic, non-irritant, odourless and tasteless.
(b) Unaffected by the oral environment, for example:
- (i) gel type materials should not imbibe water; water absorption causes swelling; the percentage water absorption should be the same as that of the denture base;
- (ii) there should be no absorption of constituents of foods and drinks;
- (iii) plasticisers (where present), should not be leached out of the materials.

(c) Mechanical properties—the set material should be soft and permanently resilient, and resistant to abrasion.
(d) Aesthetics—there should be a natural appearance, and no discolouration or staining.
(e) Other properties:
- (i) the unmixed material should have a good shelf-life;
- (ii) it should be simple to manipulate;
- (iii) it should be dimensionally stable during processing and in use;
- (iv) there should be a good bond formed between lining and denture base;
- (v) it should be easy to clean and keep clean, and be little affected by denture cleansers.

34.3.2 Classification and composition

(a) Early materials, not widely used today because of their inferior properties, include:
- (i) natural rubbers, and

(ii) poly(vinyl chloride) or poly(vinyl acetate), plasticised with dibutyl phthalate or dioctyl phthalate.

(b) Present-day materials include:

(i) Heat cured acrylics.

Powder—acrylic polymers such as poly(ethyl methacrylate) or acrylic co-polymers, and benzoyl peroxide.

Liquid—acrylic monomer (e.g. ethyl, butyl, 2-ethoxyethyl methacrylate) and plasticisers.

Alternatively these materials may be supplied as a preformed sheet, which is soaked in a monomeric material which causes it to swell, and then processed against the acrylic dough.

(ii) Self-cured acrylics

These are supplied in powder/liquid form of composition similar to the above, except that they are polymerised by a peroxide-tertiary amine system (similar to the denture repair materials etc., Section 33.4).

(iii) Heat-cured silicones

These contain a siloxane material:

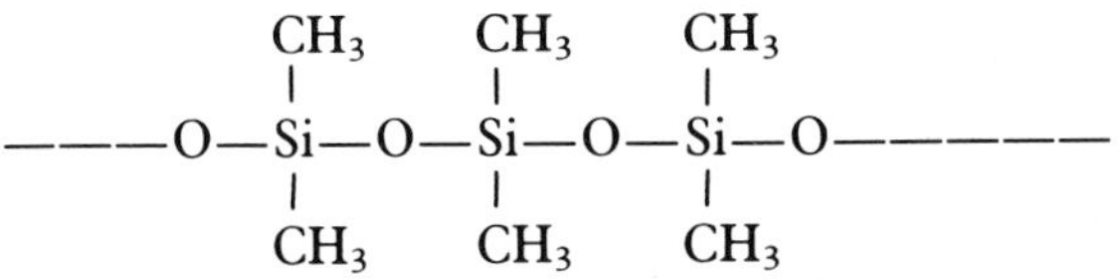

$$
\begin{array}{ccccccc}
 & CH_3 & & CH_3 & & CH_3 & \\
 & | & & | & & | & \\
---O- & Si & -O- & Si & -O- & Si & -O--- \\
 & | & & | & & | & \\
 & CH_3 & & CH_3 & & CH_3 &
\end{array}
$$

and silica as a filler. They are processed against acrylic dough. One commercial product has a methacrylate group to aid bonding with the acrylic denture base:

$$
\begin{array}{ccccl}
 & CH_3 & & & O \sim\sim \\
 & | & & & | \\
CH_2= & C & -CO_2- & & Si-O \sim\sim \\
 & & & & | \\
 & & & & O \sim\sim
\end{array}
$$

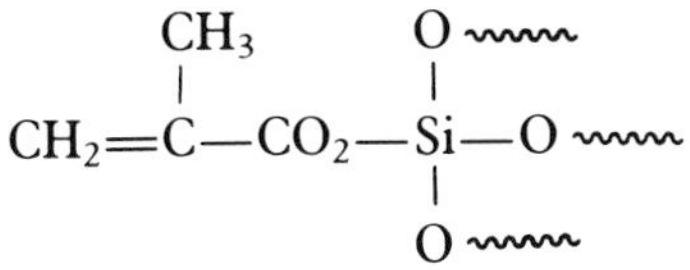

(iv) Self-cured silicones

These are similar in composition and setting to the silicone impression materials (Section 27.2). Bonding to the acrylic denture base is helped by applying a special primer to the acrylic.

34.3.3 General properties

(a) In general these materials are non-irritant and are not unpleasant in the mouth.

(b) The effect of the oral environment:

- (i) The water absorption of the heat-cured acrylic soft liners is closest to that of the acrylic denture base.
- (ii) In general the silicones have the best all-round resistance to the effects of constituents of foods and drinks—this was demonstrated in laboratory tests with olive oil and peppermint oil.
- (iii) The plasticisers of the acrylic materials are lost by being leached out into the saliva, causing hardening of the lining, and dimensional change.
- (iv) Growth of the fungus *Candida albicans* has been found to occur with some silicone materials.

(c) In terms of mechanical properties, the silicones are the most elastic, but have poorer abrasion resistance than the acrylics.

(d) The aesthetic properties of soft linings may be lost by deposits of calculus, or by use of the wrong denture cleansers.

(e) As far as other desirable properties are concerned, the following problems are sometimes encountered:

- (i) It is usually difficult to get good bonding between a self-cured silicone and the acrylic denture base.
- (ii) These materials are often adversely affected by denture cleansers, as mentioned below.

34.3.4 Conclusions

Soft linings are intended to be permanently attached to the denture. In fact their general properties are so poor that they must be considered as semi-permanent.

In practice, the following failings are commonly seen:

(a) Some materials develop a rough surface after wear, with food being embedded in the surface.

(b) Some linings split under stress and/or peel away from the denture base.

(c) There may be a change of colour due to staining and deposits of calculus.

(d) The linings may become hard due to loss of plasticiser.

(e) The surface may become bubbled if an oxygenating type of denture cleanser is used (Section 51.3.3).

(f) If a bleach is used to clean the denture (Section 51.3.3), the lining becomes white and hard.

34.4 NEW MATERIALS

Recent research has aimed at developing improved soft lining materials which will bond to denture base acrylics, yet remain permanently soft. Two approaches have been tried: (i) the use of polymerisable plasticisers, (ii) the application of powdered elastomers.

34.4.1 Polymerisable plasticisers

As mentioned above (Section 34.3.3) loss of plasticiser causes hardening of an acrylic lining. It has been shown that it can be avoided by using a component such as an alkyl maleate:

$$\begin{array}{l} \mathrm{CH{-}COOR} \\ \| \\ \mathrm{CH{-}COOR} \end{array}$$

or an alkyl itaconate:

$$\begin{array}{rl} & \mathrm{CH{-}COOR} \\ & \| \\ \mathrm{ROOC{-}} & \mathrm{CH} \end{array}$$

The maleate or itaconate will polymerise to give a low molecular weight polymer; in such a form it can plasticise the material, yet is not easily leached, in contrast to the smaller ester molecules used in conventional materials.

34.4.2 Powdered elastomers

An alternative approach is to take a powdered elastomer (e.g. butadiene-styrene and butadiene-acrylonitrile rubbers) mixed with a higher methacrylate monomer which forms a dough with the rubber. On polymerisation, a soft material without plasticisers is formed.

34.4.3 Critique

Products based on the above experimental approaches are undergoing clinical trials and show great promise.

READING REFERENCES

NOTE: Some viscoelastic parameters are discussed in the literature; knowledge of these is considered to be beyond the scope of this book.

Amin W M, Fletcher A. M, Ritchie G M 1981 The nature of the interface between polymethyl methacrylate denture base materials and soft lining materials. Journal of Dentistry 9: 336

A comprehensive study of factors influencing bonding between denture base and lining materials.

Braden M 1970 Tissue conditioners: I Composition and structure. Journal of Dental Research 49: 145

The composition and structure of five proprietary tissue conditioners.

McCabe J F 1976 Soft lining materials: composition and structure. Journal of Oral Rehabilitation 3: 273

The composition of five acrylic based materials, two of which should be classified as tissue conditioners.

Parker S, Braden M 1982 New soft lining materials. Journal of Dentistry 10: 149

This paper discusses the limitations of conventional soft lining materials and discusses the new products mentioned in Section 34.4.

Wright P S 1976 Soft lining materials; their status and prospects. Journal of Dentistry 4: 247

A comprehensive study of the composition and properties of fifteen products.

35. Partial denture casting alloys

35.1 REQUIREMENTS

(a) The material for the *connectors* of a partial denture should have the following mechanical properties:
- (i) a high modulus of elasticity, so that it is rigid in thin sections, and,
- (ii) a high proportional limit, so that permanent deformation is unlikely.

(b) For *clasp* construction, a material should have:
- (i) a high proportional limit, as above, but,
- (ii) a lower modulus of elasticity, so that the clasp is flexible enough to be withdrawn over undercuts, without either the tooth or the clasps being overstressed.

35.2 GOLD ALLOYS

35.2.1 Composition

Type IV gold alloys are used for partial denture construction; their composition is in Table 29.1.

35.2.2 Properties

The properties of these alloys are in Table 35.1 and are compared with cobalt–chromium alloys in Section 35.3.5.

35.2.3 Heat treatment

(a) Stage 1. The alloy is usually quenched after casting.

(b) Stage 2. Homogenisation is carried out (Section 10.3.2) since coring occurs with alloys containing platinum (Section 10.5.2). The alloy is heated to 700°C for 10 minutes, then quenched.
(c) Stage 3. If any cold working is done to the alloy, for example, adjustment of clasps, a stress-relief anneal is carried out (Section 9.7.4).
(d) Stage 4. Heat hardening is achieved by heating and maintaining the alloy at an elevated temperature for a sufficient time for diffusion of atoms to occur, to permit order and precipitation hardening (Section 10.4.3 and 10.4.4); this is achieved by either:

- (i) cooling the alloy slowly from 700°C,
- (ii) cooling the alloy from 450 to 250°C over 30 minutes, followed by quenching, or,
- (iii) maintaining the alloy at between 350 and 450°C for around 15 minutes, followed by quenching.

The effect of this heat treatment on the mechanical properties of these alloys can be seen in Table 35.1.

35.3 COBALT–CHROMIUM ALLOYS

35.3.1 Introduction

These alloys are hard, rigid and corrosion resistant. Besides their application for cast partial dentures, they are used for surgical implants. Because of their corrosion resistance at high temperatures, other applications have been for car sparking plugs and turbine blades. This type of alloy is often referred to as *stellite*.

35.3.2 Composition

Cobalt	35 to 65%
Chromium	20 to 35%
Nickel	0 to 30%
Molybdenum	0 to 7%
Carbon	up to 0.4%

Tungsten, manganese, silicon and iron may also be present in small quantities.

Note that cobalt is the principal constituent, hence they are termed *cobalt–chromium alloys*. Alternative names, such as chrome–cobalt, chromium–cobalt or chrome alloys are not to be preferred.

35.3.3 Effect of constituents

(a) Cobalt is a hard, strong and rigid metal.
(b) Chromium forms a solid solution with cobalt. It renders the alloy corrosion resistant, due to a *passivating* effect (Section 11.5.1).
(c) Nickel can replace some of the cobalt.
(d) Molybdenum, tungsten, manganese and silicon harden and strengthen the alloy. Molybdenum reduces the grain size.
(e) Carbon is invariably present, and it reacts with many of the other constituents to form carbides. These solidify last during cooling after casting, so appear at the grain boundaries. The carbon content of a cobalt–chromium casting depends on:
   (i) the quantity of carbon initially present before casting, and,
   (ii) pick-up of carbon from a heating flame, if this technique of melting is used (Section 35.3.4).

Control of the carbon content of these alloys is most important. The carbides that are formed embrittle the alloy, with the consequent danger of, for example, partial denture clasp fracture.

35.3.4 Manipulation

The casting technique for these alloys is similar to that of gold alloys (Ch. 43), but the following differences in manipulation should be noted:
(a) The melting point of these alloys is in the range 1250 to 1450°C, hence gypsum-bonded investments should not be used. A silica-bonded or phosphate-bonded material should be chosen (Ch. 42).
(b) Because of the high melting range, gas/air torches cannot raise the alloy temperature sufficiently to melt it. There is a choice of using either:
   (i) oxy-acetylene flame—this requires careful control to use the correct ratio of oxygen to acetylene. Too much of the former gas may result in oxidation of the alloy; too much acetylene will result in carbon pick-up by the alloy, which must be avoided (Section 35.3.3); or,
   (ii) induction heating, where the alloy is heated electrically. This method is usually preferred, as it avoids the problems mentioned above.

(c) Because of the great hardness of the alloy, special polishing and finishing techniques are required:
   (i) sand blasting is used to smooth the surface of the casting and remove adherent investment materials; and,

(ii) electrolytic polishing is then applied. The principle is the same as for electroplating, except that the appliance is made the anode of an electrolytic cell. When a current is applied, the surface layer is dissolved.

35.3.5 Comparison with gold alloys

Comparative data are presented in Table 35.1. The following points should be noted:

(a) The proportional limit of cobalt–chromium alloys is less than that of the hardened gold alloys, and the ultimate tensile strength of the former is slightly lower than that of the latter material.

(b) The cobalt–chromium alloys have a modulus of elasticity about twice that of gold alloys, that is, they are stiffer. This is very desirable for connectors (Section 35.1), and it means that sections of cobalt–chromium alloys of about half the thickness of gold alloys can be used to achieve the same degree of rigidity. Gold alloy clasps, however, are more flexible, and can be withdrawn over a greater degree of undercut (that is, a deeper undercut can be engaged) than clasps of cobalt–chromium.

(c) The cobalt–chromium alloys are more brittle (lower percentage elongation).

(d) The higher melting range, and greater hardness, of cobalt–chrium alloys, have laready been discussed (Section 35.3.4).

(e) The casting shrinkage of cobalt–chromium alloys is greater than that of the gold-containing materials, but the available investment materials appear to give satisfactory compensation for this contraction.

(f) The density of cobalt–chromium is about half that of gold. This together with the fact that cobalt–chromium dentures can be made of thinner cross-section, means that lighter dentures can be made.

35.3.6 Recent developments

An alloy containing titanium has been introduced, with 4 to 10% titanium, 5 to 15% chromium, 5 to 15% nickel, less than 3% molybdenum, small quantities of silicon, manganese, iron and carbon, the remainder being cobalt.

One advantage of such an alloy is that is has been shown to be more ductile than other cobalt–chromium alloys. However, special casting techniques are required.

Table 35.1* Properties of partial denture casting alloys

Material	Condition	Modulus of elasticity (GN/m^2)	Propor-tional limit (MN/m^2)	Ulitmate tensile strength (MN/m^2)	Elonga-tion (%)	Hardness (BHN)	Melting range (°C)	Density (g/cm^3)
Gold alloy type IV	Soft	95	360	480	15	130–150	850–950	15
Gold alloy type IV	Hard	100	585	790	10	210–230	850–950	15
Cobalt–chromium alloy	As cast	250	515	690	4	370	1250–1450	8
Silver–palladium	Soft	95	345	480	9	140–170	950–1050	12

* For details of gold alloys see Crowell, W. S. (1961) Gold alloys in dentistry. Metals Handbooks, 8th edn., vol. I, Properties and Selection of Metals, pp. 1188–1189. Metals Park, Ohio: American Society for Metals.

35.4 OTHER ALLOYS

35.4.1 Silver–palladium alloys ("white gold")

These alloys contain approximately 45% silver, 24% palladium, 15% gold, 15% copper and 1% zinc. They have been used as a less expensive substitute for alloys of high gold content. From Table 35.1 it can be seen that their proportional limit and ultimate tensile strength are inferior to type IV gold alloys. Silver–palladium alloys work harden rapidly, so that if a clasp has to be adjusted, fracture is liable to occur. Both silver and palladium dissolve oxygen when molten, leading to porosity of the casting. Heat treatment can be carried out, but this reduces the percentage elongation so much that the alloys is too brittle for clasp construction.

35.4.2 Aluminium bronze

Aluminium bronzes are alloys of copper containing up to 10% aluminium. Lesser amounts of nickel, iron and manganese are also present.

Clinical trials are being undertaken to determine how these materials will perform in service. In particular, their corrosion resistance is being studied.

READING REFERENCES

Johnson W 1957 Gold alloys for casting dentures. An investigation of some mechanical properties. British Dental Journal 102: 41

A comparison of the properties of gold and silver–palladium alloys, showing how the latter were not considered satisfactory for the construction of cast dentures.

Johnson W 1957 A comparison of cobalt–chromium alloys and yellow and white gold alloys. Dental Practitioner 8: 8

A comparison of the following properties of casting alloys for denture construction: modulus of elasticity, hardness, density, corrosion resistance, melting and casting, joining the alloys and cost.

36. The stainless steel denture base

36.1 INTRODUCTION

Stainless steel has been occasionally used as a denture base material since about 1921. Of particular importance is the 18/8 austenitic type material; for details of composition, etc., see Section 10.6.2.

36.2 CONVENTIONAL METHOD OF SWAGING

A stainless steel sheet is pressed between a die and a counter-die in a hydraulic press. Dies and counter-dies are made of low fusing alloys, such as zinc, copper–magnesium–aluminium, tin–antimony–copper, lead–antimony–tin and lead–bismuth–tin alloys.

Some problems associated with this conventional swaging procedure are:

(a) Possible dimensional inaccuracy, particularly if the contraction of the die metal or alloy is not matched by the expansion of the model.

(b) Loss of fine detail, since many stages are involved between recording the original impression and obtaining the final product.

(c) Dies and counter-dies can be damaged under hydraulic pressure; it was usually customary to use more than one die and counter-die.

(d) It was difficult to ensure a uniform thickness of the finished plate.

(e) Uneven pressure on the die and counter-die could cause wrinkling of the steel.

36.3 PROPERTIES

Despite the difficulties in swaging mentioned above, stainless steel has some merit as a denture base material:

(a) Very thin denture bases can be produced—figures of as low as 0.11 mm have been quoted, compared to about 1.52 mm for an acrylic denture.
(b) The steel is fracture resistant.
(c) Such dentures are not heavy, because of the thinness of the material, and the fact that the density of steel is not high compared to some other metallic materials (Appendix II).
(d) The corrosion resistance is good.
(e) Stainless steel can take and retain a high polish.
(f) The thermal conductivity of stainless steel is such that the sensation of temperature is rapidly transmitted to the palate. This is an advantage not shared by the polymeric denture base materials.

36.4 NEWER METHODS OF SWAGING

Because of the merits of stainless steel, new methods of swaging have been investigated, to overcome the problems outlined in Section 36.2.

36.4.1 Explosion forming

A die made using an epoxy resin is prepared from the dental impression. A stainless steel plate is placed on top of the die, with a layer of 'Plasticine' on it. A pressure-wave is produced by a small charge of high explosives. The pressure is transmitted through the 'Plasticine' on to the steel, forcing it into the requisite shape.

36.4.2 Explosion–hydraulic forming

This is similar to the above, except that water is used as the medium for transmitting the pressure wave.

36.4.3 Hydraulic forming

The apparatus for this technique is illustrated in Figure 36.1. The method is as follows:
(a) A die is placed in a metal cone and located in the pressure vessel.
(b) A sheet of stainless steel of the required thickness is placed in position over the die.
(c) A rubber diaphragm is placed over the stainless steel, and a cover plate inserted in place, and held in position by high tensile bolts.

(d) Oil is pumped into the chamber up to a pressure of around 70 MN/m^2.
(e) After the pressure has been released, the chamber is opened and the work-piece is removed and cleaned.
(f) The denture base is cut to size, and retentive tags are resistance welded into position (Section 44.3).

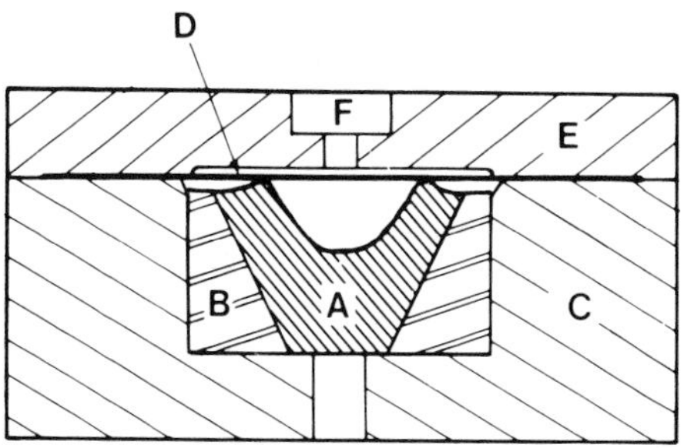

Fig. 36.1 Apparatus for hydraulic forming of stainless steel. A, die; B, metal cone; C, pressure vessel; D, sheet of stainless steel; E, cover plate; F, application of oil pressure.

(g) After polishing the denture, it can, if necessary, be reformed on the die to eliminate distortion that may have occurred during welding.

The stainless steel can be annealed by heating at 1050°C for two mintues, followed by quenching in water.

READING REFERENCE

Blair G A S Crossland B 1963 The explosive forming of stainless steel upper dentures. Denture Practitioner 13: 413

The article considers the history of the use of stainless steel as a denture base material, conventional techniques of swaging, the merits of stainless steel, and the technique of explosion forming (as mentioned in Section 36.4.1).

Bahrani A S Blair G A S Crossland B 1964 Further developments in the explosive forming of stainless steel upper dentures. Dental Practitioner 14: 499.

A description of the techniqe mentioned in Section 36.4.2.

Bahrani A S Blair G A S Crossland B 1965 Slow rate hydraulic forming of stainless steel dentures. British Dental Journal 118: 425

A fuller account of the technique described in Section 36.4.3.

37. Synthetic tooth materials

37.1 ACRYLIC TEETH

These are manufactured by:
(a) Dough moulding, using permanent metal moulds, but otherwise similar to the method of processing heat cured acrylic denture base materials.
(b) Injecting into a metal mould polymer powder that has been softened by heating.

The former method is the more widely used one today.

The following points are of practical importance:
(a) The teeth will bond chemically with the acrylic denture base, providing that the tooth surface to be bonded is clean and free and of wax.
(b) The presence of monomer, either on fabrication or repair of the denture, can cause crazing (Section 33.3.4). For this reason, most acrylic teeth are cross-linked, which makes them more resistant to solvent action.
(c) The abrasion resistance of acrylic teeth is not ideal, and wear of teeth in service frequently occurs.

The properties of acrylic and porcelain teeth are compared in Section 37.2.2.

37.2 PORCELAIN TEETH

37.2.1 Introduction

Porcelain can also be used for the construction of teeth; its composition and properties are discussed in Chapter 28.

37.2.2 Comparison with acrylic teeth

This is given in Table 37.1.

Table 37.1 Comparison of acrylic and porcelain teeth.

Property	Acrylic	Procelain
Mechanical properties	Not as brittle, but poor abrasion resistance	Brittle; more resistant to abrasion
Thermal expansion	Same as acrylic denture base	Much lower than acrylic (see Appendix II); causes stresses in acrylic denture base
Aesthetics	Can be excellent	Can be excellent
Density	1.18g/cm^3	2.35g/cm^3
Retention to denture base	Chemical bonding if proper manipulation observed (Section 41.1)	Mechanical bonding by pins or undercut holes
Adjustment	Can be ground and then easily polished	More difficult to grind and difficult to polish
In service	(i) Considered to transmit less forces to the mucosa (ii) No clicking on contact with the opposing teeth	(i) Considered to transmit more forces to the mucosa (ii) Clicking occurs on contact with the opposing teeth

37.3 RECENT DEVELOPMENTS

The use of glass-ceramics (Section 12.5) for artificial teeth has been suggested, and the claims made:

(a) Glass-ceramic teeth can be produced by a glass-moulding procedure in which there is little shrinkage during the moulding process. Hence teeth produced by this method can be as accurate as the mould used in their production and accurate cusp angles which do not alter during the processing of the teeth can be predicted at the moulding stage. In contrast conventional porcelain may show a volume shrinkage of 30 to 40% on firing.

(b) The transverse strength of glass-ceramics is of the order of twice that of conventional porcelain.

(c) Glass-ceramics are non-porous and impervious to fluids.

(d) If the material wears, it maintains a polished surface.

READING REFERENCES

MacCulloch W T 1968 Advances in dental ceramics. British Dental Journal 124: 361

This paper includes a discussion of porcelain teeth, with reference to historical aspects, problems of manufacture, and new types of porcelain.

SECTION VII

Orthodontic appliances

38. Materials in orthodontics

38.1 INTRODUCTION

Orthodontic appliances are employed to cause tooth movement for the treatment of malocclusion. An appliance is composed of *active* and *reactive* components. An active component applies a force to a tooth which is to be moved. This force should not be large enough to affect adversely the periodontal tissues, nor should it be too small. A reactive component anchors the appliances to teeth which are not to be moved. Appliances may be classified as either removable or fixed.

(a) Removable appliances usually consist of a polymeric framework. This supports the active part which may consist of springs or rubber bands to apply a continuous force, or adjustable screws for the application of intermittent forces.

(b) Fixed appliances are secured in place by one or both of two techniques:

- (i) By using bands which are cemented around the clinical crown of a tooth.
- (ii) By direct bonding of brackets to acid-etched enamel.

38.2 ORTHODONTIC BASE POLYMERS

These are usually autopolymerising acrylic resins, similar to those used for denture repair (Section 33.4). Recent analyses have shown that the main constituents of these materials are as follows:

(a) Powder—predominately poly (methyl methacrylate), some products with lesser amounts of polystyrene, poly (ethyl methacrylate)

or poly (butyl methacrylate). At least one product is mainly poly (ethyl methacrylate).
(b) Liquid—methyl methacrylate, with 0 to 6% ethylene glycol dimethacrylate.

In addition, peroxide and amine components will be present in powder and liquid respectively.

The materials are formulated to facilitate their handling by the technician. These resins are in general softer and less rigid than denture materials.

38.3 ALLOY SYSTEMS

Since inert, corrosion resistant alloys are required for oral use, only a limited range of materials can be used, as detailed below.

38.3.1 Stainless steel

The method of production of wires has been discussed in Section 9.3.2. Figure 9.7 shows the type of fibrous structure that results from such cold-working. As well as a change in structure, the properties of the alloy are altered; cold working increases the tensile strength and hardness, but reduces the ductility.

Dental stainless steel wires are made from the austentic material (Section 10.6.2). During the working of the wire to the required form in the dental laboratory, further work hardening occurs. If a considerable amount of such working is necessary the ductility may be reduced to the point where fracture occurs. To avoid this risk it is necessary to choose a material which will withstand the required degree of working.

Three grades of stainless steel wire are usually required: ‘soft’, ‘half-hard’ and ‘hard’. If much cold working is to be carried out, a softer material should be selected, as it will work harden during manipulation. Conversely, a harder material can be selected if there is to be little cold-working.

With stainless steel wires it is not possible to apply heat treatment to restore the ductility of the wire during the working procedure. This is because:
(a) A minimum temperature of around 500°C is necessary to produce any degree of stress relief annealing. However, if some wires are heated for a prolonged period in the temperature range 500–900°C, a reaction occurs between chromium and carbon, with the formation of chromium carbide and its precipitation at the grain

boundaries. There are two reasons for avoiding this in practice:

(i) The alloy becomes more brittle due to slip interference of the precipitated carbide.

(ii) The corrosion resistance is reduced because there is less chromium left in the grains to produce the required passivating effect.

The above phenomenon is called *weld decay*. It can be avoided by either:

(i) Having an alloy of very low carbon content, so that carbides will not be precipitated. In practice it is difficult and expensive to completely remove carbon from steel; or

(ii) By using a *stabilised stainless steel*—this contains small quantities of either titanium or columbium. These constituents form carbides more readily than chromium, leaving the latter metal in solid solution.

(b) Full restoration of ductility necessitates heating the wire to a temperature above 950°C, when recrystallisation occurs. This gives a fine equiaxed grain structure, but destroys the fibrous structure of the wire, on which its 'springiness' depends.

38.3.2 Cobalt chromium

The composition and properties of such materials are discussed in relation to their use for cast partial dentures (Ch. 35).

The wrought materials can be heat-treated by an age hardening process, though the wires are usually pre-treated by the manufacturer.

38.3.3 Nickel-chromium

Wires are supplied in an alloy containing 80% nickel and 20% chromium. These wires are also used in the manufacture of heating elements because of their comparatively high electrical resistivity.

38.3.4 Nickel-titanium

These alloys contain nickel and titanium in the ration 55/45 by weight, giving the intermetallic compound NiTi. For orthodontic use, 1.6% cobalt is included in the formulation.

38.3.5 Beta-titanium

Titanium can exist in an α–form (hexagonal close packed structure) below 885°C and a β–form (body centred cubic structure) at higher temperatures. With the incorporation of alloying elements, α–titanium is stable at room temperature. A typical composition of such an alloy (mass %) is 79% Ti, 11% Mo, 6% Zr, 4% Sn. Titanium has excellent corrosion resistance.

38.3.6 Gold alloys

The function of alloying elements on the properties of gold are discussed in Section 10.5.2.

Gold alloy wires may be of the following types:

(a) Simple ternary alloys of gold, copper and silver
(b) Platinised alloys, with 10 to 20% platinum and palladium
(c) Highly platinised alloys, with up to 50% platinum and palladium

As with stainless steel wires, these materials have a fibrous structure. Sufficient heating to cause recrystallisation must be avoided if the resilience of the wire is to be retained. The more highly platinised alloys have higher recrystallisation temperatures, so are indicated for use when soldering is to be carried out.

38.4 METALLIC COMPONENTS

38.4.1 Wires

The alloys listed above can all be used for orthodontic wires, nickel-titanium and β–titanium being the most recent. Wires can also be used as components of partial dentures, e.g. wrought rests and clasp arms.

In Chapter 39, some comparative properties of materials are considered. Stainless steel is the most widely used alloy of choice. Owing to economic resons, gold wires are seldom used.

Chapter 44 discusses the principles of joining metals by soldering and welding. Note that these techniques are inapplicable to nickel-titanium alloys, which have to be joined by mechanical crimping.

38.4.2 Brackets, bands and screws

Prefabricated components such as brackets, bands and screws are usually made from stainless steel.

Brackets for direct bonding techniques (see below) are designed to bond mechanically to the resin; this is achieved either by a metal mesh on, or by perforation in, the bracket. Polymeric brackets (e.g.

polycarbonate) have not proved to be particularly successful, owing to their inadequate strength properties.

Bands are cemented to the crowns of teeth, using, for example, a zinc phosphate cement.

38.5 ELASTIC MODULES

Elastic modules can be made either from natural rubber, or from synthetic polyester-urethane elastomers. These modules exhibit stress relaxation, owing to their viscoelastic nature (Section 5.7.1). Thus, the force exerted by a module will decrease as a function of time.

38.6 DIRECT BONDING MATERIALS

38.6.1 Materials

The bonding resins are usually filled dimethacrylates, similar in principle to composite restorative materials (Ch. 19). These resins bond mechanically to the brackets (see above) and to acid etched enamel. The procedures for acid etching should be followed carefully (Section 20.4).

38.6.2 Critique

(a) Problems are sometimes encountered in de-bonding brackets.
(b) Some advantages of direct bonding techniques include:
  (i) greater ease in the maintenance of good oral hygiene
  (ii) better aesthetics
  (iii) the ability for precise placement of brackets
  (iv) the ability to bond on to unerupted and partially erupted teeth.

39. Some biomechanical principles

39.1 TOOTH MOVEMENT

Tooth movement can be achieved by the applicaton of a force to the tooth by an orthodontic appliance. In studying forces, it is necessary to specify the magnitude of the force, and the direction and point of application.

Tooth movement may be classified into the following five types:
(a) Tipping movement, where force is applied to a single point on the crown of the tooth
(b) Rotational movements, achieved by applying a force couple. Two equal (and opposite) forces F, separated by a distance d produce a moment M = Fd. For example, 2 forces of 0.3 N, 4 mm apart, produce a moment of 1.2 N mm
(c) Translation, or bodily, movement can occur if a force is applied to a large area of the crown of the tooth
(d) Extrusion of a tooth from its socket can be achieved
(e) Intrusion can also be carried out

The magnitude of the applied force is important. Severe force can damage periodontal tissues. The correct force depends on which type of movement is required, and also on the geometry of the tooth roots. For bodily movements, forces of up to 3 N have been quoted; other procedures require typically 0.25 to 0.5 N.

39.2 DESIRABLE MECHANICAL PROPERTIES

Separate consideration must be given to the requirements for active and reactive components (see Section 38.1).

Reactive components, which anchor the appliance to teeth which are not to be moved, should not deform. Thus high values of both yield stress and modulus of rigidity are important.

Active components must ideally meet the following criteria:
(a) Great flexibility is required. Thus a more flexible component

will be able to apply lower and a more constant force over a greater distance. Note that flexibility is a function both of mechanical properties and the geometry of the material (see below).
(b) High resilience is required; the material should be able to store and release elastic energy.

39.3 COMPARATIVE MECHANICAL PROPERTIES OF WIRES

From Table II.5 (Appendix II), it can be seen that, in general, the chromium-containing alloys (stainless steel, nickel-chromium and cobalt-chromium) have higher moduli of elasticity than gold and titanium alloys. The flexibility of the modern titanium alloys is a useful property, as they can apply an active force to a tooth over a greater distance than a stainless steel wire of similar geometry.

39.4 INTRODUCTION TO FORCE MECHANICS

(a) Basically a wire in an appliance can be considered as a beam. From an orthodontic viewpoint, three parameters need to be considered.

- (i) the rigidity, often referred to as the load-deflection rate
- (ii) the maximum load, or allowable working load, related to the elastic limit
- (iii) the maximum deflection—related to the maximum amount of elastic strain.

(b) Flexure of a cantilever beam

(i) Flexural rigidity $= \dfrac{E \cdot \pi \cdot r^4}{4}$,

where E = modulus of elasticity
and r = radius of the wire

The load-deflection rate also depends on the length L of the wire; it is universally proportional to L^3

For a rectangular wire, load-deflection rate is proportional to bh^3, where h is the dimension of the wire in the direction of bending

Example: Doubling the modulus will double the rigidity. Doubling the radius has a significantly greater effect on rigidity. Consider two wires, of the same material, of modulus E, one with radius x, one with radius 2x

Flexural rigidity of first wire $= \dfrac{E \cdot \pi \cdot x^4}{4}$

$$\text{Flexural rigidity of second wire} = \frac{E \cdot \pi \cdot 16x^4}{4}$$

Wire 2 has a rigidity 16 times greater than wire 1.

(ii) Allowable working load.
This is proportional to the elastic limit. For a circular wire, it is proportional to R^3 and 1/L. For a rectangular wire, it is proportional to bh^2.

(iii) Maximum deflection depends on the elastic limit divided by modulus of elasticity. For a circular wire, this parameter is proportional to 1/r, and to L^2. For a rectangular wire, it is proportional to 1/h.

Note. The above discussion is designed to introduce the subject, showing how mechanical properties and geometrical design are both important. Many other factors can be studied from the references below, such as the use of braided wires, loops, etc.

(c) Torsion of a wire—this is a twisting action applied to a wire. The load-deflection rate is proportional to 1/L, where L is the length is torsion.

Note. In practice, the loading pattern of components of orthodontic appliances can be complex, involving tension, compression, bending and torsion.

READING REFERENCES

Burstone C J 1975 In: Graber T M, Swain BF (eds) Current orthodontic concepts and techniques 2 edn. Saunders, Philadelphia Vol I

An extensive discussion of the biomechanics of tooth movement.

Burstone C J Goldberg A J 1980 Beta titanium: a new orthodontic alloy. American Journal of Orthodontics 77: 121

Kusy R P 1981 Comparison of nickel-titanium and beta titanium wire sizes to conventional orthodontic arch wire materials. American Journal of Orthodontics 79: 625

These papers compare the properties of a number of wires of different types.

SECTION VIII

Laboratory materials and procedures

40. Model and die materials

40.1 INTRODUCTION

A *model* is a replica of the teeth and/or the associated supporting bony tissues of one jaw, which is prepared from an impression. A *die* is a model of a single tooth, again prepared from an impression.

Model and die materials should have the following properties:
(a) Mechanical properties–high strength, to reduce the likelihood of accidental breakage, particularly of teeth from a model, and should be as hard as possible, so that the surface will not be damaged during carving of a wax pattern.
(b) Ability to reproduce fine detail and sharp margins.
(c) Dimensional accuracy and stability–should show little dimensional change on setting, and should remain stable.
(d) Compatibility with impression materials—there should be no interaction between surface of impression and model or die.
(e) Good colour contrast with other materials being used, for example, inlay wax or porcelain.
(f) Cheapness and ease of use.

Models and dies for dental use are frequently prepared from plaster of Paris, or from hard plaster materials, known as dental stones. Both these materials have calcium sulphate hemihydrate, $(CaSO_4)_2$, H_2O (sometimes written $CaSO_4$, $\frac{1}{2}H_2O$) as their main constituent. This material is discussed next (Section 40.2) followed by consideration of alternative die materials (Section 40.3).

40.2 CALCIUM SULPHATE HEMIHYDRATE

40.2.1 The hydrates of calcium sulphate

These are listed in Table 40.1

40.2.2 Dental gypsum products

(a) Dental plaster has *calcined* calcium sulphate hemihydrate as its main constituent, together with chemicals to control the setting time (Section 40.2.6).
(b) Impression plaster is as above, with, for example, added potassium sulphate, borax and colouring agents (Sections 25.1 and 40.2.6).
(c) Model and die materials are based on *autoclaved* calcium sulphate hemihydrate, plus additives to adjust the setting time (Section 40.2.6), and pigments, to distinguish the material from plaster, which is white.
(d) Some dental casting investment materials contain autoclaved calcium sulphate hemihydrate, to act as a binder (Ch. 42).

40.2.3 The setting reaction of calcium sulphate hemihydrate

When hemihydrate is mixed with water, the dihydrate is formed, as follows:

$$(CaSO_4)_2, H_2O + 3H_2O \rightarrow 2CaSO_4, 2H_2O$$

This is the reverse of the reaction whereby hemihydrate is formed. From the above equation it can be calculated that 100 g of hemihydrate require about 18.6 ml water to give complete hydration. In practice, however, more water than this is used when mixing plaster or stone, to give a smooth workable mix.

On mixing the hemihydrate with water, the following things are believed to occur (though there still is considerable dispute in the scientific literature about the nature of the setting reaction):
(a) Some hemihydrate dissolves, giving Ca^{2+} and SO_4^{2-} ions, the solubility of hemihyrate in water at room temperature is about 0.8%.
(b) At this temperature, the solubility of the dihydrate is only about 0.2%; the dissolved hemihydrate forms the dihydrate in solution, which is then supersaturated. Crystal growth of the dihydrate from this solution then occurs.

(c) The following factors are also important in relation to this reaction:

(i) Crystal growth occurs on nuclei of crystallisation; in this case nuclei may be crystals of gypsum initially present as an impurity in the hemihydrate crystals.

(ii) Diffusion, or movement, of the Ca^{2+} and SO_4^{2-} ions to these nuclei, also appears to be important (Section 40.2.8).

(iii) As the dihydrate crystallises, so more hemihydrate dissolves and the process continues.

40.2.4 The setting process

The following factors can be observed during the setting reaction:

(a) Initially the mix or hemihydrate and water can be poured (if the correct water/powder ratio is used, Section 40.2.5).

(b) The material becomes rigid, but not hard ('initial set')—at this stage the material can be carved but not moulded.

(c) The so-called 'final set' follows, when the material becomes hard and strong. However, at this stage the hydration reaction is not necessarily complete, nor has optimum strength and hardness necessarily been achieved.

(d) Heat is given out during setting, since the hydration of the hemihydrate is exothermic.

(e) Dimensional changes also take place:

(i) A setting expansion can be observed. The linear expansion is in the range 0.3 to 0.4% for most plasters and 0.05 to 0.3% for dental stones. This expansion is caused by the outward thrust of the growing crystals of dihydrate.

(ii) The above expansion is, in fact, apparent. The expanded set material contains crystals of dihydrate and pores. The volume of crystals of the set material is less than the initial volume of the hemihydrate. The magnitude of this reduction in volume of the crystalline material can be calculated from the molecular weights and specific gravities of hemihydrate, water and dihydrate, and is approximately 7%.

(iii) If mixed plaster is placed under water at the initial set stage, a greater expansion on setting occurs; this is *hygroscopic expansion* and is sometimes used to expand gypsum bonded investment materials (Section 42.4.3).

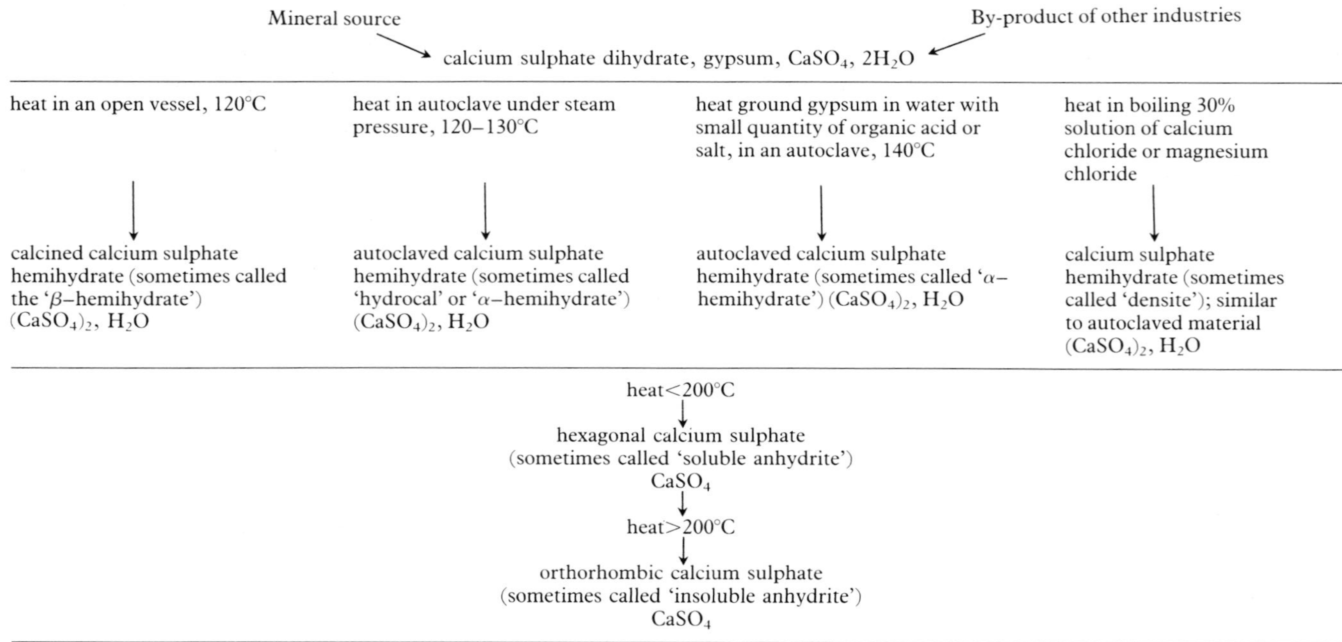

Table 40.1 Hydrates of calcium sulphate

Mineral source → calcium sulphate dihydrate, gypsum, $CaSO_4$, $2H_2O$ ← By-product of other industries			
heat in an open vessel, 120°C	heat in autoclave under steam pressure, 120–130°C	heat ground gypsum in water with small quantity of organic acid or salt, in an autoclave, 140°C	heat in boiling 30% solution of calcium chloride or magnesium chloride
↓	↓	↓	↓
calcined calcium sulphate hemihydrate (sometimes called the 'β–hemihydrate') $(CaSO_4)_2$, H_2O	autoclaved calcium sulphate hemihydrate (sometimes called 'hydrocal' or 'α–hemihydrate') $(CaSO_4)_2$, H_2O	autoclaved calcium sulphate hemihydrate (sometimes called 'α–hemihydrate') $(CaSO_4)_2$, H_2O	calcium sulphate hemihydrate (sometimes called 'densite'); similar to autoclaved material $(CaSO_4)_2$, H_2O

heat$<$200°C
↓
hexagonal calcium sulphate
(sometimes called 'soluble anhydrite')
$CaSO_4$
↓
heat$>$200°C
↓
orthorhombic calcium sulphate
(sometimes called 'insoluble anhydrite')
$CaSO_4$

40.2.5 Differences between calcined and autoclaved hemihydrate

Though these two materials are chemically identical, they differ in the following ways:

(a) Manufacture—see Table 40.1

(b) Particle size and shape:

  (i) Calcined hemihydrate particles are larger; irregular and porous (Fig. 40.1 (a)).

  (ii) The particles of the autoclaved material are smaller, regular and non-porous (Fig. 40.1 (b)).

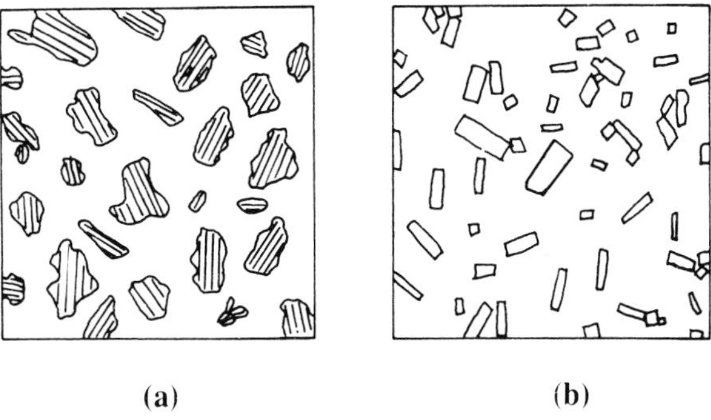

Fig. 40.1 Particles of calcium sulphate hemihydrate. (a) The calcined material (× 100). (b) The autoclaved material (× 100).

(c) Water/powder ratio—theoretically this is 0.186 (Section 40.2.3). However, neither hemihydrate, when mixed with water to this ratio, will give a smooth workable mix. The ratios that are used are:

  (i) Calcined hemihydrate (as in plaster) 50 to 60 ml/100g.

  (ii) Autoclaved hemihydrate (as in stone) 22 to 35 ml/100g.

The reason for the difference is that the porous particles of a calcined material soak up a considerable amount of water.

(d) The set material—this consists of a network of interlocking dihydrate crystals; the spaces between these crystals are initially occupied by the excess water used in mixing the material (this water will contain calcium sulphate in solution). The greater the quantity of excess water, the more porous (or less dense) is the set material; thus the porosity of set plaster is greater than the porosity of set stone.

(e) Mechanical properties of the set material—strength and hardness depend on the density of the material; thus stone is harder and stronger than plaster.

(f) Applications. Where strength and hardness are required, autoclaved hemihydrate, as in stone, is the material of choice. Examples are models for construction of dentures, dies for crowns, bridge and inlay work, and binders for casting investments (Ch. 42). When mechanical properties are not of primary importance, plaster can be used. Examples—mounting models, and some orthodontic study models.

N.B.—In the literature a distinction is sometimes made between 'model' and 'die stones', or 'stones' and 'improved stones' or 'type I' and 'type II stones'. In fact it is probably not necessary to make such a distinction, since there is little or no difference between stones available for model and die construction.

40.2.6 The effects of additives

Nearly all acids and salts, when added to a mix of plaster or stone, affect the setting:

(a) The setting time may be increased for decreased:

(i) Accelerators

Example (1). Potassium sulphate is believed to accelerate by increasing the rate of solution of calcium sulphate hemihydrate.

Example (2). Gypsum accelerates by providing nuclei for crystal growth of further dihydrate.

(ii) Retarders

Examples. Potassium citrate and borax; these either reduce the rate of dissolution of hemihydrate, or are adsorbed on to nuclei of crystallisation, thus 'poisoning' these nuclei, and rendering them ineffective.

(b) The setting expansion may be altered:

(i) Increased expansion—for example, calcium acetate can give over 1% linear setting expansion.

(ii) Decreased expansion—for example, potassium sulphate can reduce the linear setting expansion down to 0.05%.

(c) The strength of the material is usually reduced by additives (but see Section 40.2.11).

40.2.7 Manipulation

(a) Storage—closed containers, to prevent reaction with moisture from the atmosphere, which can cause formation of the dihydrate

which can accelerate the setting (Section 40.2.6 and 40.2.8).
(b) Contamination—keep free from traces of set gypsum and other impurities.
(c) Correct water/powder ratio (Section 40.2.5)—for example, if stone is mixed with too much water, the set material may be as weak as plaster.
(d) Avoid incorporation of air in mix—sift powder on to the water, and mix the slurry in such a manner as to avoid trapping air in the material.
(e) Mixing time of one minute is usually sufficient to give a smooth lump-free slurry.
(f) Vibration is usually used in casting a model or die from an impression; this helps the slurry to flow well into the impression and helps to eliminate air bubbles. Over vibration should be avoided as this may cause distortion of some impression materials.
(g) A separating agent is applied to a stone die before preparation of a wax pattern on the die—this facilitates removal of the pattern from the die. Unfortunately these agents can soften the surface of the die.

40.2.8 Setting time

This is usually measured as the time taken for the setting material to become sufficiently rigid to withstand the penetration of a needle of known diameter under a known load. Two such pieces of apparatus are known as *Vicat* and *Gillmore* needles.

The setting time depends on:
(a) The composition of the plaster or stone, as supplied by the manufacturer:

- (i) Gypsum, if present (for example, due to incomplete dehydration during the manufacturing process) will accelerate the setting (Section 40.2.6).
- (ii) Hexagonal calcium sulphate, if present, will hydrate rapidly.
- (iii) Orthorhombic calcium sulphate, which can result from gross overheating of the gypsum during manufacture, reacts very slowly with water (known as 'dead-burnt' plaster).
- (iv) Other impurities may be present, which either occurred in the gypsum starting material, or were introduced during the manufacturing process.
- (v) Added accelerators and/or retarders—see Section 40.2.6.

(b) The physical form of the plaster or stone—during manufacture grinding is usually carried out after the dehydration process. This accelerates the setting:

(i) Since some of the ground crystals can act as nuclei for the crystal growth on setting.

(ii) Grinding increases the surface area of the hemihydrate exposed to water, thus increasing the rate of solution of the hemihydrate.

Table 40.2 The effect of temperature on the setting time of dental stone

Temperature °C	Time for complete hydration of a dental stone at a water/powder ratio 0.3 (minutes)
5	65
25	75
30	60
35	50
40	45
45	40
50	55

(c) Temperature of the mix—this has very little effect up to 50°C for example, Table 40.2 gives results for one batch of dental stone. This is in contrast to most chemical reactions, which are accelerated considerably by an increase in temperature. This can be explained by assuming that the rate of reaction depends on the rate of random diffusion of Ca^{2+} and SO_4^{2-} ions to the growing dihydrate crystals. The rate of diffusion of ions in solution depends not only on the nature of the ions, but also on (i) temperature and (ii) the concentration of ions.

(i) Temperature—it can be shown that the rate of diffusion of Ca^{2+} and SO_4^{2-} ions at 50°C is very approximately double the rate at 5°C.

(ii) Concentration—the rate of diffusion of ions is directly proportional to their concentration. The solubility of hemihydrate is approximately 0.8 and 0.4% at 5 and 50°C respectively. Thus at higher temperatures the rate of diffusion is reduced, owing to a decrease in concentration.

Factors (i) and (ii) above are opposite to each other and approximately equal in magnitude—hence temperature has only a comparatively small effect on the rate of reaction within the range 5 to 50°C. At higher temperatures, retardation of hydration occurs, and at 100°C there is no hydration—at approximately this temperature both hemihydrate and dihydrate have the same solubility.

(d) Water/powder ratio. This has very little effect on the rate of hydration of the hemihydrate, although an increase in water content of a slurry gives a slower setting time as measured by the Vicat or Gillmore needle test. The reason is, that at a higher water/powder ratio, there are fewer growing dihydrate crystals per volume of mixed material. So in the more dilute slurries, more crystal growth has to occur before there is enough crystal contact to give sufficient rigidity to withstand the penetration of a setting time needle.
(e) Time of mixing. An increase in the mixing time can accelerate the set. Mixing can break up some of the formed dihydrate crystals, thus forming more nuclei of crystallisation.

40.2.9 Strength

This depends on:
(a) The material that is used—for example, autoclaved or calcined hemihydrate (Section 40.2.1) and the additives present (Section 40.2.6).
(b) The water/powder ratio (Section 40.2.5 and 40.2.7)—see Table 40.3.

Table 40.3 The strength of plaster and stone

Material	Compressive strength (MN/m^2)
Plaster, water/powder ratio 0.6 after one hour	10
Plaster, water/powder ratio 0.6 dried to constant weight at 45°C	21
Stone, water/powder ratio 0.25 after one hour	30
Stone, water/powder ratio 0.25 dried to constant weight at 45°C	72

(c) The dryness of the set material—see Table 40.3. For optimum properties, the plaster or stone should be left to hydrate for at least one hour (and perferably longer), and then dried to constant weight at 45°C.

40.2.10 Critique of model and die materials based on calcium sulphate hemihydrate

(a) Mechanical properties are not ideal—fracture of teeth from stone models can occur with careless handling; also stone dies are not always sufficiently hard to resist abrasion during the carving of a wax pattern.

(b) These materials have the ability to reproduce fine detail and sharp margins.
(c) The dimensional accuracy and stability are good—the small linear setting expansion (Section 40.2.4) is not considered to be a significant source of error in most dental procedures.
(d) Compatibility with impression materials—some of these materials cause a slight softening of the stone surface. Impression plaster has to be treated with a separating agent before casting up a model in dental stone (Section 25.1.2).
(e) Colour contrast—dental stones usually contain pigments.
(f) Dental stones are inexpensive and easy to use.

40.2.11 Recent developments

Two techniques are being investigated to produce dental stones with improvement in abrasion resistance and other mechanical properties: (a) Impregnation of the gypsum by a polymer—a polyester, polystyrene, acrylics and epoxy-resin have been suggested for this purpose. (b) Incorporation of wetting agents such as lignosulphonates (derived from lignin, one of the main constituents of wood) such additives can reduce the water requirement of a stone, and enable the production of a harder stronger and more dense set gypsum.

In addition, these additives retard the setting time and increase the setting expansion. Both of these effects can be overcome by the incorporation of potassium sulphate (Section 40.2.6).

40.3 ALTERNATIVE DIE MATERIALS

40.3.1 Silicophosphate cement—similar to the filling and cementing material (Section 18.2)

(a) Advantage: harder than die stone.
(b) Disadvantage: shrinkage on setting, loss of water on standing.

40.3.2 Amalgam—similar to the restorative material (Ch. 22):

(a) Advantage: produces a hard die, reproduces fine details and sharp margins.
(b) Disadvantages: can only be packed into a rigid (for example, composition) impression; long time to reach maximum hardness; high thermal conductivity, so can cool a wax pattern rapidly, which

may lead to distortion of the pattern—this can be overcome by warming the die; a separating agent is needed as with stone dies.

40.3.3 Polymers and filled polymers

These are either self-curing acrylic materials, or polymeric materials (for example, epoxy resins, polyesters and epimines) with fillers (either metallic or ceramic fillers).
(a) Advantage: more abrasion resistant and not as brittle as die stones.
(b) Disadvantage: shrinkage on polymerisation may be a source of inaccuracy—fillers reduce this shrinkage.

40.3.4 Metal sprayed dies

A bismuth–tin alloy, which melts at 138°C can be sprayed directly on to an impression to form a metal shell, which can then be filled with dental stone.
(a) Advantage: a metal coated die can be obtained rapidly from elastomeric impression materials.
(b) Disadvantage: the alloy is rather soft; care is needed to prevent abrasion of the die.

40.3.5 Electroplated dies

Some impression materials can be electroplated—for example, impression composition can be copper plated, and elastomeric materials can be silver plated (see Section 11.6).
(a) Copper plating.
The following general technique is used:

- (i) The surface of the impression is rendered conductive by coating it with fine particles of copper or graphite.
- (ii) The coated impression is made the cathode (negative electrode) of a plating bath, with an anode (positive electrode) of copper.
- (iii) The electrolyte is an acid solution of copper sulphate (about 250g/litre) together with organic constituents (for example alcohol or phenol) which are believed to increase the hardness of the deposited metal.
- (iv) A current is passed, causing slow dissolution of the anode, and movement of copper ions from anode to cathode, so plating the impression. A current of 5 to 50 mamp/cm^2 of

cathode surface is applied for approximately 10 hours.

(v) Dental stone is then cast into the plated impression; when the stone has set, the metal covered die can be removed from the impression.

(vi) This technique is often not considered suitable for the elastomeric materials—it is believed that they are not dimensionally stable in an acid solution.

(b) Silver plating.

Polysulphide and silicone impression materials can be silver plated by the same general technique as above, except:

(i) The impression is coated with silver or graphite powder.

(ii) The anode is silver.

(iii) The electrolyte is an alkaline solution of silver cyanide (with other constituents such as potassium cyanide and potassium carbonate).

As above, the current and time for plating must be adequately controlled according to the instructions supplied with the plating kit.

Precaution. If any acid (for example, pickling acid, or acid copper sulphate solution) comes in contact with the alkaline cyanide solution, HCN gas will be given off—this is an obvious toxic hazard. The cyanide solution should be kept in a fume cupboard, with no acids nearby. Because of this risk, silver plating is not often used.

40.3.6 Ceramic die materials

Two ceramic die materials are available:

(a) A material for the production of dies on which porcelain restorations are to be fabricated, without the use of a platinum foil matrix. To form the dies heating to over 1000°C is necessary.

(b) A ceramic material, supplied as a powder and liquid, and mixed to a putty-like consistency. After 1 hour the material is removed from the impression and fired at 600°C for 8 minutes to produce a hard strong die.

READING REFERENCES

Combe E C Smith D C 1964 Some properties of gypsum plasters. British Dental Journal 117: 237

A comparison of the available dental stones for the construction of models and dies

Newman A Williams J D 1969 Die materials for inlay, crown and bridge work. British Dental Journal 127: 415

A very comprehensive review of the various types of die material

Spratley M H Combe E C 1973 A comparison of some polymer-containing die materials Journal of Denistry 1: 158

A comparison of properties of three filled polymer materials with a dental stone

Combe E C Grant A A 1973 The selection and properties of materials for dental practice 6-dental alloys and associated materials. British Dental Journal 134: 240

One section of this paper deals with the selection of die materials

41. Waxes and baseplate materials

41.1 INTRODUCTION

Waxes were first used in dentistry in the early eighteenth century for the purpose of recording impressions of edentulous mouths. Although superseded by other impression materials, waxes are still employed in large quantities in various clinical and laboratory procedures.

The construction of many dental appliances requires the use of waxes with specific and often markedly different physical properties. In order to obtain these requirements, dental waxes are usually blended from both natural and synthetic materials.

41.2 BASIC CONSTITUENTS OF DENTAL WAXES

The basic constituents of dental waxes come from three main sources:

(a) mineral,
(b) insect, and
(c) vegetable.

The structure and properties of the most important materials are classified in Table 41.1. Since the properties of these naturally occurring materials cannot be controlled, synthetic waxes (e.g. nitrogenous derivatives of fatty acids) or polymers of ethylene oxide may offer advantages.

41.3 PHYSICAL PROPERTIES OF WAXES

The most frequently quoted physical property of waxes is their melting point. While this may be of importance in industry it does not have the same significance in dentistry where blends of waxes are employed. The important physical properties of waxes used in dentistry, apart from ease of manipulation, are:
(a) solid–solid transition temperature, are:
(b) thermal expansion and contraction;
(c) flow, and
(d) internal stress.

41.3.1 Solid–solid transition temperature

As the temperature of a wax is raised, a solid–solid transition occurs where the stable crystal lattice form (orthorhombic in most dental waxes) commences to change to a hexagonal form which is present below the melting point of the wax. It is during this progressive change from one lattice type to the other that waxes are able to be manipulated without flaking, tearing or becoming unduly stressed.

The existence of this solid–solid transition point and the temperature at which it occurs not only allows waxes to be manipulated satisfactorily, but also determines much of their physical behaviour and suitability for various clinical and laboratory procedures. Waxes which should remain rigid in the mouth must have a solid–solid transition temperature above 37°C.

41.3.2 Thermal expansion and contraction

The coefficient of thermal expansion of waxes is higher than that of any other dental material. This is a potential source of error in dental procedures, since a pattern will shrink appreciably on cooling from its solidification temperature to room temperature. It can be shown that on cooling from 37 to 20°C, a linear shrinkage of almost 0.6% can occur for a wax with a coefficient of thermal expansion of $350 \times 10^{-6}/°C$ (Section 6.5).

41.3.3 Flow

Waxes deform when subjected to a load for a period of time. This plastic deformation or percentage 'flow' depends on temperature and is found to be low when the temperature of the wax is below the

Table 41.1 Classification of naturally occurring waxes

Type	Example	Source	Structure	Properties
(a) Mineral	Paraffin wax	Obtained during the distillation of crude petroleum	Straight-chained hydrocarbon Polycrystalline	Brittle at ambient temperature
	Microcrystalline wax or ceresin	As above	Branch-chained hydrocarbon Polycrystalline	Less brittle than paraffin wax, due to their oil content
(b) Insect	Beeswax	Honeycombs	Less crystalline than paraffin wax—more amorphous material	When blended with paraffin wax, (i) at room temperature makes it less brittle, (ii) at higher temperature (e.g. mouth temperature) reduces the flow of the wax
(c) Vegetable	Carnauba wax	South American palm trees	—	Hard, lustrous, tough wax. Blended with paraffin wax to harden it and raise its solid–solid transition temperature (see Section 41.3.1)
	Candelila wax	Plants	—	Similar to carnauba
	Resins and gums	Trees	—	Used to add adhesive qualities to waxes

solid–solid transition temperature (i.e. when the materials are in the stable crystal lattice form).

The flow property of waxes and wax mixtures increases as their temperature is raised above the transition temperature.

It is important in an inlay wax for use in the direct technique (41.4.3) that there should be:
(a) a large flow about 5°C above mouth temperature, so that good detail of the cavity will be obtained, and
(b) negligible flow at 37°C, so that no distortion will occur on removal of the pattern from the cavity.

41.3.4 Internal stresses

Waxes have low thermal conductivity, so making it difficult to achieve uniform heating. If a wax is moulded or adapted to shape without adequate heating to above the solid–solid transition temperature, considerable stresses will be set up in the material. If the wax is subsequently warmed, relief of the stresses will occur, resulting in distortion.

41.4 DENTAL APPLICATIONS OF WAXES

41.4.1 Modelling wax

This is used as a pattern material (Section 42.1), and for the registration of jaw relationships, in the construction of dentures. The desirable properties are:
(a) It should be easy to mould when softened, and not tear, flake or crack.
(b) It should be easy to carve.
(c) It should be capable of being melted and solidified a number of times without change of properties.
(d) No residue of wax should be left after applying boiling water and detergent to the mould formed about the wax.

The exact compositions of available modelling waxes are not usually revealed by the manufacturers, but suitable materials can be prepared using mixtures of such waxes as paraffin wax and beeswax, with a small quantity of a harder and tougher wax such as carnauba.

A range of materials of different softening temperatures is available.

In the manipulation of the materials it is important that the wax is evenly heated throughout its whole bulk and adapted to shape before cooling, to minimise subsequent distortion due to relief of internal stresses.

Modelling waxes used for clinical procedures should show little or no dimensional change when they are heated to mouth temperature and subsequently cooled to room temperature.

41.4.2 Sheet casting wax

Sheet casting wax is supplied in sheets which have been rolled to a precise thickness. When such wax is being manipulated, care must be taken not to make it thinner. This can be avoided by heating the wax in hot water and using moist cotton-wool to adapt it to shape. It is important that both clasps and connectors of cast metallic dentures should be of the correct thickness.

Ready-formed polymeric components are available to simplify the waxing-up of a cast partial denture.

Both casting waxes and polymeric components should burn out from the mould without leaving any residue.

41.4.3 Inlay wax

Inlay wax is used for the preparation of inlay patterns, either:
(a) in the mouth, by the *direct technique*, or,
(b) on a model or die cast up from an impression—the *indirect technique*.

For use in the former application, it is important that the wax should:
(a) have as low as thermal contraction as possible, though inevitably this must be high (Section 41.3.2),
(b) have the correct flow properties (Section 41.3.3), and,
(c) be coloured (usually blue or green) to contrast with the oral tissues.

In addition, all inlay waxes should:
(a) be easy to carve without chipping or flaking, and,
(b) burn out of the mould without leaving any residue.

The constituents of inlay waxes are similar to modelling waxes (Section 41.4.1). The proportion of harder waxes is increased, however, to produce a blend capable of meeting the more stringent requirements of an inlay wax.

41.4.4 Carding and boxing-in-wax

This is a wax with a high flow value at room temperature and is easily mouldable without the need for heating. It is used by manufacturers to attach artificial teeth to the mounts on which they are supplied, and is also used in the dental laboratory to 'box-in' impressions prior to casting up.

41.4.5 Sticky wax

This is an adhesive brittle wax, usually made of beeswax and some naturally occurring resins. It should show no flow at room temperature. It is used in the dental laboratory for a variety of applications where temporary joining of articles is required, for example, joining together metal parts prior to soldering and joining fragments of a broken denture prior to the repair procedure. It should be easily removed by boiling water and should show minimal shrinkage on cooling to prevent movement of the parts to be joined.

41.4.6 Impression waxes

These are dealt with in Section 25.4. Impression, corrective and disclosing waxes are all characterised by their high degree of flow at mouth temperature.

41.5 THERMOPLASTIC BASEPLATE MATERIALS

These may be made of:
(a) wax, similar to modelling wax (Section 41.4.1),
(b) shellac, or shellac with aluminium, or,
(c) a polymer such as polystyrene.

Baseplate materials should be:
(a) readily adaptable to the required shape,
(b) rigid and exhibit little flow at mouth temperature, and,
(c) should not distort on standing, or in use.

42. Investment materials

42.1 INTRODUCTION

When a restoration or appliance is being made by a 'lost wax' process, the wax pattern is embedded in an investment material. The wax is then removed from this mould, and the space which it occupied is filled by the material of which the restoration or appliance is to be made. For example:

(a) A wax pattern of a denture, in which the teeth have been set up in embedded in a two-part mould, made of plaster of Paris or dental stone (or a mixture of the two) contained in a two-part metal container (a *flask*). The wax is removed by means of boiling water and detergent, leaving the teeth embedded in the set gypsum. The space formerly occupied by the wax is subsequently filled with the polymeric denture base material (Ch. 33).

(b) The wax pattern of an inlay or other cast restoration is embedded in a heat-resistant investment material, which is capable of setting to a hard mass. The wax is removed from such a mould usually by burning out, before casting the molten alloy.

This chapter is primarily concerned with the latter materials, since details of plaster and stone are dealt with in Chapter 40.

42.2 REQUIREMENTS FOR INVESTMENT MATERIALS

All investment materials contain:

(a) A refractory substance—a material that will not decompose or

disintegrate on heating, and
(b) A binder—a material which will set and bind together the particles of the refractory substance.

In addition the following properties are desirable:
(a) The mould must expand to compensate for the shrinkage on cooling of the alloy.
(b) The powder should be of a fine particle size to ensure a smooth surface on the casting.
(c) The mixed unset material should have a smooth consistency.
(d) The material should have a suitable setting time.
(e) The set material should be permeable to allow air to escape as the molten alloy enters the mould.
(f) The strength of the material should be sufficient to withstand the force of the molten alloy entering the mould.

42.3 TYPES OF INVESTMENT MATERIAL

Three types are available. They all contain silica (SiO_2) as the refractory constituent. The chief difference between them is the type of binder used, as follows:
(a) Gypsum-bonded investments are widely used for gold alloys, but are unsuitable for alloys which melt at temperatures approaching 1200°C (Section 42.4).
(b) Phosphate-bonded materials are used for casting cobalt–chromium alloys, since they can withstand higher temperatures (Section 42.5).
(c) Silica-bonded investments are an alternative to the phosphate-bonded materials for high temperature casting (Section 42.6).

42.4 GYPSUM-BONDED INVESTMENTS

42.4.1 Constituents

(a) Silica is present in one of its allotropic forms (for example, cristobalite or quartz) to:
   (i) act as a refractory, and,
   (ii) to provide mould expansion by thermal expansion and inversion (Sections 12.6 and 42.4.3).

(b) Autoclaved calcium sulphate hemihydrate, for the following purposes:
   (i) to react with water and on hydration (Section 40.2.3) to bind the silica together,

(ii) to impart sufficient strength to the mould, and
(iii) to contribute to the mould expansion by the setting expansion which occurs (Section 40.2.4).

(c) A reducing agent such as powdered charcoal, to reduce any oxide formed on the metal.

(d) Modifying chemicals such as boric acid or sodium chloride, to inhibit shrinkage on heating (Section 42.4.3).

42.4.2 Manipulation

(a) The mixing of an investment material is similar to that of dental stone (Section 40.2.7). Use of the correct water/powder ratio is important to ensure that the correct strength, setting time and expansion are obtained.

(b) Before investing the wax pattern, it is washed with a non-foam detergent to remove any oil or grease, and to facilitate the wetting of the pattern by the investment mix.

(c) The casting ring is usually lined with a wet asbestos strip. This does two things:

(i) it facilitates mould expansion (as outlined in the next section), since it can be compressed as expansion occurs, whereas a rigid ring on its own cannot do this.
(ii) it contributes to the hygroscopic expansion (Section 42.4.3).

(d) Investing the pattern may be done:

(i) under vacuum, to prevent trapping air on the surface of the pattern, or
(ii) painting investment material on to the pattern with a brush before carefully inserting it into the filled casting ring.

(e) The mould is heated through 150 to 200°C; this dries out the excess water and burns off the wax. The mould is then slowly heated to above the temperature of inversion—usually to 700°C. It is held at this temperature for 30 minutes to ensure that the wax is completely burnt out.

42.4.3 Dimensional changes of the mould

(a) Setting expansion is caused by the crystal growth of gypsum (Section 40.2.4).

(b) Hygroscopic expansion—in one technique the investment is immersed in water after setting has begun. A greatly increased setting expansion occurs (the *hygroscopic expansion*, Section 40.2.4) so less thermal expansion is required. Increased hygroscopic expansion is obtained in the following cases:

(i) when a lower water/powder ratio is used,
(ii) for an investment material of greater silica content,
(iii) if water of higher temperature is used, and
(iv) for longer immersion in water.

(c) Thermal expansion. The thermal expansion of silica is discussed in Section 12.6. Investment materials containing cristobalite and quartz show rapid expansions between 200–300°C and 500–600°C respectively, due to displacive transformation of the silica (Fig. 42.1).

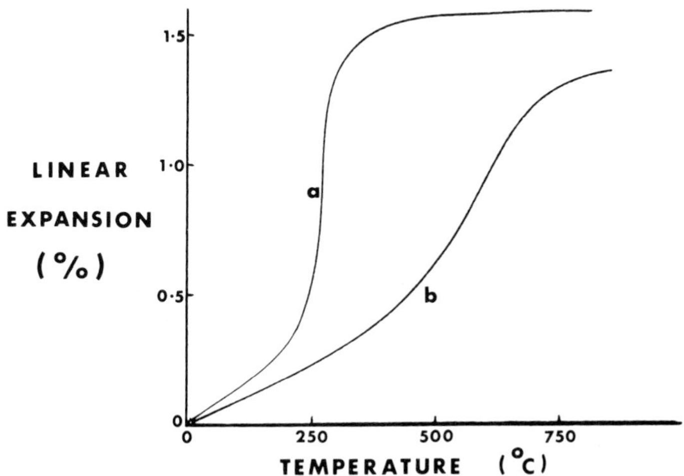

Fig. 42.1 Thermal expansion of investments, (a) containing cristobalite, (b) containing quartz.

The amount of thermal expansion therefore depends on:

(i) the temperature,
(ii) the quantity of silica in the material,
(iii) the allotropic form of silica used; for example, the thermal expansion of cristobalite is greater than that of quartz at most temperatures (Fig. 12.1), and
(iv) the water/powder ratio—thicker mixes have greater thermal expansion.

(d) Shrinkage on heating. This occurs due to the dehydration of the set gypsum in two stages:

(i) $2CaSO_4, 2H_2O \rightarrow (CaSO_4)_2, H_2O + 3H_2O$
(ii) $(CaSO_4)_2, H_2O \rightarrow 2CaSO_4 + H_2O$

The investment shrinkage is eliminated or reduced by the presence of small quantities of additives such as sodium chloride or boric acid.

42.4.4 Other properties

(a) The total expansion of the mould is generally sufficient to compensate for the shrinkage on cooling of gold alloys (about 1.5% by volume).
(b) The investments containing finer particles of silica and calcium sulphate hemihydrate give smoother surfaces on the finished casting.
(c) Gypsum bonded investments are easy to manipulate giving a smooth consistency mix.
(d) The setting time of these materials can be easily controlled, as for stone and dental plaster (Section 40.2.8).
(e) The set investment is porous, as is set gypsum (Section 40.2.5)—this helps to prevent back-pressure porosity in castings (Table 43.3).
(f) The strength of these materials, when set, if mixed at the correct water/powder ratio, is sufficient to withstand the forces of the molten alloy as it enters the mould. The autoclaved hemihydrate is used in preference to the calcined material for this reason (Section 40.2.9).

42.4.5 Limitations

Above around 1200°C, a reaction can occur between calcium sulphate and silica:

$$CaSO_4 + SiO_2 \rightarrow CaSiO_3 + SO_3$$

The sulphur trioxide gas that is evolved:
(i) causes porosity in the casting, and
(ii) contributes to the corrosion of the casting.

For this reason gypsum bonded investments are not used for the higher fusing dental alloys, such as cobalt–chromium. In this case phosphate- or silica-bonded materials are chosen.

42.5 PHOSPHATE-BONDED INVESTMENTS

42.5.1 Composition and setting

Magnesium oxide can react with a phosphate such as an ammonium phosphate in an aqueous system as follows:

$$MgO + NH_4H_2PO_4 \rightarrow MgNH_4PO_4 + H_2O$$

The crystals of the magnesium ammonium phosphate bind together the particles of the silica refractory.

42.5.2 Manipulation

These materials are mixed with water, similar to gypsum-bonded investments. However, the following differences in manipulation should be noted:
(a) Because of the strength of the set material, metal casting rings are not needed. In their place, plastic rings can be used; they are removed after the material has set, but before the investment is heated.
(b) The investment is heated in 1000 to 1100°C.

42.5.3 Properties

(a) Expansion. The setting reaction is accompanied by an expansion, analogous to the crystal growth of gypsum. Also, thermal expansion occurs on heating.
(b) Porosity. A set phosphate-bonded material shows a certain degree of porosity, again similar to the gypsum containing investments.
(c) Strength. The set material increases in strength during heating, possibly due to chemical interaction between silica and the binder, giving complex silicophosphates.

42.6 SILICA-BONDED INVESTMENTS

42.6.1 Setting reactions

(a) Stage 1; hydrolysis

Ethyl silicate can be hydrolysed to silicic acid, with liberation of ethyl alcohol:

$$Si(OC_2H_5)_4 + 4H_2O \rightarrow Si(OH)_4 + 4C_2H_5OH$$

In practice, a polymerised form of ethyl silicate is used, yielding a sol of poly(silicic acid).

(b) Stage 2; gelation

The sol is mixed with cristobalite or quartz, then gel formation is made to occur under alkaline conditions by adding magnesium oxide. There is a slight shrinkage at this stage.

(c) Stage 3; drying

On heating, considerable shrinkage occurs and there is loss of alcohol and water, leaving a mould made of silica particles tightly packed together.

As an alternative to the above, simultaneous hydrolysis and gel formation can occur, when an amine such as piperidine is incorporated.

42.6.2 Properties

(a) Dimensional changes

There is a large amount of thermal expansion, due to the very large percentage of silica in the final material. This expansion is usually sufficient to compensate for:

(i) the setting shrinkage of the investment material, and,
(ii) the casting shrinkage of the alloy.

(b) Porosity. The particles of the set material are packed so closely together that the porosity is negligible. Air spaces or vents must be left in the investment to permit escape of air from the mould.

READING REFERENCES

Earnshaw R 1960 Investments for casting cobalt–chromium alloys, Part I. British Dental Journal 108: 389

Earnshaw R 1960 Investments for casting cobalt–chromium alloys, Part II. British Dental Journal 108: 429

These two papers give a great wealth of information on silica and phosphate bonded investments, particularly their chemistry and their dimensional changes.

43. Principles of casting; faults in casting

43.1 GENERAL METHOD OF CASTING

This can be illustrated by considering the procedure used in the casting of an inlay in a gold alloy. The wax pattern (Ch. 41) has a sprue pin attached to it. The pattern is then invested (Ch. 42). After setting of the investment material this pin is removed to provide a channel for the molten alloy to enter the mould. Attached to the sprue pin and the casting ring is a crucible former (or sprue base), which can be made of rubber or other polymers, or wax, or copper (Fig. 43.1).

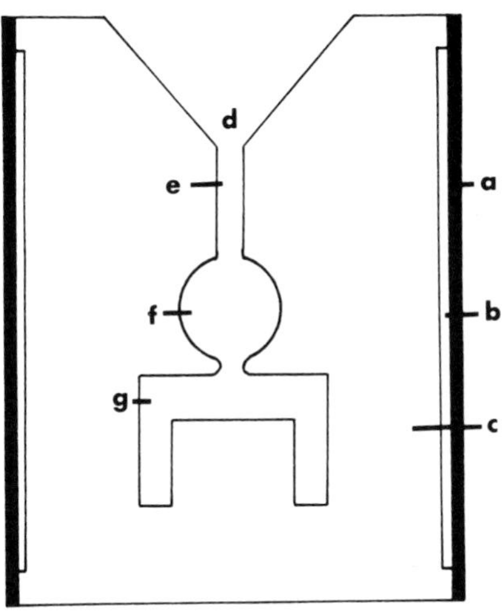

Fig. 43.1 Cross section through an inlay casting mould, after removal of crucible former, sprue and wax. (a) Casting ring, (b) asbestos lining, (c) investment material, (d) crucible former, (e) sprue, (f) reservoir, (g) inlay mould.

It is important that the correct diameter of sprue is used—this should be related to the size of the casting. A very small inlay can have a sprue of 1.3 mm diameter; for most inlays it is 2.0 mm, and for very large crowns 2.6 mm. In some cases a *reservoir* may be needed (Fig. 43.1). This is a piece of wax attached to the sprue about 1 mm away from the pattern. It can help to avoid porosity due to shrinkage. If the space occupied by the wax of the reservoir is of greater cross-section than the casting, the alloy that fills it will solidify later than in the main casting, and provide a reservoir of molten alloy to fill the space caused by shrinkage.

After removal of the sprue pin and the crucible former, the investment is heated in a furnace to burn out the wax and expand the mould. The alloy is melted by air/gas torches. The molten alloy is usually forced into the mould by a centrifugal method. As an alternative, air or steam pressure can be used.

Castings of larger dimensions than inlays—for example, the metal frameworks of partial dentures, usually necessitate the use of multiple sprues to ensure that the mould will be filled with the molten alloy before solidification of any part commences.

When the casting is to be made in cobalt–chromium alloy, melting may be by an oxy-acetylene torch, or by an electrical method, known as induction heating.

43.2 FAULTS IN CASTING

A casting may be dimensionally inaccurate (Table 43.1); have a rough surface (Table 43.2); or be porous (Table 43.3).

Additionally, a casting can be contaminated:

(a) Due to oxidation, caused by:

- (i) overheating the alloy,
- (ii) use of oxidising zone of flame, or,
- (iii) failure to use flux.

(b) Due to sulphur compounds, caused by breakdown of investment if over-heated.

An incomplete casting will result if:

(a) insufficient alloy is used,

(b) the alloy is not able to enter thin portions of the mould,

(c) the mould is too cold, causing premature solidification of the alloy,

(d) the sprues are blocked by foreign matter, such as particles of flux or investment or unburnt wax,

(e) there is back pressure of gases in the mould—see Table 43.3,

(f) the alloy is not fully molten, or
(g) too low a casting force is used.

Table 43.1 Dimensional errors in castings

Problem	Cause	Method of avoiding fault
Casting too large	Excessive mould expansion	(i) Use correct temperature (ii) Use correct type of investment material
Casting too small	Too little mould expansion	Heat the mould sufficiently
Distorted casting	Distorted wax pattern	Correct handling of wax (Section 41.3.4)

Table 43.2 Rough surfaces and fins on castings

Problem	Cause	Method of avoiding fault
Rough surface	(i) Investment breakdown	Avoid overheating mould and alloy
	(ii) Air bubbles on wax pattern	Correct use of wetting agent, or correct vacuum investing technique
	(iii) Weak surface of investment	Avoid use of too high water/powder ratio of investment; Avoid dilution of the investment material from application of too much wetting agent
Fins on casting	Cracking of investment material	Avoid too rapid heating of investment

Table 43.3 Porosity

Problem	Cause	Method of avoiding fault
(a) Irregular voids	Shrinkage on cooling of alloy	(i) Use sprues of correct thickness (ii) Place sprues at bulkiest section of the pattern (iii) Reservoir sufficiently near the pattern to be effective
(b) Irregular voids	Inclusion of particles of investment material	Heat mould upside down so that particles fall out of the mould
(c) Spherical voids	Occluded gases in the molten alloy	Avoid overheating and prolonged heating of the alloy
(d) Rounded margins; regular large voids	Back pressure effect; air unable to escape from mould	(i) Use sufficient casting force (ii) Use investment of adequate permeability (iii) Avoid presence of residue of wax in mould (iv) Place pattern no more than 6–8 mm away from end of casting ring
(e) Porosity	Turbulent flow of molten alloy into mould	Correct placement of sprues

READING REFERENCE

Skinner E W 1965 Casting technics for small castings. Dental Clinics of North America, March, p 225

44. Soldering and welding

44.1 DEFINITIONS

Soldering is the joining of metals by the fusion of an intermediary alloy which has a lower melting point. *Brazing*, a term used industrially, is a soldering operation at temperatures above about 500°C. In dentistry such a distinction is not usually made.

Welding is a process in which the parts themselves are joined together, by the application of heat and/or pressure.

44.2 SOLDERING

44.2.1 Desirable properties of dental solders

(a) The fusion temperature must be at least 50 to 100°C lower than the melting temperature of the alloys to be joined.
(b) The solder should be as strong as the alloys being soldered.
(c) The molten material should flow freely and wet the components well.
(d) Good tarnish and corrosion resistance are necessary.
(e) The colour of the solder should be similar to that of the metals being joined.

44.2.2 Gold solders

(a) Composition—gold, silver and copper, with lesser quantities of zinc and tin. Gold contributes to the corrosion resistance. Zinc and tin help to lower the melting range by the formation of eutectic alloys (Section 10.4.5).

(b) Fusion range limits—between 750 to 900°C.
(c) Applications—suitable for most dental gold alloys.

44.2.3 Silver solders

(a) Composition—these are silver copper alloys; zinc and cadmium may also be present to lower the fusion temperature.
(b) Fusion range limits—600 to 750°C.
(c) Applications—used for base metal alloys, and particularly useful for stainless steel; their lower fusion temperature reduces the likelihood of weld decay (Section 38.3.1).

44.2.4 Fluxes

(a) Functions of a flux:
  (i) to protect the alloy surfaces from oxidation during soldering;
  (ii) to dissolve metallic oxides as they are formed.
(b) Materials. These may be either borax or fluorides such as potassium fluoride. The latter flux is used particularly for the chromium-containing alloys, as it can dissolve the passivating oxide film.
(c) Precaution. Some fluoride-containing fluxes evolve toxic fluorides when heated; avoid inhaling such fumes.

44.2.5 Practical points in soldering

(a) It is essential that the metallic parts to be joined are thoroughly clean.
(b) A solder of the correct fusion temperature should be selected.
(c) The reducing zone of the flame is used.
(d) The flame should be removed from the solder as soon as it flows.
(e) Immediately after soldering the work is quenched in water.

44.2.6 Investment soldering

This is used when very accurate alignment of the parts to be joined is required. The principles outlined in the previous section also apply here. The alignment is achieved by securing the parts together with sticky wax. After embedding in a refractory investment material, the wax is removed using boiling water and detergent, before soldering is carried out.

44.2.7 Soldering failures

These can usually be attributed to:
(a) Failure to clean the parts.
(b) Improper fluxing.
(c) Poor flow of solder if not sufficiently heated.
(d) Overheating of solder—a pitted joint of low strength may result.

44.3 WELDING

One example of welding (gold foil) is referred to in an earlier chapter (Ch. 23). Most other metals require higher temperatures to give successful welded joints. The most common method of achieving such *hot-welding* in dentistry is by the application of *resistance welding* or *spot welding*. The following principles are involved:
(a) The pieces to be joined are pressed firmly together between two electrodes, usually made of copper. Grooved electrodes are available to give good contact with orthodontic wires.
(b) An electric current is passed through the electrodes and the pieces of metal.
(c) If the parts to be joined are relatively poor conductors of electricity they will heat up more than the electrodes when the current is passed.
(d) If sufficient heat is generated in the portion of metal in contact with the electrodes, and if enough pressure is applied, a welded joint is formed.
(e) Either the magnitude of the current, or the time which it is passed, may be varied to give the desired optimum conditions.
(f) A current of 250 to 750 amperes is usually used, for a time of between 1/25th and 1/50th of a second.
(g) Too low a current, or too short a time, results in a weak joint; conversely, too much heating may thin the metal unduly.

This technique is not used:
(a) for gold alloys which are good conductors of electricity;
(b) for butt-joints.

Spot-welding is very successful for the formation of overlapping joints of stainless steel or other chromium-containing alloys.

45. Abrasion and polishing

45.1 INTRODUCTION

It is important that all dental restorations and appliances should have a smooth surface. Food debris will be deposited on rough surfaces, from which it will be difficult to remove. Apart from poor oral hygiene, deposits can be a factor in causing corrosion of metallic materials (Section 11.3.2). Also, patients cannot often tolerate rough surfaces in the mouth.

A rough surface is made smooth by a process known as *abrasion* in which hard sharp particles of *abrasive* are moved over the surface. Each particle of abrasive acts as a fine tool, cutting a groove in the surface of the article under treatment. The surface is thereby smoothed, but a series of scratches will be left, the dimensions of which will be dependent on the particle size of the abrasive. In any finishing process it is usual for a series of abrasives of increasing fineness to be used. The article should be washed well when changing from one abrasive to another. The work is moved continuously so that the scratches are produced in all directions.

The abrasive particles must be harder than the surface being abraded. These particles may be bonded together, as in a grinding wheel, disc or strip, or they may be carried across the surface by a brush or buff.

Unlike abrasion, *polishing* does not cut grooves in a material, but rather reduces irregularities. With some materials, particularly thermoplastic polymers, the surface flows to fill in any scratches, as it becomes heated.

45.2 ABRASION

45.2.1 Factors influencing the efficiency of abrasives

These include:
(a) The hardness of the abrasive particles; for example, diamond is the hardest material, whereas pumice, garnet, etc., are relatively mild abrasives (Section 45.2.3).
(b) The shape of the abrasive particles; particles with sharp edges will obviously be more efficient than those with obtuse angles.
(c) The particle size of the abrasive; larger particles will be able to cut deeper grooves.
(d) The mechanical properties of the abrasive; if the material breaks it should form a new cutting edge. Thus brittleness can be an advantage.
(e) The rate of movement of the abrasive particles—slower abrasion produces deeper scratches.
(f) The pressure applied to the abrasive—too great a pressure may fracture an abrasive cutting instrument and increase the heat of friction that is evolved.
(g) The properties of the material that is being abraded—a brittle material can be abraded rapidly, whereas a malleable and ductile material (for exmaple, pure gold) will flow instead of being removed by the abrasive.

45.2.2 Generation of heat

The amount of heat generated depends on the factors enumerated in the previous section. Cooling is often required, for example:
(a) In the cutting of tooth structure at high speeds, a water spray is required.
(b) In abrading polymeric materials, excessive heat should be avoided as it can cause stress relief and warpage.

45.2.3 Materials

(a) Diamond is the hardest known abrasive; its particles can be embedded in a ceramic or metallic binder, as in dental burs (Section 46.4).
(b) Tungsten carbide is used mainly for the construction of burs (Section 46.3) and abrasive wheels.
(c) Silicon carbide may be supplied as a powder, or bonded with rubber to form the stones and wheels used in the dental laboratory.

(d) Alumina is used similarly to silicon carbide.
(e) Emery is a mixture of alumina and iron which is supplied as an abrasive coating on cloth or paper.
(f) Sand (silica)—this is used:
   (i) in the familiar sandpaper,
   (ii) in abrasive paper discs, and
   (iii) in sandblasting procedures, particularly for cobalt–chromium alloys.
(g) Garnet is a milder abrasive, containing magnesium aluminium silicate, and used as a coating for paper discs.
(h) Cuttle-fish bone has similar uses to garnet.
(i) Pumice is prepared by crushing pumice-stone, a porous volcanic rock. It is used as a suspension in water, particularly in the finishing of acrylic resins.
(j) Tripoli is a ground porous rock, which is mixed with a wax to form a 'brick' of material.

45.3 POLISHING

45.3.1 Materials

(a) Whiting (or precipitated chalk) is used as a suspension in water for polishing plastics, such as acrylic.
(b) Zinc oxide in alcohol can be used for polishing amalgam restorations.
(c) Iron(III) oxide (rouge) is supplied in a soap base for polishing gold alloys. It is contra-indicated for polishing all chromium-containing alloys, as it can contaminate the surface and facilitate corrosion.
(d) Chromium oxide is also used in a soap base, and is supplied for polishing stainless steel and cobalt–chromium alloys.

45.3.2 Electrolytic polishing

This is the reverse procedure to electroplating (Sections 11.6 and 40.3.5). The alloy to be polished is made the anode of an electrolytic cell. As the current is passed, some of the anode is dissolved leaving a bright surface. This is an excellent method for polishing the fitting surface of a cobalt–chromium alloy denture; so little material is removed that the fit of the denture is virtually unaltered.

45.4 BURNISHING

Burnishing is a technique used to adapt the margins of a gold inlay. The instrument for this procedure can be made either of stainless steel or a chromium plated alloy. The instrument should not contain copper, which can become incorporated into the surface of the gold.

The ability of an alloy to be burnished may depend on:

(a) high percentage elongation,
(b) low proportional limit and proof stress, and
(c) a slow rate of work hardening

SECTION IX

Miscellaneous materials

46. Dental instruments

46.1 INTRODUCTION

In this chapter, the main topic considered is the materials from which dental instruments are made. The design and clinical usage of burs are considered to be beyond the scope of this book.

46.2 STEEL

For an introduction to the metallurgy of carbon steels, see Section 10.6

46.2.1 Burs

Steel burs are made of the hyper-eutectoid alloy, which, on slow cooling, consists of pearlite and cementite. Because of the cementite that is present, hyper-eutectoid steels are harder than hypo-eutectoid alloys, and so are preferred for greater efficiency in cutting hard dental tissues. Steel burs usually contain manganese and molybdenum, which also contribute to the hardness of the alloy.

Steel burs can cut dentine effectively, but their blades are quickly blunted in cutting enamel. Their properties are contrasted with tungsten carbide burs in Section 46.3.

46.2.2 Other instruments

Hyper-eutectoid steels are used in the production of cutting instruments and amalgam condensers.

Hypo-eutectoid steels, which are less brittle than the above, are used for dental forceps.

N.B. Care must be taken in sterilizing steel burs and instruments; if this is done by a wet method (steam or chemical sterilisation), a corrosion inhibitor should be used, such as sodium nitrite or dicyclohexylammonium nitrite. Also, two pieces of steel should not come in contact with each other in the steriliser, as electrolytic corrosion may occur (Section 11.3).

46.3 TUNGSTEN CARBIDE

Burs made of tungsten carbide particles, embedded in a matrix of cobalt (5 to 10%) are available as an alternative to steel ones. These are made by a process of powder metallurgy (Section 9.3.3). They are moulded to their approximate shape, then sintered, and soldered to a steel shaft. They are then accurately ground using diamond instruments.

Tungsten carbide has the following properties in contrast to steel:
(a) It is considerably harder, so is much more efficient in cutting enamel.
(b) It is very rigid, with a high modulus of elasticity.
(c) It is not as resilient or tough as steel, and being more brittle, cannot be used in thin sections.

The following are important practical points in the use of tungsten carbide burs:
(a) Care must be taken in handling them—they should not be dropped or subjected to sudden stresses. They should be applied to, and removed from, enamel and dentine while rotating at full speed.
(b) A bur must be symmetrical about its axis of rotation, particularly for high speed cutting. Otherwise there will be excessive vibration and the stresses from the eccentric rotation will be liable to fracture the bur.
(c) If chemical sterilisation is to be carried out, it is important that the agent used should not dissolve, attack or corrode (i) the cobalt matrix, (ii) the solder, or (iii) the steel shaft. For these reasons halogenated phenols, iodine and hydrogen peroxide are contraindicated.

Other chemical sterilising methods can be used with success.

Tungsten carbide tipped hand instruments are also available. It is important that no bending stresses should be applied to these, as they are liable to fracture.

46.4 DIAMOND

Diamond is even harder than tungsten carbide. Burs and abrasive wheels are made which have diamond chips bonded to the surface of a metallic shaft. A ceramic bonding agent is frequently used.

READING REFERENCE

American Dental Association 1981 Dentists' desk reference: materials, instruments and equipment, 1st edn.

Section III of this work is devoted to instruments. The seven chapters of this section deal comprehensively with selection, design and usage of equipment.

47. Prefabricated pins and posts

47.1 PINS

47.1.1 Applications

Prefabricated pins can be used as (a) aids for the retention of amalgam and composite restorations, (b) in some instances, for the retention of bridges and splints and (c) to provide rotation resistance in crown post systems.

47.1.2 Requirements

(a) Pins should be securely retained in the dentine.
(b) There should be adequate bonding (mechanical attachment and/or chemical bonding) between the pin and the restorative material.

47.1.3 Types

The following types of pin have been used:
(a) Threaded pins are most frequently used. These are self-tapping pins that shear off at a predetermined portion, or unscrew from a bur shank.
(b) Other pins include:
  (i) A cemented pin of smaller diameter than the channel into which it is to be placed. Space is thus available for the cement, which is attached to the pin mechanically, because of grooves in the pin.
  (ii) In contrast to the above, a friction locked pin is larger than the channel in the dentine. In placing the pin, the dentine is deformed elastically.

47.1.4 Materials

Pins may be made of stainless steel or titanium alloy. Some pins are gold plated to aid bonding to an amalgam restoration.

47.1.5 Properties

Table 47.1 gives some data for the axial retention of pins in dentine and restorative materials. Greater retention is usaully obtained with greater diameter of pin. Gold plating appears to aid bonding to amalgam in some cases.

Table 47.1* Resistance to axial force of various pin systems

	Outside diameter (mm)	Force to remove from dentine (N)	Force to remove from a composite** (N)	Force to remove from dental amalgam (N)
Stainless steel	0.77	122	166	169
Stainless steel	0.63	70	141	137
Stainless steel	0.77	95	181	192
Stainless steel	0.61	84	115	121
Stainless steel	0.78	84	172	168
Stainless steel	0.57	51	106	89
Gold plated	0.78	282	209	310
Gold plated	0.62	198	188	245
Gold plated	0.61	65	118	117
Titanium	0.76	99	160	186
Titanium	0.6	79	102	91

* Data from Segal A J M Sc. thesis, University of Manchester, 1983.
** Conventional macro-filled two paste composite

It must be realised that the presence of pins in a restoration does not give reinforcement of the material, and may, in some instances, reduce tensile strength. Pins should be regarded merely as aids to retention.

Pins induce stress in dentine, which may cause portions of remaining tooth to fracture. Placing pin holes may:

(a) Cause pulpal damage by heat,
(b) Perforate the pulp chamber, or
(c) Perforate the periodontal ligament.

47.2 CROWN POSTS

47.2.1 Application

Crown posts are used to attach an aritificial tooth crown to the root of a tooth to reinforce the remaining supragingival tooth structure.

47.2.2 Types

In addition to cast gold posts some systems are available where prefabricated posts are supplied. Reamers of matching size are supplied with the posts, so that the post fits the reamed post space.

Posts may be made of:

(a) Brass
(b) Gold
(c) Nickel–cobalt–chromium alloy
(d) Platinum–iridium
(e) Stainless steel
(f) Titanium alloy

The available types include:

(a) Parallel-sided smooth posts
(b) Parallel-sided roughened posts
(c) Parallel-sided threaded posts with taps
(d) Parallel-sided coarse threaded self-tapping posts
(e) Tapered smooth posts
(f) Tapered threaded posts.

48. Fluoride containing materials

48.1 INTRODUCTION

It is well established that topical or systemic use of fluorides can reduce the incidence of caries. The strongly electronegative fluoride ions may displace weaker ions (e.g. hydroxyl ions) in tooth enamel, thus strengthening it chemically, and may also affect bacterial plaque activity. A number of fluoride containing materials are discussed elsewhere—e.g. dental cements (some polycarboxylates, Section 17.3.1; glass-ionomers, Section 18.3) and some dentifrices (Section 51.1). Also, the presence of 1 part per million of fluoride in drinking water has a beneficial caries reducing effect. Below, some further sources of fluoride are considered.

48.2 FLUORIDE SOLUTIONS

The following are available for application by the clinician:
(a) Sodium fluoride solution, typically 2%.
(b) 8% stannous fluoride solution; this solution is not stable, so fresh material has to be prepared for each treatment. Application of the solution to interproximal areas is achieved by the use of unwaxed dental floss. Stannous fluoride should not be used where there are inflamed or injured gingivae.
(c) Acidulated phosphate fluoride (APF) solutions contain 1.23% fluoride ion concentration and orthophosphoric acid. The acidic environment (pH = 3) enhances fluoride uptake by enamel.

48.3 FLUORIDE GELS

Acidulated phosphate fluoride gels are available. There is a considerable difference in rheological properties between commercial products. Not all are true gels; some products containing, for example, sodium carboxymethyl cellulose, are viscous fluids. Other products are true gels with thixotropic properties.

It must be emphasised that the large quantities of fluoride in gels can present a possible toxic hazard, especially for young patients. Particular care must be taken to ensure that the gel is not swallowed.

Gels are often used with special trays, to ensure that the fluoride is in contact with the enamel for the required period of time. These trays may be made of:

(a) Wax,
(b) Poly (vinyl fluoride), with or without foam inserts,
(c) Alginate impression materials,
(d) Vacuum moulded splint materials,
(e) An air filled rubber membrane contained in a plastic tray. The membrane contains a disposable paper insert in which the gel is placed. The membrane helps to keep the paper in close contact with the enamel.
(f) A foam–plastic composition; these trays are disposable.

48.4 MOUTH RINSES

Sodium fluoride and APF solutions may be self-administered. In this case, materials are less concentrated than the solutions discussed in Section 48.2, since they are designed to be used more frequently. Research has indicated that, for example, monthly use of 0.2% fluoride or daily use of 0.05% solutions are beneficial in reducing the incidence of caries.

48.5 VARNISHES

The object of using varnishes containing fluoride is to keep the fluoride ions in contact with enamel for longer periods than is possible with other topical fluoride application techniques.

48.6 FLUORIDE CONTAINING PROPHYLAXIS PASTES

The following types of prophylaxis paste have been used:

(a) Stannous fluoride—pumice,
(b) Stannous fluoride—zirconium silicate,
(c) APF—silicon dioxide.

The use of pastes is not an adequate substitute for other techniques of fluoride application.

48.7 PRECAUTIONS

Early symptoms of acute fluoride poisoning appear at about 3 mg per kg body weight; 50 mg per kg body weight is a lethal dose.

49. Mouth protectors

49.1 USES

(a) To prevent injuries to both hard and soft tissues of the oral cavity of players engaged in contact sports.
(b) May also be used as a vehicle for topical fluoride application.
(c) Used in the treatment of bruxism.
(d) Suggested for haemostatic splints.

49.2 REQUIREMENTS

(a) Clinical requirements include: no toxic ingredients; no objectionable taste or odour; adequate retention; minimal thickness; no encroachment on airway.
(b) Required mechanical properties: adequate resilience; high impact strength.
(c) Other properties: ease of use; low cost.

49.3 MATERIALS

The following materials have been used:
(a) Poly (vinyl acetate–ethylene) co-polymer,
(b) Poly (vinyl chloride),
(c) Rubber,
(d) Plasticised acrylic,
(e) Polyurethane.

49.4 TYPES

Mouth protectors can be classified as:
(a) Stock protectors. These are supplied in different sizes, ready to use. They are commonly fabricated from rubber or poly (vinyl chloride). Some are available made from poly (vinyl acetate–ethylene) co-polymer or polyurethane.

(b) Mouth-formed protectors. These can be of two types:

  (i) A plastic rim which can be lined with a resilient polymer similar to tissue conditioners (Section 34.2).

  (ii) A thermoplastic material, which after heating is moulded in the mouth to the required shape.

(c) Custom-made protectors. These can be made from soft vinyl or soft acrylic-type polymers. Alternatively soft vulcanised rubber, or a self-curing latex rubber can be employed.

It is generally recognised that, of the above types, stock protectors are the least satisfactory.

READING REFERENCE

Nicholas N K 1969 Mouth protection in contact sports. New Zealand Dental Journal 65: 14

A review and comparison of the various types of mouth protectors

Going R E Loehman R E Chan M S 1974 Mouthguard materials: their physical and mechanical properties. Journal of the American Dental Association 89: 132

This paper contains considerable information on the available commercial materials, including composition, requirements, and properties. The authors have measured properties relating to the durability, stability, and ability to protect from trauma.

50. Radiographic materials

50.1 CONSTITUENTS OF RADIOGRAPHIC FILMS

50.1.1 Emulsion

The emulsion of a film consists of:

(a) Silver halides:

(i) Silver bromide, AgBr, is the most commonly used halide. It is prepared by precipitation from the reaction of silver nitrate and potassium bromide solutions:

$$AgNO_3 + KBr \rightarrow AgBr + KNO_3$$

(ii) Silver chloride, AgCl, can be used for an emulsion with rapid development properties, but it has less sensitivity to electromagnetic radiation (Section 50.2.1) than a silver bromide emulsion.

(iii) In addition to silver bromide, silver iodide, AgI, is usually present in small quantities in an X-ray emulsion to increase the sensitivity of the emulsion.

The average grain size of the silver halides affects the sensitivity of the film. The grain size distribution affects the exposure latitude, that is, the ability of the film to record a wide range of exposures.

(i) The greater the average grain size, the greater will be the sensitivity of the film.

(ii) A wider range of grain sizes gives greater exposure latitude.

(b) Gelatin has the following functions, among others:

(i) to prevent the silver halide precipitate from forming a sludge during manufacture.

(ii) to form a transparent layer when it is coated on to the film base.
(iii) to swell in the presence of aqueous solution, and so absorb processing chemicals during developing, fixing, etc.
(iv) to prevent reaction between halide and silver atoms in the exposed film (Section 50.2.1)

(c) Additives in the emulsion may include:
(i) sensitising dyes, to improve the sensitivity of the film to certain parts of the electromagnetic spectrum.
(ii) agents to prevent growth of bacteria, etc.
(iii) chemicals to improve the mechanical properties of the gelatin, to prevent it from becoming too brittle when dry.
(iv) an agent to prevent formation of bubbles as the emulsion is being coated on the base.
(v) a chemical to improve the ability of the film to be stored without deterioration.

50.1.2 Base

The film base is made of a clear plastic, such as a polyester. The base is coated with an adhesive, then with the emulsion, on both sides. The emulsion is coated with a protective layer to prevent abrasion.

50.1.3 Packaging

The film is wrapped between sheets of black paper to prevent exposure to light. A thin sheet of lead foil is present on the side of the film away from the X-ray tube, to prevent scattered X-ray from fogging the film.

50.2 PRODUCTION OF THE RADIOGRAPHIC IMAGE

50.2.1 Action of electromagnetic radiation on film

On exposure to radiation such as visible light or X-rays, the silver halides are decomposed; the halogens formed react with the emulsion but metallic silver is left in each grain forming a latent image. The amount of decomposition of the silver halides depends on the exposure time and wavelength of the radiation.

50.2.2 Developing the film

The latent image is converted to a visible one by treatment of the film with a developer. The principal constituent of a developer is a reducing agent which will convert silver halides to silver. The grains of halide containing nuclei of metallic silver are reduced preferentially. A negative is produced which inverts the light and dark portions of the original image.

Developers are aqueous solutions including the following constituents:

(a) Reducing agents (e.g. hydroquinone) which should have high selectivity, that is, be able to reduce the exposed crystals of silver halide much more rapidly than the unexposed ones.

(b) An alkaline constituent is present, since the developer works too slowly at low pH levels. During development, hydrogen ions are liberated, so reducing the pH. Thus a buffer is included in the developer solution. Examples: sodium carbonate with sodium bicarbonate; sodium hydroxide with boric acid.

(c) A preservative (e.g. sodium sulphite) to retard oxidation of the developing agents.

(d) A restrainer, or anti-foggant (e.g. potassium bromide) is included, otherwise the developer would reduce unexposed grains of silver halide, giving 'fogging' of the film.

The following factors influence the time required to give proper development:

(a) Temperature of solution.

(b) Agitation during development.

(c) Composition and age of the developing solution.

Developing solutions may deteriorate or age due to:

(a) Oxidation.

(b) Increase in bromide concentration, causing reduction in developing rate.

(c) Fall in pH.

(d) Reduction in concentration of sodium sulphite.

50.2.3 Rinsing, fixing, washing, drying

(a) Rinsing—the developed film is rinsed to remove excess developer.

(b) Fixing—this process is the removal of the unexposed silver halide which has not been reduced by the developer. This prevents further development of the film. Fixing agents such as sodium or ammonium thiosulphate are used; these form soluble silver complexes which are removed from the film.

(c) Washing is carried out to remove all the fixing chemicals from the film.

(d) Drying is the final stage in the preparation of a radiograph.

Note: Automatic X-ray film processors are available, the most rapid of which can produce an X-ray for inspection in about 90 seconds.

50.3 INTENSIFYING SCREENS

The intensifying screens used in contact with radiographic films are usually coated with calcium tungstate crystals. This material glows blue-violet when it is activated by radiation. An advantage of using intensifying screens is that a lower radiation dose is required.

50.4 PROPERTIES OF X-RAY FILMS

50.4.1 Optical density

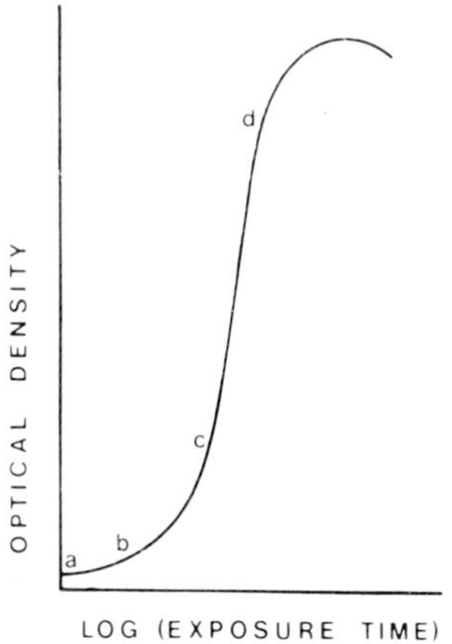

Fig. 50.1 Characteristic curve of an X-ray film: (a) basic fog, (b) threshold value, (c)–(d) approximately linear portion.

The optical density D of a film is given by:

$$D = \log_{10} I_i / I_t$$

where I_i is the intensity of the incident light and I_t is the intensity of the light transmitted by the film.

50.4.2 Characteristic curves

A characteristic curve for film is obtained by plotting D against the logarithm of the exposure time (Fig. 50.1). From this curve the following can be observed:
(a) When an unexposed film is developed, a small optical density is present, known as *basic fog*.
(b) The threshold value of the exposure is given by point b—the minimum exposure time to give an optical density measurably greater than basic fog.
(c) An approximately linear portion of the curve is observed (not always true for modern film emulsions).

From such characteristic curves, the following data for films can be obtained.
(a) The contrast of the film.
(b) The exposure latitude.
(c) The sensitivity.

50.5 FAULTS

If the film is too dark, it may be due to:
(a) Fogging of the film before development.
(b) Overexposure.
(c) Overdevelopment.

Similarly, too pale a film will result from underexposure or underdevelopment.

50.6 XERORADIOGRAPHY

The technique of xerography is widely used on document-copying machines. It has been suggested for applications in radiology.

In the xerographic process, an electrostatically charged sheet of a photoconductor (e.g. amorphous selenium) has a positive charge uniformly distributed over one surface. The other surface is in contact with an earthed conducting material. When the selenium is exposed to electromagnetic radiation, its electrostatic charge is conducted into the earthed material. The extent to which this happens is related to the intensity of exposure. A latent image is produced by the radiation. When a negatively charged powder is applied to the latent image, the powder is attracted to areas of the photoconductor where there is residual positive charge—that is, to areas least affected by the radiation. In this way an image is produced.

Some advantages of xeroradiography, when compared to conventional radiographic techniques, have been claimed:

(a) Both hard and soft tissues are clearly defined on a xeroradiograph.

(b) A lower dose of radiation is required.

(c) From an economic viewpoint, no silver salts are required, and darkroom facilities are not necessary.

READING REFERENCES

Smith N J D 1973 Radiography and radiology for the dental practitioner. 2— Materials and Processing. British Dental Journal 134: 491

A discussion of dental X-ray films, methods of processing and faults that can occur.

Chong M P Docking A R 1965 The sensitometric properties of dental X-ray films. Australian Dental Journal 10: 354

An investigation of the characteristic properties of seven dental X-ray films.

Kodak Ltd (1968) Fundamentals of radiographic photography

A series of five booklets dealing briefly, yet comprehensively, with all aspects of radiographic photography.

Binnie W H Stacey A J Davis R Cawson R A 1975 Applications of xeroradiography in dentistry Journal of Dentistry 3: 99

The authors trace briefly the history of the applications of xeroradiography, the principles involved and the advantages of the technique.

51. Dentifrices, mouthwashes, denture cleansers and denture adhesives

51.1 DENTIFRICES

The materials available to the public usually contain a number of constituents, including:

(a) Abrasives. The properties of the abrasive used are most important. Too harsh an abrasive will remove enamel; too mild an abrasive may fail to remove all deposits from the teeth. The following substances have been suggested as suitable abrasives: precipitated calcium carbonate, precipitated apatite, dibasic calcium phosphate ($CaHPO_4$ and $CaHPO_4$, $2H_2O$), sodium metaphosphate, $Na_3\ (PO_3)_3$, and hydrated alumina (Al_2O_3, $3H_2O$).

(b) Surface-active agents. Synthetic detergents can be incorporated to improve the ability of the dentifrice to wet the tooth surface.

(c) A humectant is included (e.g.glycerol) to retain moisture when the material is exposed to air. This is to avoid hardening of the paste.

(d) A binder, usually a colloid, is included to prevent separation of solid and liquid constituents.

(e) A flavouring agent (e.g. spearmint or peppermint) is included.

(f) A fluoride may be present, e.g. stannous fluoride or sodium monofluorophosphate (Na_2PO_3F).

(g) Minor components can include preservatives, astringents and oxidising agents.

51.2 MOUTHWASHES

51.2.1 Functions

Mouthwashes can be used for a number of purposes:

(a) To remove or destory bacteria.

(b) To act as an astringent.

(c) To deodorise.
(d) To have a therapeutic effect by relieving infection or preventing dental caries.

51.2.2 Constituents

(a) The following types of constituents have been employed as antibacterial agents:
 (i) phenolic compounds;
 (ii) quaternary ammonium compounds;
 (iii) essential oils, such as oil of peppermint and oil of wintergreen.
(b) Zinc chloride, zinc acetate and aluminium potassium sulphate are examples of astringent ingredients.
(c) Other ingredients include ethanol, dyes, sweetening agents, surface active agents.
(d) Water is the chief constituent of mouthwashes. Some products are supplied as concentrates, to be used after dilution.

51.3 DENTURE CLEANSERS

51.3.1 Deposits on dentures

If soft food debris clings to a denture, it can easily by removed by light brushing or rubbing, followed by rinsing. The hard deposits of calculus that can form on dentures are much more difficult to remove. The composition of these calcareous deposits varies from person to person, but essentially they consist of:
(a) An inorganic portion, shown to contain calcium phosphate, calcium carbonate and lesser quantities of other phosphates.
(b) An organic portion which bonds the deposit to the denture and is between 15 and 30% of the total deposit—this consists of mucoproteins.

51.3.2 Requirements of cleansers

Ideally a material should have the following characteristics:
(a) Non-toxic, easy to remove and leaving no traces of irritant material.
(b) The ability to attack or dissolve both the organic and inorganic portions of denture deposits.
(c) Harmless to all materials used in the construction of dentures,

Table 51.1 Properties of denture cleansers

Cleanser	Chief constituents	Comments
(a) Abrasive cleansers		
(1) Powder	Abrasives such as calcium carbonate	Abrasion of polymeric denture base materials and teeth
(2) Paste	Abrasive agents and/or acids	(i) Abrasion of polymeric materials (ii) Can be difficult to remove paste completely from denture
(b) Dilute mineral acids	3–5% hydrochloric acid	Dissolves inorganic components of denture deposits, but corrosion of some alloys may occur (a corrosion inhibitor may be present)
(c) Oxygenating cleansers	Sodium percarbonate or perborate with an alkaline detergent, e.g. trisodium phosphate	(i) Do not easily remove heavy deposits (ii) Harmful to soft lining materials
(d) Hypochlorite solutions	Dilute sodium hypochlorite	Can solubilise mucoproteins, but, (i) May cause bleaching (ii) Can corrode base metal alloys (iii) May leave an odour on dentures
(e) Enzyme cleansers	Proteolytic enzymes	Developed in attempts to break down the organic components of denture cleansers

including denture base polymers and alloys, acrylic and porcelain teeth and resilient lining materials.
(d) Not harmful to clothing, etc., if accidentally splashed or spilled.
(e) Stability on storage.
(f) Preferably bactericidal and fungicidal.

51.3.3 Classification and limitations of materials

The available types of material, their chief active constituents, and their main disadvantages are summarised in Table 51.1.

51.3.4 Results of a survey

Among the results which emerged in a survey of denture cleansing routines based on 1000 patients, were the following:
(a) Method of cleansing:

steeping and brushing dentures	about 30%
brushing alone	about 50%
steeping alone	about 20%

(b) Materials of choice—the oxyenating cleansers appear to be the most popular.
(c) Frequency of cleaning—about 50% clean their dentures only once, or less than once a day.
(d) Satisfaction with cleaning method—although only 17.5% claimed to be dissatisfied with their denture cleansing routine, almost 70% had dentures that were stained, either on the palate or round the teeth.
(e) The need exists for new and improved materials, particularly for those patients who have problems keeping their dentures clean.

51.4 DENTURE ADHESIVES

51.4.1 Uses

Adhesives are bought in large quantities by denture wearers, in attempts to improve the retention and function of their dentures. Denture adhesives may also be used in the following cases:
(a) As an aid in retention during the construction phase of a denture.
(b) As an aid to the retention of dentures and special appliances such as obturators, where there are physical limitations to the degree of retention that can otherwise be achieved.
(c) As a vehicle to aid application of drugs to the oral mucosa.

51.4.2 Constituents

The available proprietary products each contain some of the following constituents:
(a) Gelatin, pectin or a gum which will swell and become softer in the presence of water.
(b) Cellulose materials to act as thickening agents.
(c) Hexachlorophene or other antibacterial agents.
(d) A constituent such as sodium lauryl sulphate to reduce the surface tension.
(e) A filler such as magnesium oxide.
(f) A flavouring agent such as peppermint oil.

READING REFERENCES

Gershon S D Rader M 1972 Dentifrices. In: Balsam M S, Sagarin E (eds) Cosmetics: Science and Technology, 2nd edn. Wiley-Interscience, New York, vol 1, ch 14

This is a most extensive and comprehensive literature review of dentifrices, including discussion of functions, therapeutic dentifrices, dentifrice ingredients and formulations.

Rosenthal M W 1972 Mouthwashes. In: Balsam M S, Sagarin E (eds) Cosmetics: science and technology, 2nd edn. Wiley–Interscience, New York, vol 1, ch 15

This chapter gives extensive details about the constituents, formulation and functions of mouthwashes

Council on Dental Materials, Instruments and Equipment of the American Dental Association 1983. Denture cleansers. Journal of the American Dental Association 106: 77

A critical appraisal of denture cleansers, including comments on adverse effects, and safety in use of, such products

Stafford G D 1970 Denture adhesives—a review of their uses and compositions. Dental practitioner 21: 17

This paper gives the constituents, uses and disadvantages of denture adhesives

52. Surgical applications of materials

52.1 INTRODUCTION

In this chapter materials have been selected for brief discussion if they fulfil at least one of three criteria:
(a) Materials used in dental implants (Section 52.3).
(b) Some examples of medically used materials, (e.g. in orthopaedic surgery) where the materials are similar to those used in dentistry (Sections 52.4 and 52.5).
(c) Splint materials (Section 52.6).

52.2 REQUIREMENTS OF IMPLANT MATERIALS

(a) Biological requirements—should not be carcinogenic; should not give an allergic or prolonged inflammatory response.
(b) Chemical properties—inert and corrosion resistant.
(c) Mechanical properties—sufficient strength to resist the forces encountered in service. In instances where the implant is subject to stresses, resistance to fatigue failure is very important.
(d) Other properties:
   (i) capable of being sterilised, and
   (ii) economic and easy to use.

52.3 DENTAL IMPLANTS

52.3.1 Purpose

To provide an abutment for the support of prostheses, crowns, bridges, etc.

52.3.2 Types

Dental implants may be classified as:
(a) Endosseous implants—inserted into mandibular or maxillary bone. The implants may be metallic or ceramic (see Section 52.3.3).
(b) Subperiosteal implants—placed subperiosteally on the surface of the mandible or maxilla.
(c) Intramucosal implants, part of which are inserted beneath the mucosal tissues.

52.3.3 Materials

(a) Metallic materials: cobalt–chromium or titanium alloys.
(b) Other materials: vitreous carbon, porous alumina (Al_2O_3) or porous calcium aluminium silicate ($CaAlSiO_3$).

Some of the above materials are still being tested experimentally. As a general principle, the ceramic materials are very inert, but may be suspect because of their poor mechanical properties.

52.4 METALLIC IMPLANTS

Many metallic materials are unsuitable for use. For example, pure gold, though biologically inert, has poor mechanical properties. On the other hand, steel may have excellent mechanical properties, but is not corrosion resistant.

Today, the following alloys are used, either routinely or experimentally:
(a) Cobalt–chromium alloys (e.g. 'Vitallium', a Co—Cr—Mo alloy): excellent mechanical properties and good corrosion resistance (Section 35.3).
(b) Stainless steel (surgical grade); also, excellent mechanical properties, though not as inert in the body as cobalt–chromium.
(c) Titanium—inert material, and titanium alloys.
(d) Tantalum—inert, and sufficiently ductile to be drawn into a wire, hence its use as a suture material and for abdominal wall repair.

52.5 BONE CEMENTS

Autopolymerising acrylic resin (Section 33.4) has been used for the cementation of hip prostheses. For example, in the Charnley technique, a hip prosthesis made for stainless and high density polyethylene is cemented with an acrylic dough.

Recently acrylic and polycarboxylate cements have been suggested for use with dental implants.

52.6 SPLINT MATERIALS

Splints are used in the treatment of traumatised teeth and fractured jaws. They may be made of alloys or polymers:
(a) Cast sterling silver, 92.5% silver, 7.5% copper is used. These alloys may tarnish and become black, but can be kept clean by meticulous attention to oral hygiene.
(b) Acrylic splints are sometimes fabricated—both heat-curing and autopolymerising acrylics may be used.

READING REFERENCES

Taylor A R 1970 Endosseous dental implants. Butterworth, London

Chapter 2 of this book is devoted to a consideration of implant materials—the requirements of materials, and a discussion of both metallic and non-metallic materials.

Ludwigson D C 1964 Today's prosthetic metals. Journal of Metals. March, p 226

This article gives a history of the use of metal prostheses.

Zarb G A, Melcher A H, Smith D C 1972 Cementation of dental implants: Rationale and preliminary observations. Journal of the Canadian Dental Association, 38: 328.

Preliminary observations on the use of acrylic and polycarboxylate cements for dental implants.

Williams D F, Roaf R 1973 Implants in surgery. Saunders, London

This book describes the properties of all implant materials, the design of implants and the clinical uses of implants in orthopaedics, cardiovascular surgery and plastic and reconstructive surgery.

APPENDICES

I. The SI units

I.1 INTRODUCTION

The letters 'SI' are an abbreviation for 'Système International d'Unités' At least 30 countries have decided to adopt this system, and it is likely to be used throughout the world in the near future.

I.2 BASIC UNITS

Six basic units of this system are listed in Table I.1. The first four of these are of particular relevance to the subject matter of this book.

Table I.1 Basic SI units

Physical quantity	Name of SI unit	Unit symbol
Length	metre	m
Mass	kilogram	kg
Time	second	s
Electric current	ampere	A
Temperature*	kelvin	K
Luminous intensity	candela	cd

*In this book temperatures are expressed in degrees Celsius
°C = K − 273.15

I.3 DERIVED SI UNITS

A number of units have been derived from the basic units. A list of those used in this book is in Table I.2.

I.4 PREFIXES FOR SI UNITS

Prefixes can be used to form decimal multiples and sub-multiples of SI units. These are listed in Table I.3.

I.5 USE OF SI UNITS

In this book, SI units are used throughout with two exceptions

where existing units are retained for convenience. These exceptions are:
(a) The Angstrom (1 Å = 10^{-10} m) has been retained as the unit in which atomic diameters are expressed (as in Table 10.1).
(b) Densities are expressed in g/cm^3 instead of kg/m^3.

Table I.2 Derived SI units

Physical quantity	Name of SI unit	Unit symbol
Area	square metre	m^2
Volume	cubic metre	m^3
Force	newton	N = kgm/s^2
Pressure, stress	newton per square metre	N/m^2
Work, energy, quantity of heat	joule	J = Nm
Power	watt	W = J/s
Thermal conductivity	watt per metre degree Kelvin	W/mK

Table I.3 Prefixes for SI units*

Factor by which the unit is multiplied	Prefix	Symbol
10^{12}	tera	T
10^{9}	giga	G
10^{6}	mega	M
10^{3}	kilo	k
10^{2}	hecto	h
10	deca	da
10^{-1}	deci	d
10^{-2}	centi	c
10^{-3}	milli	m
10^{-6}	micro	μ
10^{-9}	nano	n
10^{-12}	pico	p
10^{-15}	femto	f
10^{-18}	atto	a

* Note: It is recommended that prefixes used are those representing 10 raised to a power which is a multiple of 3.

I.6 CONVERSION FACTORS

Table I.4 gives a useful list of conversion factors.

Table I.4 Conversion factors

Unit	SI equivalent
Angstrom, Å	10^{-10} m
*British thermal unit, Btu	1.055 kJ
*calorie, cal	4.186J
dyne	10^{-5} N
foot, ft	0.3048 m
gram/cubic centimetre, g/cm^3	1000 kg/m^3
inch, in	25.4 mm
*kilogram-force/square centimetre, kgf/cm^2	98.1kN/m^2
*kilogram-force, kgf	9.81 N
*ounce, oz	0.02835 kg
*ounce, fluid, fl oz	28.41 cm^3
*pound, lb	0.454 kg
*poundal, pdl	0.1383 N
*pound-force, lbf	4.448 N
*pound-force/square inch, lbf/in^2 or p.s.i.	6.895 kN/m^2
square inch	645.16 mm^2

* approximate values

II. Physical and mechanical properties of dental materials

Table II.1 Density of some dental materials

The density of a material is the ratio of its mass to its volume. It is dependent on both temperature and pressure, and the values shown below are those at 20°C and 760 mmHg (293 K and 101.32 kN/m^2).

Material		Density, g/cm^3
Pure metals		
	Chromium	7.1
	Cobalt	8.9
	Copper	8.9
	Gold	19.3
	Mercury	13.6
	Molybdenum	10.2
	Nickel	8.9
	Palladium	12.0
	Platinum	21.4
	Silver	10.5
	Tin	7.3
	Titanium	4.5
	Zinc	7.1
Alloys		
	Cobalt–chromium	8
	Inlay gold	17
	Nickel–chromium	8
	Partial denture gold	15
	Silver–palladium	12
	Silver–tin amalgam	11
	Stainless steel	8
Non-metals		
	Aluminous porcelain	2.8
	Fused porcelain	2.4
	Acrylic resin	1.2

Table II.2 Physical properties of enamel and dentine

	Enamel	Dentine
Coefficient of thermal expansion ($\times 10^{-6}$/°C)	11.4	8.3
Thermal conductivity (W/mK)	0.88	0.59
Density (g/cm^3)	2.2	1.9
Hardness (KHN)	300	70
Compressive strength (MN/m^2)	200	300
Tensile strength (MN/m^2)	35	60

Table II.3 Physical and mechanical properties of restorative materials

Material	Coefficient termal expansion ($\times 10^{-6}$/°C)	Thermal conductivity (W/mk)	Tensile strength (MN/m²)	Compressive strength (MN/m²)
Filling materials				
Acrylic resin	81	0.2	30	70
Amalgam	25	23	60	300
Composite materials	28	—	40	200
Silicate	8	0.8	15	200
Lining cements				
Zinc oxide–eugenol	—	0.5	—	15
Resin-bonded zinc oxide–eugenol	—	—	—	38
EBA cements	—	—	—	90
Zinc phosphate	—	1.3	5	100
Zinc polycarboxylate	—	—	14	90
Ceramic materials				
Porcelain	7	1.5	70	280
Aluminous porcelain	—	—	150	—

Table II.4 Mechanical properties of dental casting alloys

Material	Condition	Modulus of elasticity GN/m^2	Proportional limit MN/m^2	Ultimate tensile strength MN/m^2	Elongation %	Hardness BHN
Gold alloys						
Type I	As cast	75	85	200	25	40– 75
Type II	As cast	75	160	345	24	70–100
Type III	Soft	75	195	365	20	90–140
Type III	Hard	80	290	445	10	120–170
Type IV	Soft	95	360	480	15	130–150
Type IV	Hard	100	585	790	10	210–230
Silver–palladium alloy	Soft	95	345	480	9	140–170
Cobalt–chromium alloy	As cast	250	515	690	4	370
Nickel–chromium alloy	As cast	200	100	500	30	300

Table II.5 Mechanical properties of wrought dental alloys

Material	Conditions	Modulus of elasticity GN/m^2	Proportional limit MN/m^2	Ultimate tensile strength MN/m^2	Elongation %	Hardness BHN
Cobalt–chromium	Work hardened	240	1000	1800	2	250
Gold alloy	Work hardened	95	550	825	3	220
Nickel–chromium	Work hardened	210	900	1350	1	225
Stainless steel (18Cr; 8Ni)	Soft	200	280	620	50	170
	Medium hard	200	1050	1250	6	250
	Hard	230	1450	1700	1	350
Titanium	Work hardened	100	500	750	30	200
Titanium alloy (6Al; 4V)	Work hardened	120	1100	1200	12	300

III. Formulae of some polymers and related compounds of dental interest

These are listed in alphabetical order:
1. *Agar*—see polysaccharides (no. 36).
2. *Alginates*—see polysaccharides (no. 36).
3. *Alginic acid*—see polysaccharides (no. 36).
4. *Bakelite.* This name is given to condensation polymers, formed by the reaction between phenol and formaldehyde:

$$C_6H_5OH + H_2C{=}O \longrightarrow C_6H_4(OH)CH_2OH$$

(phenol) (formaldehyde)

$$C_6H_4(OH)CH_2OH + C_6H_4(OH)CH_2OH \longrightarrow C_6H_4(OH)CH_2C_6H_3(OH)CH_2OH + H_2O$$

Further condensation reactions can occur, to yield a complicated three-dimensional network of molecules.
5. *Benzoin methyl ether*—used to initiate polymerisation of composite resins by the use of ultraviolet light

$$C_6H_5{-}CH(OCH_3){-}C({=}O){-}C_6H_5$$

6. *Benzoyl peroxide*—an initiator used in the polymerisation of methyl methacrylate and aromatic dimenthacrylates (Section 8.3.1):

$$C_6H_5{-}COO{-}OOC{-}C_6H_5$$

7. *BIS-GMA*—an aromatic dimethacrylate used in many composite restorative materials:

$$CH_2{=}C(CH_3){-}C({=}O){-}O{-}CH_2{-}CH(OH){-}CH_2{-}O{-}C_6H_4{-}C(CH_3)_2{-}C_6H_4{-}O{-}CH_2{-}CH(OH){-}CH_2{-}O{-}C({=}O){-}C(CH_3){=}CH_2$$

A similar dimethacrylate, but without hydroxy groups has been used

$$CH_2{=}C(CH_3){-}C({=}O){-}O{-}CH_2{-}CH_2{-}O{-}C_6H_4{-}C(CH_3)_2{-}C_6H_4{-}O{-}CH_2{-}CH_2{-}O{-}C({=}O){-}C(CH_3){=}CH_2$$

8. *Bisphenol-A.* This chemical has the formula:

$$HO{-}C_6H_4{-}C(CH_3)_2{-}C_6H_4{-}OH$$

For examples of its use, see BIS-GMA (no. 7) epimine compounds (no. 14), epoxy compounds (no. 15) and polycarbonates (no. 30).

9. *Bisphenol-A dimethacrylate.* An aromatic dimethacrylate used in some composite filling materials as a diluent monomer for BIS-GMA (no. 7). Formula:

$$CH_2{=}C(CH_3){-}C({=}O){-}O{-}C_6H_4{-}C(CH_3)_2{-}C_6H_4{-}O{-}C({=}O){-}C(CH_3){=}CH_2$$

10. *Bowen's resin*—a name given to BIS-GMA (no. 7).

11. *Dibutyl phthalate.* This is a plasticiser for poly(methyl methacrylate), and has the formula:

$$C_6H_4(COOC_4H_9)_2$$

12. *N, N-dihydroxyethyl-p-toluidine.* This compound produces free radicals on interaction with benzoyl peroxide, similar to dimethyl-p-toluidine (no. 13)

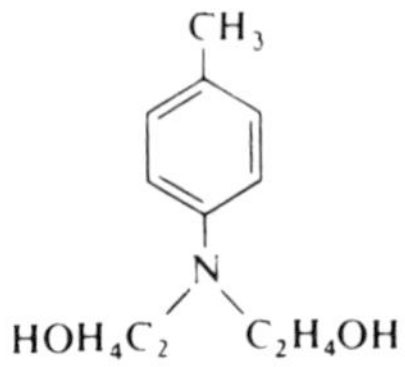

CH_3

$HOH_4C_2 \quad C_2H_4OH$

13. Dimethyl-p-toluidine. This is a tertiary amine of formula:

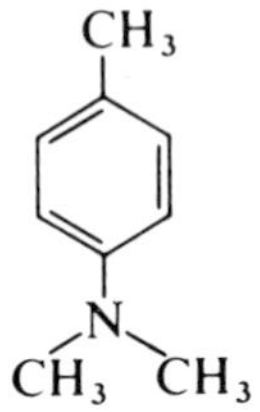

CH_3

N

$CH_3 \quad CH_3$

It can be used as an activator for 'self-cured' acrylics (Section 8.3.1).

14. Epimine compounds contain the group:

N

$CH_2{-}CH_2$

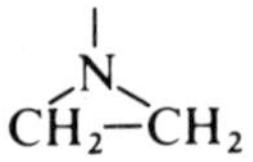

For example, the compound:

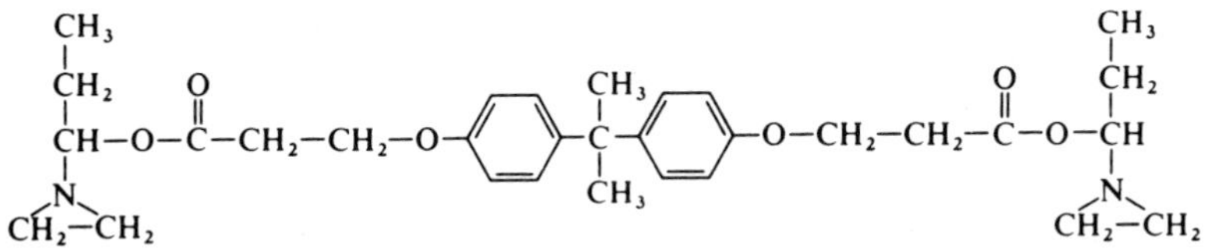

CH_3 CH_3

CH_2 O CH_3 O CH_2

$CH{-}O{-}C{-}CH_2{-}CH_2{-}O{-}C{-}O{-}CH_2{-}CH_2{-}C{-}O{-}CH$

N CH_3 N

$CH_2{-}CH_2$ $CH_2{-}CH_2$

is a constituent of temporary crown and bridge materials (Section 32.4). Bisphenol-A (see no. 8) is a starting product in the synthesis of such polymers.

Also, the compound:

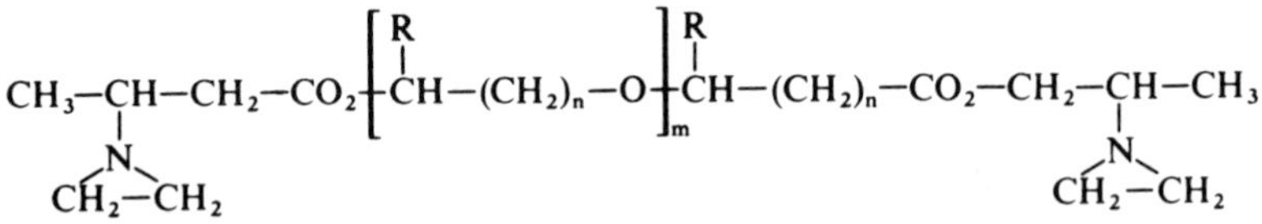

$$CH_3{-}\underset{\substack{|\\ N\\ CH_2-CH_2}}{CH}{-}CH_2{-}CO_2{-}\left[\overset{R}{\overset{|}{C}}H{-}(CH_2)_n{-}O\right]_m{-}\overset{R}{\overset{|}{C}}H{-}(CH_2)_n{-}CO_2{-}CH_2{-}\underset{\substack{|\\ N\\ CH_2-CH_2}}{CH}{-}CH_3$$

is a constituent of a polyether impression material (Section 27.3).

15. Epoxy compounds contain the group:

$$-\overset{|}{C}\overset{O}{\diagdown\!\!\diagup}\overset{|}{C}-$$

Such compounds can react with bisphenol-A (see no. 8) as follows:

$$2\,Cl-CH_2-\underset{\diagdown O \diagup}{CH-CH_2} + HO-C_6H_4-C(CH_3)_2-C_6H_4-OH$$

(epichlorohydrin) (bisphenol-A)

$$\downarrow NaOH$$

$$Cl-CH_2-\overset{OH}{\overset{|}{C}H}-CH_2-O-C_6H_4-\underset{CH_3}{\overset{CH_3}{C}}-C_6H_4-O-CH_2-\overset{OH}{\overset{|}{C}H}-CH_2-Cl$$

$$\downarrow NaOH$$

$$\overset{O}{CH_2-CH}-CH_2-O-C_6H_4-\underset{CH_3}{\overset{CH_3}{C}}-C_6H_4-O-CH_2-\overset{O}{CH-CH_2} + 2HCl$$

This latter compound (or polymers of it) are frequently used as starting products in the preparation of other polymers. Such epoxides can react, for example, with amines:

$$2\,R-\overset{O}{CH-CH_2} + R'-NH_2 \longrightarrow R-\overset{OH}{\overset{|}{C}H}-CH_2-\overset{R'}{\overset{|}{N}}-CH_2-\overset{OH}{\overset{|}{C}H}-R$$

Thus amines can be used to link two epoxy containing molecules together. Glycidyl methacrylate is another important epoxy compound:

$$CH_2=\underset{CH_3}{\underset{|}{C}}-\overset{O}{\overset{\|}{C}}-O-CH_2-\overset{O}{CH-CH_2}$$

This can also react with bisphenol-A as above.

16. Glycidyl methacrylate—see epoxy compounds (no. 15).

17. Gutta percha—see polyisoprene (no. 32).

18. Hydroquinone is a stabiliser for acrylic monomers:

$$HO-C_6H_4-OH$$

(1,4-dihydroxy-benzene)

This monomethyl ether of hydroquinone may be used for the same purpose:

$$HO-C_6H_4-OCH_3$$

19. Hydroxyethyl methacrylate (HEMA) has the formula:

$$CH_2{=}C(CH_3)-COO-CH_2-CH_2-OH$$

HEMA—methyl methacrylate co-polymers have been suggested as denture base materials (Section 33.6).
20. 2-hydroxy-4-methoxybenzophenone is a constituent of some composite restorative materials, to improve their colour stability:

$$C_6H_5-C({=}O)-C_6H_3(OH)-O-CH_3$$

21. Itaconic acid. An aqueous solution of a co-polymer of acrylic acid and itaconic acid is used for glass-ionomer cement liquids (Section 18.3.2). Itaconic acid has the formula:

$$CH_2{=}C(COOH)-CH_2-COOH$$

22. Lauryl mercaptan has the formula:

$$CH_3(CH_2)_{11}\ SH$$

It is used as an activator for self-cured acrylics (Section 8.3.1). Its systematic chemical name is 1-dodecanethiol.
23. Mercaptan—this is an organic compound with the formula R-SH (a thio-alcohol). Examples—lauryl mercaptan (no. 22), and polymers supplied for use as impression materials (Section 27.1.1).

24. NPG-GMA. This is the abbreviated name for the reaction product of N-phenyl glycine (no. 27) and glycidyl methacrylate (no. 16). Formula:

$$HO-\overset{O}{\overset{\|}{C}}-CH_2-\underset{|}{\overset{C_6H_5}{N}}-CH_2-\overset{OH}{\overset{|}{C}}H-CH_2-O-\overset{O}{\overset{\|}{C}}-\overset{CH_3}{\overset{|}{C}}=CH_2$$

25. Nylon—see Section 8.2. This type of polymer is prepared by the reaction between a di-acid and a di-amine as follows:

$$n[H_2N-(CH_2)_6-NH_2] + n[HO-\overset{O}{\overset{\|}{C}}-(CH_2)_4-\overset{O}{\overset{\|}{C}}-OH]$$

(hexamethylene diamine) (adipic acid)

$$\longrightarrow H\left[HN-(CH_2)_6-NH-\overset{O}{\overset{\|}{C}}-(CH_2)_4-\overset{O}{\overset{\|}{C}}\right]_n OH + nH_2O$$

Many other nylon polymers are available, using different acid and amine starting materials.

26. Phenol-formaldehyde polymers—see bakelite (no. 4).

27. N-Phenylglycine: (see no. 24)

$$HO-\overset{O}{\overset{\|}{C}}-CH_2-NH-C_6H_5$$

28. Poly(acrylic acid)—see Table 8.1.

29. Polyamides—see proteins (no. 41).

30. Polycarbonates—see Section 8.2. They are produced either by the reaction of bisphenol-A with diphenyl carbonate:

$$nHO-C_6H_4-\overset{CH_3}{\underset{CH_3}{\overset{|}{\underset{|}{C}}}}-C_6H_4-OH + nO=C(O-C_6H_5)_2$$

(bisphenol-A) (diphenyl carbonate)

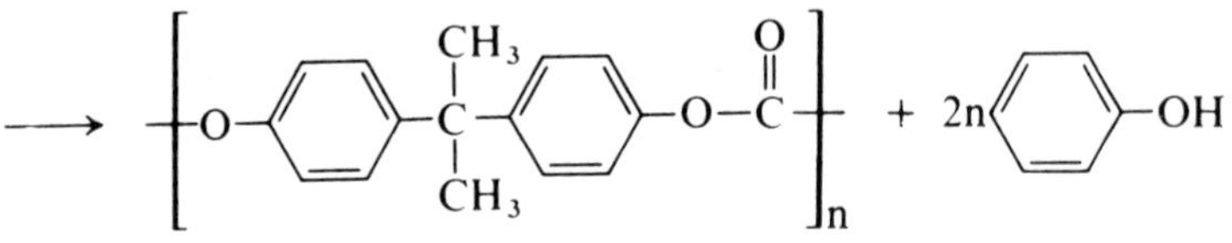

$$\rightarrow \left[-O-C_6H_4-C(CH_3)_2-C_6H_4-O-\overset{O}{\overset{\|}{C}}- \right]_n + 2n\,C_6H_5-OH$$

or by the reaction of bisphenol-A with phosgene:

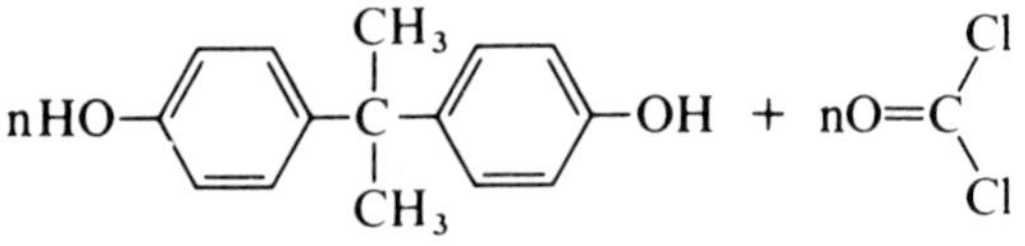

$$n\,HO-C_6H_4-C(CH_3)_2-C_6H_4-OH + n\,O{=}CCl_2$$

(bisphenol-A) (phosgene)

$$\xrightarrow{NaOH} \left[-O-C_6H_4-C(CH_3)_2-C_6H_4-O-\overset{O}{\overset{\|}{C}}- \right]_n + 2n\,NaCl$$

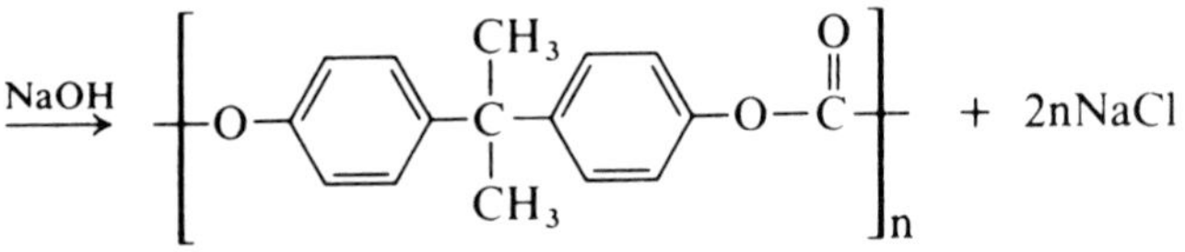

31. Polyethylene—see Table 8.1.

32. Polyisoprene. Natural rubber and gutta percha are both polyisoprenes. Isoprene has the formula C_5H_8 or:

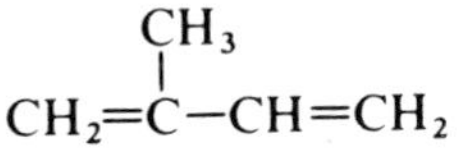

$$CH_2{=}\overset{CH_3}{\overset{|}{C}}-CH{=}CH_2$$

Polyisoprene occurs in two isomeric forms: (*isomers* are compounds with the same molecular formula, but having a different mode of arrangement of atoms):

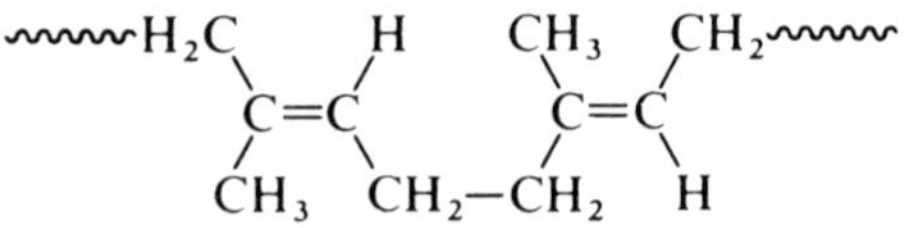

$$\sim H_2C(CH_3)C{=}CH-CH_2-CH_2-C(CH_3){=}CH-CH_2\sim$$

gutta percha (*trans*-isomer)

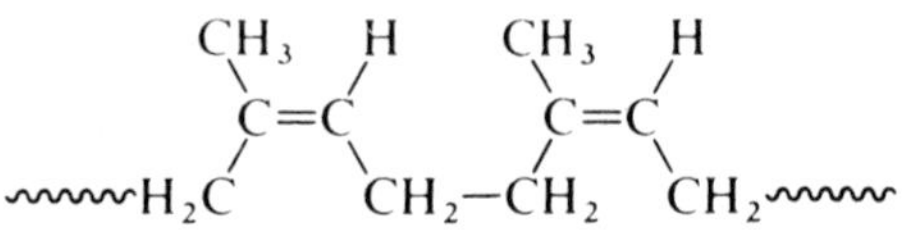

$$\sim H_2C(CH_3)C{=}CH-CH_2-CH_2-C(CH_3){=}CH-CH_2\sim$$

natural rubber (*cis*-isomer)

33. *Poly(methacrylic acid)*—see Table 8.1.
34. *Poly(methyl methacrylate)*—see Table 8.1 for formula, and Section 8.3 for its formation by polymerisation
35. *Polypeptides*—see proteins (no. 41).
36. *Polysaccharides* are naturally occurring polymers which are carbohydrates, that is, have the general formula $C_x(H_2O)_y$. Agar and algnic acid, both extracted from seaweed, are related to this class of compound.
37. *Polystyrene*—see Table 8.1.
38. *Polysulphides.* The formation of these is discussed in Section 8.2.
39. *Polythene*—see Table 8.1.
40. *Poly(vinyl chloride)*—see Table 8.1.
41. *Proteins* (or polyamides, or polypeptides) are naturally occurring polymers with the structure:

$$-NH-\underset{\displaystyle H}{\overset{\displaystyle R}{\underset{|}{\overset{|}{C}}}}-\overset{\displaystyle O}{\overset{\|}{C}}-NH-\underset{\displaystyle H}{\overset{\displaystyle R}{\underset{|}{\overset{|}{C}}}}-\overset{\displaystyle O}{\overset{\|}{C}}-$$

where R is an organic group.
42. *PVC*—poly(vinyl chloride)—see Table 8.1.
43. *Rubber*—see polyisoprene (no. 32).
44. *Silicones*—see Section 8.2 and no. 45.
45. *Siloxane*—the chemical name given to silicone polymers, with alternating silicon and oxygen atoms in the polymer chain.
46. *p–Toluene sulphinic acid.* This has the formula:

$$CH_3-C_6H_4-SO_2H$$

It can provide free radicals to initiate the polymerisation of methyl methacrylate (Section 8.3.1). It is, however, an unstable compound, being readily oxidised in air to p-toluene sulphonic acid:

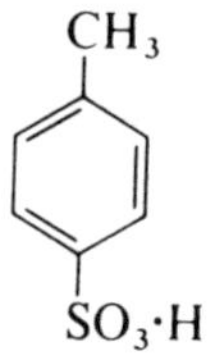

$$CH_3-C_6H_4-SO_3{\cdot}H$$

This latter compound cannot initiate free radical polymerisation.

47. *Tributyl boron.* Formula: $(C_4H_9)_3B$.

48. *Triethylene glycol dimethacrylate*—a low viscosity diluent monomer used in composite restorative materials

$$CH_2{=}C(CH_3)-C(=O)-O-(CH_2)_2-O-(CH_2)_2-O-(CH_2)_2-O-C(=O)-C(CH_3){=}CH_2$$

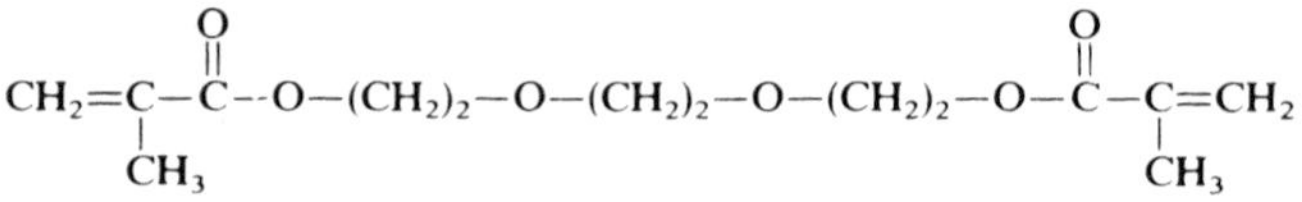

49. *Urethane dimethacrylate*—an alternative monomer to BIS-GMA (no. 7):

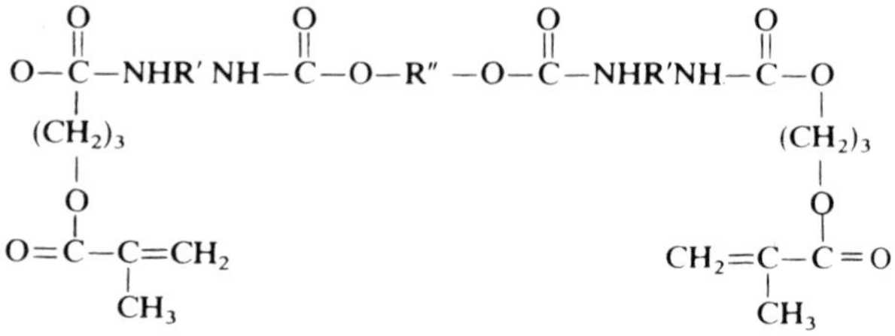

$$CH_2{=}C(CH_3)-C(=O)-O-(CH_2)_3-O-C(=O)-NHR'NH-C(=O)-O-R''-O-C(=O)-NHR'NH-C(=O)-O-(CH_2)_3-O-C(=O)-C(CH_3){=}CH_2$$

where R′ and R′′ are different radicals.

50. *Vinyl silanes* are used as coupling agents in composite restorative materials. Example—gamma-methacryloxypropyltrimethoxy silane:

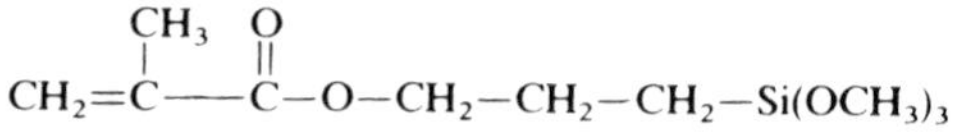

$$CH_2{=}C(CH_3)-C(=O)-O-CH_2-CH_2-CH_2-Si(OCH_3)_3$$

51. *Visible light activation* of composites uses the reaction between an ∝-diketone and an amine in the presence of light of the appropriate wavelength:

$$Ar_2C = O \underset{}{\overset{\text{light}}{\rightleftharpoons}} (Ar_2C = O)$$

(ketone) (ketone in excited state)

$$\downarrow \quad RCH_2CH_2NR_2$$

(amine)

$$(Ar_2C = O)^{\bullet -} \; (RCH_2—CH_2—NR_2)^{\bullet +}$$

$$\downarrow$$

$$Ar_2\dot{C}—OH + R\,CH_2\,\dot{C}H\,N\,R_2$$

(two free radicals formed)

Index